A Manual for Operation Theater Technicians

A Manual for Operation Theater Technicians

Previously known as
Textbook for Operation Theater Technicians

As per the Latest Syllabus and Guidelines of
'Diploma in Operation Theater Technicians'

Second Edition

Neelam Rai MSc (N) PhD
Principal
Savitri Hospital and Paramedical Institute
School and College of Nursing
Gorakhpur, Uttar Pradesh, India

Arpit Ravindra Lal MSc (N)
Assistant Professor
Savitri Hospital and Paramedical Institute
School and College of Nursing
Gorakhpur, Uttar Pradesh, India

Forewords
Pratiksha John
Asif Masood

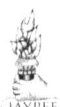

JAYPEE BROTHERS MEDICAL PUBLISHERS
The Health Sciences Publisher
New Delhi | London

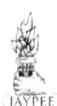

Jaypee Brothers Medical Publishers (P) Ltd.

Headquarters
Jaypee Brothers Medical Publishers (P) Ltd.
EMCA House
23/23-B, Ansari Road, Daryaganj
New Delhi - 110 002, India
Landline: +91-11-23272143, +91-11-23272703
+91-11-23282021, +91-11-23245672
Email: jaypee@jaypeebrothers.com

Corporate Office
Jaypee Brothers Medical Publishers (P) Ltd
4838/24, Ansari Road, Daryaganj
New Delhi 110 002, India
Phone: +91-11-43574357
Fax: +91-11-43574314
Email: jaypee@jaypeebrothers.com

Overseas Office
J.P. Medical Ltd.
83 Victoria Street, London
SW1H 0HW (UK)
Phone: +44 20 3170 8910
Email: info@jpmedpub.com

EU GPSR Authorised Representative
Logos Europe, 9 rue Nicolas Poussin
17000, La Rochelle, France
Phone: +33 (0) 6 67 93 73 78
E-mail: Contact@logoseurope.eu

Website: www.jaypeebrothers.com
Website: www.jaypeedigital.com

© 2023, Jaypee Brothers Medical Publishers (P) Ltd.

The views and opinions expressed in this book are solely those of the original contributor(s)/author(s) and do not necessarily represent those of editor(s) and publisher of the book.

All rights reserved. No part of this publication may be reproduced, stored or transmitted in any form or by any means, electronic, mechanical, photocopying, recording or otherwise, without the prior permission in writing of the publishers.

All brand names and product names used in this book are trade names, service marks, trademarks or registered trademarks of their respective owners. The publisher is not associated with any product or vendor mentioned in this book.

Medical knowledge and practice change constantly. This book is designed to provide accurate, authoritative information about the subject matter in question. However, readers are advised to check the most current information available on procedures included and check information from the manufacturer of each product to be administered, to verify the recommended dose, formula, method and duration of administration, adverse effects and contraindications. It is the responsibility of the practitioner to take all appropriate safety precautions. Neither the publisher nor the author(s)/editor(s) assume any liability for any injury and/or damage to persons or property arising from or related to use of material in this book.

This book is sold on the understanding that the publisher is not engaged in providing professional medical services. If such advice or services are required, the services of a competent medical professional should be sought.

Every effort has been made where necessary to contact holders of copyright to obtain permission to reproduce copyright material. If any have been inadvertently overlooked, the publisher will be pleased to make the necessary arrangements at the first opportunity.

Inquiries for bulk sales may be solicited at: jaypee@jaypeebrothers.com

A Manual for Operation Theater Technicians

First Edition: 2017

Second Edition: **2023**

ISBN: 978-93-5696-264-4

Dedicated to

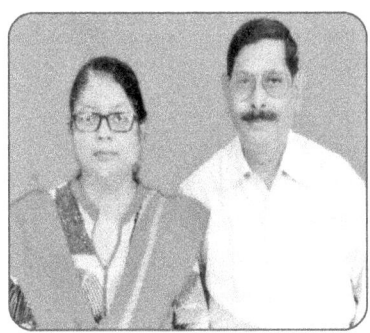

Mrs and Mr DR Lal

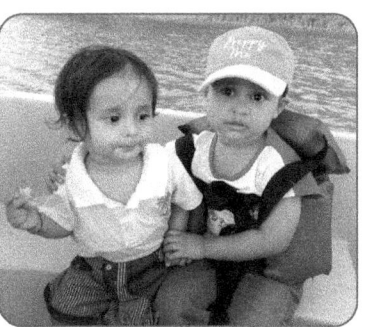

Vaishnavi and Shivansh

Foreword

In the fast-paced realm of healthcare, where lives are saved and miracles happen every day, there is a group of professionals who often remain unseen, yet their impact is profound. The Operation Theater Technicians are the unsung heroes of the surgical world, and it is with great pleasure that I introduce this book, a celebration of their expertise, dedication, and invaluable contributions.

Within the pages of this book, you will embark on a captivating journey into the realm of Operation Theater Technicians—a field where precision, teamwork, and unwavering commitment reign supreme. This book serves as a testament to their exceptional skills and unwavering dedication, while also recognizing the tremendous efforts of the authors who have meticulously captured the essence of their profession.

Ms Neelam Rai and Mr Arpit Ravindra Lal, whose passion for the subject matter shines through in every word, have crafted a remarkable resource that pays homage to the invaluable work of Operation Theater Technicians. Their expertise and deep understanding of this specialized field are evident throughout the book, making it an invaluable asset for both aspiring technicians and seasoned professionals alike.

Ms Neelam Rai and Mr Arpit Ravindra Lal, bring a wealth of experience and insight to this project, having dedicated themselves to the art and science of surgical support for many years. Their combined expertise, gained through years of hands-on experience and continuous learning, is evident in the comprehensive coverage of topics ranging from aseptic techniques and surgical equipment to patient care and safety. Their ability to distil complex concepts into easily digestible information ensures that readers will gain a profound understanding of the role and responsibilities of Operation Theater Technicians.

Beyond their technical proficiency, the authors' commitment to compassionate patient care is a recurring theme in this book. They recognize that beyond the surgical suite, there are individuals in vulnerable situations who seek comfort and reassurance. Through their insightful guidance, they emphasize the importance of empathy, effective communication, and the human touch in every interaction, reminding us that the heart is just as vital as the hands in the world of healthcare.

I commend Ms Neelam Rai and Mr Arpit Ravindra Lal, for their dedication to sharing their knowledge and expertise with others. Their passion for the field of Operation Theatre Technology is evident, and their commitment to advancing the profession shines through in the meticulous research and practical insights presented in this book. As authors, they serve as beacons, guiding readers on a path of continuous learning and growth.

I would also like to express my gratitude to the Operation Theatre Technicians who tirelessly strive for excellence in their work. Your skills, knowledge, and unwavering dedication make a significant difference in the lives of countless patients. This book stands as a testament to your invaluable contributions, and I hope it serves as a source of inspiration and recognition for your remarkable work.

It is with great pleasure that I introduce this book, an extraordinary testament to the world of Operation Theatre Technicians and the authors who have brought their stories to life. May this book ignite curiosity, foster learning, and inspire a new generation of professionals who will continue to push the boundaries of excellence in surgical support.

Ms Pratiksha John
MSc Nursing
Department of Paediatrics
Savitri Hospital and Paramedical Institute,
Gorakhpur, Uttar Pradesh, India

Foreword

It is a great pleasure and privilege that I write this foreword for *A Manual for Operation Theater Technicians* written by Ms Neelam Rai and Mr Arpit Ravindra Lal. This book is a suitable guide to help the teachers and students alike in the Paramedical as well as Nursing education.

This book is well written and structured so that it is straightforward for the readers. Text has been presented in very simple language, which is an added attraction of this book. I really congratulate them for their enthusiasm and hard work in writing and bringing out this book.

Having read this book in its entirety, I recommend it to both students and teachers, and qualified surgical assistants. I am very sure that this book will go into several editions and prints as it readily deserves.

Asif Masood
MCh (Plastic Surgery)
Savitri Hospital and Research Center
Gorakhpur, Uttar Pradesh, India

Preface to the Second Edition

An OT Technician plays a vital role in aligning the entire perioperative event for its smooth flow and functioning. The responsibility of an OT Technician starts from preoperative period, continues throughout the intraoperative period and follows till the postoperative care until the patient gets discharged. The objective of perioperative care is to provide better conditions for patients before, during and after the operation.

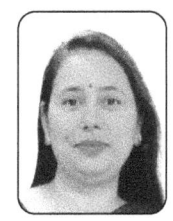

This edition of *A Manual for Operation Theater Technicians* which was previously known as *Textbook for operation Theater Technicians* is exclusively designed to meet the requirements of the new syllabus that was implemented sometime

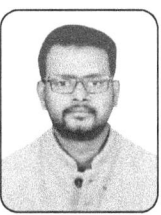

after the last edition was published. This edition is authored strictly to fall in line with the new syllabus and we as authors feel grateful to all our buyers who somehow adjusted with the previous edition after a sudden syllabus change. We are aware of the difficulties faced by the students as there were no books available in the market for this particular course as per the updated syllabus, therefore, We, being a little connected with the Paramedical courses, took this as a burden to bring out this book.

This will suffice as a systematic and top quality material for OT Technician students and others associated with Operation Theater and would help the readers to understand the importance and role of OT Technicians/Nurses in Operation Theater in the entire perioperative period. This book would provide a wide coverage of all the important topics that are included in the curriculum as well as many other paramedical courses.

About this book, it is divided into two parts. First part covers two chapters and the second part contains four chapters. This book can be extensively used by the whole teaching community. We hope the readers find a very relatable text. We will be considerate and appreciative to the analytical comments and suggestions for any further improvement.

Neelam Rai
Arpit Ravindra Lal

Preface to the First Edition

An OT Technician plays a vital role in aligning the entire perioperative events for its smooth flow and functioning. The responsibility of an OT Technician starts from preoperative period, continues in the intraoperative period and follows the postoperative until discharge. The goal of perioperative care is to provide better conditions for patients before operation, during operation and after operation.

Textbook for Operation Theater Technicians is designed to provide a systematic and quality material for OT Technician students and other medical students. It helps to understand the essentials in the operation theater and the role of OT Technician/nurse in the entire perioperative period. This book provides wide coverage of those topics, which are included in the curriculum of paramedical students. This book is divided into two parts. First part covers nine chapters whereas second part covers six chapters which contain meaningful diagrams and pictures. This book can also be used as reference by teachers. We hope the readers will find a very readable text. We will always appreciate the analytical comments and suggestions for further improvement of this book.

Neelam Rai
Arpit Ravindra Lal

Acknowledgments

I am grateful to the Lord Almighty Who strengthened me and showed His blessing upon me to complete this task with positive spirit and enthusiasm. I take this opportunity to express my heartfelt regards to my teachers and lovable parents who have brought me up.

I am indebted to Dr Brijesh Kr Jaiswal, Managing Director, Savitri Hospital and Paramedical Institute, Gorakhpur, Uttar Pradesh, India, for his support.

My sincere thanks to all the faculty members of Savitri Hospital and Paramedical Institute for their valuable cooperation. I feel proud and privileged to mention some of my colleagues' name here for their inexpressible help and motivation, without them this assignment would not have been possible; Ms Rekha Umale, Ms Smitha Sunny, Ms Monica, Mr Vijay Raj Yadav, Ms Anjali Nathaniel and Mr Shiju Thomas.

I put across my deep gratitude to my lovable husband for his intense care and concern which assisted me in accomplishing this task. Credit also goes to my sweet children for their love and smile that used to relax me after my tiresome work.

I gratefully thank Shri Jitendar P Vij (Group Chairman), Mr Ankit Vij (Managing Director), Shri Jitendar P Vij (Group Chairman), Mr Ankit Vij (Managing Director), Mr MS Mani (Group President), Dr Madhu Choudhary (Director-Educational Publishing), Ms Pooja Bhandari [Director-Production (Books and Journals)], Ms Sunita Katla (Executive Assistant to Group Chairman and Publishing Manager), Ms Samina Khan (Executive Assistant to Director-Educational Publishing), for their all-round support as and when needed.

I also acknowledge the help of Dr Upma Tomar (Development Editor), Mr Rajesh Sharma (Production Coordinator), Ms Seema Dogra (Cover Visualizer), Mr Narsingh Kumar (Proofreader), Mr Jagvir Singh (Typesetter), Sumit Kumar (Graphic Designer), and wish to thank all others of M/s Jaypee Brothers Medical Publishers (P) Ltd, New Delhi, India, who worked for this project.

Contents

PART I

1. **General Anatomy and Physiology** 3
   - General Orientation about the Parts of Human Body *3*
   - Various Terms Used in Anatomy *5*
   - Structure of Cell, Cell Organelles and their Functions *10*
   - Cell Structure *10*
   - Cell Cycle *17*
   - Human Tissues, Types, Structure and Function *21*
   - **Osteology:** Skeletal System *26*
   - Ribs and Sternum *28*
   - Pectoral Girdle and Upper Limb *28*
   - Pelvic Girdle and Lower Limb *29*
   - Types of Bones *30*
   - Arthrology Joints: Types, Basic Structure *35*
   - Myology *38*
   - Anatomical Spaces *44*
   - Histology Skin and Appendages *45*
   - **Alimentary System:** GIT *47*
   - Process of Food Ingestion, Digestion, Absorption and Defecation *52*
   - Respiratory System *56*
   - Breathing Mechanism, Different Respiratory Volumes *62*
   - Respiratory Volume *65*
   - Lung Capacities *67*
   - Urinary System *68*
   - Process of Urine Formation *71*
   - Reproductive System *73*
   - Female Reproductive System *76*
   - Endocrine System *80*
   - **Nervous System:** Structure of Brain and Spinal Cord *86*
   - **Blood:** Composition and Functions *94*
   - Pathophysiology *99*
   - Clinical Significance *100*
   - Structure and Functions of Sensory Organs: Eye, Ear, Nose, Tongue Special Senses *101*

- Cardiac System *107*
- Lymphatic System *117*

2. **Pathology, Pharmacology and Microbiology** **121**
    - Inflammation *121*
    - Healing *126*
    - Apoptosis *129*
    - Necrosis *130*
    - Shock *133*
    - Disorders of Blood Coagulation System *137*
    - Disorders of Immune System of Body *142*
    - Immune Disorders *146*
    - Disease Transmission and Prevention of Infection *150*
    - Sterilization *154*
    - **Bacteria:** Virus and Fungi *157*
    - Routes of Drug Administration *159*
    - Adverse Effects and Side Effects of Drugs *162*
    - Side Effects of Drugs *165*
    - Analgesics *168*
    - Drugs Used in Cough and Expectoration *171*
    - Drugs for Cough *171*
    - Drugs Used in Bronchial Asthma and COPD *172*
    - Drugs Used in Gastrointestinal Tract *174*
    - Basic Idea of Antimicrobials *192*
    - Basic Idea of Antihistamine and Corticosteroids *204*
    - Drug Used in Treatment of Anemia *205*
    - Anesthetics Agent *209*
    - Muscle Relaxant *219*

PART II

3. **Surgical Anatomy** **225**
    - Structure of Anterior Abdominal Wall including Clinical Anatomy of Hernia *227*
    - Structure of Posterior Abdominal Wall *236*
    - Structure of Thoracic Wall *240*
    - Meninges and Scalp *246*
    - Surface Anatomy and Bony Landmarks *251*
    - Concept of Mediastenum *260*
    - Skin as Sensory Organ *268*
    - Applied Ocular Anatomy *276*
    - Major Muscles of Body *281*

4. **Basics of OT Techniques, CSSD Techniques and Anesthesia Technique** **286**
   - Handwashing and Surgical Scrubbing *286*
   - Preoperative Preparation of Patient including Surgery Site *295*
   - Postoperative Care including Dressing *298*
   - Methods of Sterilization and Basic Functioning of CSSD *302*
   - Central Sterile Supply Department *304*
   - Various Positions Used in Different Surgeries *309*
   - Anesthesia, Boyle's Machine and Anesthesia Work Station *312*
   - Gases Used in Anesthesia *319*
   - Triage of Patients *321*
   - Details of Hand Instruments Used in Common Surgeries *323*
   - Preanesthetic Checkup *337*
   - Skin Preparation *341*
   - Infection Control in OT *347*
   - Basic Ideas of Different IV Fluids *366*
   - Needles, Sutures and Knots *371*
   - Cauterization (Cautery) *378*

5. **Hand Hygiene and Prevention of Cross Infection** **382**
   - Hand Hygiene and Method of Handwashing *382*
   - Prevention of Cross Infection *384*
   - Stages of Infection *385*
   - Nature of Infection *386*
   - Chain of Infection *387*
   - Universal Precaution *390*
   - Asepsis *393*
   - Hand Hygiene *397*
   - Personal Protective Equipment *399*
   - Biomedical Waste Management *403*

6. **Basic Life Support (BLS) and Cardiopulmonary Resuscitation** **408**
   - Code Blue *408*
   - Resuscitation Techniques or Basic Life Support *410*
   - Procedure of CPR *413*
   - Advanced Trauma Life Support (ATLS) *416*

Index 419

Paramedical Council Syllabus

DETAILS OF CURRICULUM FOR FIRST YEAR DIPLOMA IN OPERATION THEATER TECHNICIAN

Paper 1st—theory	Topics	Hours
1. General anatomy and physiology (cytology, histology, osteology and only basics of all organs systems of body).	1. General orientation about part of human body. Various term use in anatomy, total numbers of bones, their names and locations, basic idea about organizations of body from cell to organ systems.	06 Hours
	2. Structure of animals cell organelles and their functions.	06 Hours
	3. Human tissue—types structure and functions.	10 Hours
	4. Osteology—name, location, identification and basic details of all bone (details of skull bone is not required).	20 Hours
	5. **Joint:** Types, basic structure and example.	06 Hours
	6. Skin and appendages.	02 Hours
	7. **Git:** Locations, gross structure, various part and their functions	30 Hours
	8. **Respiratory tract:** Location, gross structure, various part and their functions, details of breathing mechanism.	30 Hours
	9. **Urinary tract:** Gross structure, various part and their functions (microscopic structure is not required) process of urine formation and voiding.	20 Hours
	10. **Male reproductive system:** Only gross structure and function of different part (microscopic structure is not required).	10 Hours
	11. **Female reproductive systems:** Only gross structure and function of different part (microscopic structure is not required). Menstrual cycle.	10 Hours
	12. **Endocrine system:** Hormones secreted by pituitary thyroid, parathyroid, pancreas, adrenal cortex, adrenal medulla, gonads and functions of different hormones. (Details of structures of these glands not required).	20 Hours

Paper 1st—theory	Topics	Hours
	13. Gross structure of brain and spinal cord function of different part of brain and spinal cord (details not required).	30 Hours
	14. Blood compositions of functions details about of plasma, RBCs, WBCs, platelets, clotting system.	30 Hours
	15. Gross structure and functions of sensory organs—eye, ear, nose, tongue. (Details not required).	20 Hours
	16. Basic gross structure of heart, vessels opening into heart and leaving the heart arterial and Venous tree of body.	20 Hours
	17. **Lymphatic systems:** Structure and functions.	10 Hours
	18. **Immune systems:** Components and various mechanism of defences	20 Hours
2. Only basic of relevant pathology, pharmacology (including ansesthetic agent) and microbiology.	1. Basic steps of acute and chronic inflammation and healing of wound.	05 Hours
	2. Basics of necrosis and apoptosis.	02 Hours
	3. Basics of shock.	02 Hours
	4. Basics of disorders of blood coagulation systems.	08 Hours
	5. Basics of disorders of immune system of body.	05 Hours
	6. Modes of disease transmission and prevention of infection.	05 Hours
	7. Sterilization and methods of sterilization in hospitals.	10 Hours
	8. Basic idea about types of bacteria, virus, fungi.	20 Hours
	9. Routes of drug administration.	02 Hours
	10. Adverse effects and side effects of drugs.	02 Hours
	11. **Basic idea of analgesics:** Opioid and NSAIDs.	02 Hours
	12. Basic idea of drugs used in cough and expectoration.	01 Hours
	13. Basic idea of drugs used in bronchial asthma and COPD.	02 Hours
	14. Basic idea of drugs used in GIT.	03 Hours
	15. Basic idea of antimicrobials.	20 Hours
	16. Basic idea of anti H-1 histaminase and corticosteroids.	01 Hours
	17. Drug used in anemia.	02 Hours
	18. Anaesthetic agent (local and general).	25 Hours
	19. Muscle relaxants.	05 Hours

Paper 2nd Theory	Topics	Hours
1. Detailed Surgical Anatomy.	1. Detailed structure of anterior abdominal wall including clinical anatomy of hernia.	10 Hours
	2. Detailed structure of posterior abdominal wall.	03 Hours
	3. Detailed structure of thoracic wall.	03 Hours
	4. Concept of meninges and scalp.	03 Hours
	5. Surface anatomy and important bony landmarks.	13 Hours
	6. Concept of mediastinum.	03 Hours
	7. Skin as sensory organ.	03 Hours
	8. Applied ocular anatomy.	02 Hours
	9. Location of major muscles of body.	10 Hours
2. Basics of OT techniques and anesthesia techniques.	1. Hand wash and surgical scrubbing.	03 Hours
	2. Pre-operative preparation of patient including surgery site.	07 Hours
	3. Post-operative care including dressing.	05 Hours
	4. Basic idea of various methods of sterilization and basic functioning of CSSD.	15 Hours
	5. Various positions used in different surgeries.	15 Hours
	6. Types of anesthesia, Boyle's machine and anesthesia work station.	10 Hours
	7. Gases used in anesthesia.	08 Hours
	8. Triage of patients.	02 Hours
	9. Diagram and details of hand instrument used in common surgeries.	40 Hours
	10. Pre anesthesia checkup.	03 Hours
	11. Infection control in OT.	05 Hours
	12. Basic idea of different IV fluids.	05 Hours
	13. Needles, sutures and knots.	15 Hours
	14. Cautery.	05 Hours
3. Hand hygiene and prevention of cross infection.	1. Detailed structure of anterior abdominal wall including clinical anatomy of hernia.	15 Hours
	2. Detailed structure of posterior abdominal wall.	15 Hours
4. Basic life support (BLS) and cardiopulmonary resuscitation (CPR).	1. Code blue.	05 Hours
	2. Details of basic life support (BLS) and cardiopulmonary resuscitation (CPR).	35 Hours

PAPER I

Section Outline

1. General Anatomy and Physiology 3
2. Pathology, Pharmacology and Microbiology 121

CHAPTER 1

General Anatomy and Physiology

Chapter Outline

- General Orientation: Parts of Human Body
- Cell Structure and Functions
- Human Tissue
- Osteology
- Joints
- Skin and Appendages
- GIT
- Respiratory Tract
- Urinary Tract
- Male Reproductive System
- Female Reproductive System
- Endocrine System
- Brain and Spinal Cord
- Blood
- Sensory Organs
- Cardiac System
- Lymphatic System

GENERAL ORIENTATION ABOUT THE PARTS OF HUMAN BODY

Introduction

Anatomy is the study of the structure or the makeup of the body and the relationship between them.

They are many specialties in the study of anatomy:
- Gross anatomy
- Microscopic anatomy
- Development anatomy
- Embryology

Gross Anatomy

- It studies the body structure without microscope.
- Systematic anatomy studies the functions of the organs and its relationship within a system.
- Regional anatomy studies the parts of the body according to the regions.
- Systematic and regional anatomy is used to study gross anatomy.

Microscopic Anatomy

❖ Microscopic anatomy is also known as histology.
❖ To study the tissues that form different organs of the body a microscope is used.

Physiology

❖ Physiology is the study of the functions or work of the parts of the body.
❖ Anatomy and physiology are always studied to together so that one received a complete understanding of the human body.

Branches of Human Anatomy

Sl. No.	Branches	Definition
1.	Cytology	The scientific study of structure and function of cell
2.	Histology	The study of the microscopic structure of the Tissue
3.	Embryology	It is the branch of biology and medicine concerned with the study of embryos and their development
4.	Systemic anatomy	It is the study of specific system of the body
5.	Morphology	Study of the forms, shapes and structure of the body
6.	Organology	It is the human body organs
7.	Myology	The study of structure, arrangement and functions of the body muscles
8.	Osteology	The study of the structure and functions of the skeleton and their bony structure
9.	Genetics	The study of genes, genetics variations and heredity in the living organism
10.	Neurology	It is the branch of medicine that deals with the anatomy, function and disorder of the nervous system
11.	Microscopic anatomy	It is the study of the structure that cannot be seen with the necked eyes. Its need microscope
12.	Macroscopic anatomy (Gross anatomy)	It is the study of the structure that can be seen with the naked eye. Or It is the study of the structure that can be examined without the use of a microscope
13.	Regional anatomy	The study of anatomy based on regions or divisions of the body and emphasizing the relations between various structure like muscles and nerves and arteries, etc.

Contd...

Contd...

Sl. No.	Branches	Definition
14.	Surface anatomy	It is the study of the external features of the body
15.	Teratology	It is the scientific study of congenital abnormalities and abnormal formations
16.	Radiological Anatomy	It is the study of the structure of human body that includes the use of several imaging techniques, such as radiography, ultrasonography, echocardiology, radioisotope studies, CT scanning and MRI
17.	Applied anatomy	It is the direct application of the facts of human anatomy medicine and surgery

VARIOUS TERMS USED IN ANATOMY

Anatomical position (Fig. 1.1) is that of the body standing upright with the feet at shoulder width and parallel, toes forward. The upper limbs are held out to each side and the palms of the hands face forward **(Figs. 1.2A to C)**.

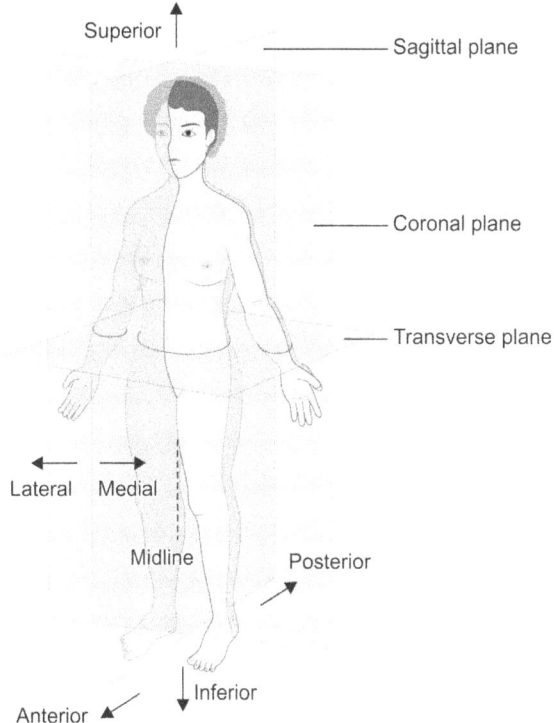

Fig. 1.1: Anatomical position.

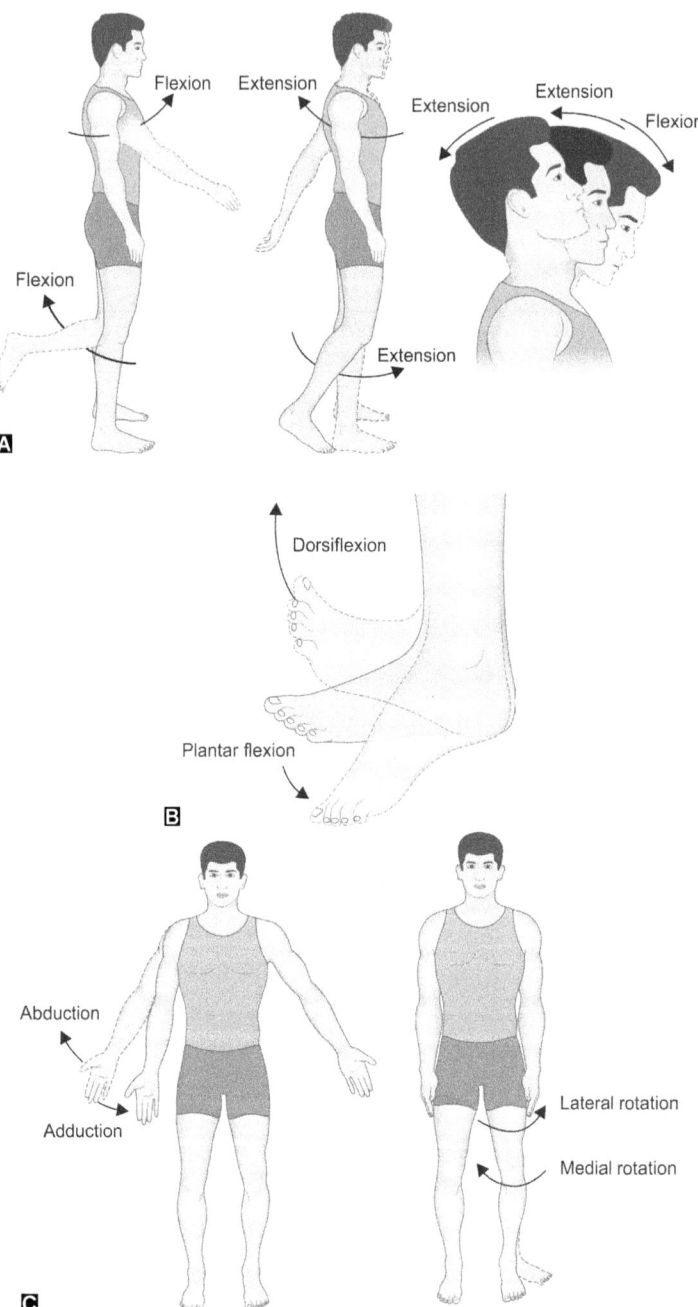

Figs. 1.2A to C: Range of motion.

Sl. No.	Anatomical terminology	Definition
1.	Superior (Cranial)	A position above or higher than part of the body proper.
2.	Inferior (Caudal)	A position below or lower than another part of the body.
3.	Anterior (Ventral)	The front or direction towards the front of the body. The toes are anterior to the foot.
4.	Posterior (Dorsal)	The back or direction toward the back of the body. The popliteus is posterior to the patella.
5.	Lateral	The side or direction toward the side of the body.
6.	Proximal	A position in a limb that is nearer to the point of attachment or the trunk of the body.
7.	Distal	A position in a limb that is farther from the point of attachment or the trunk of the body.
8.	Medial	The middle or direction toward the middle of the body.
9.	Superficial	A position closer to the surface of the body. The skin is superficial to the bones.
10.	Deep	A position farther from the surface of the body. The brain is deep to the skull.
11.	Peripheral	Away from the central part of the body. For example, Femoral artery is peripheral from the brain and the spinal cord.
12.	Plantar	Bottom of the foot is supported by the plantar fascia.
13.	Visceral	The internal organs deep within the chest or abdomen.
14.	Coronal section (Frontal plane)	A vertical plane that divided the body into dorsal and ventral portions.
15.	Sagittal section	A vertical plane that is parallel to the mid plane.
16.	Horizontal	A section horizontally through the central.

Commonly Used Terms of Movement

Sl. No.	Term	Meaning	Example
1.	Flexion	Bending or decreasing the angle between body parts	Flexing the elbow joint
2.	Extension	Straightening or increasing the angle between body parts	Extending the knee joint

Contd...

Contd...

Sl. No.	Term	Meaning	Example
3.	Abduction	Moving away from the median plane	Abducting the upper limb
4.	Adduction	Moving toward the median plane	Adducting the lower limb
5.	Rotation	Moving around the long axis	Medial and lateral rotation of UL
6.	Circumduction	Circular movement combining flexion, extension, abduction circumduction of upper limb	For example, bowling
7.	Eversion	Moving the sole of the foot away from the median plane	
8.	Inversion	Moving the sole of the foot toward the median plane	For example, as if to remove the thorn
9.	Supination	Rotating the forearm and hand laterally, palm faces anteriorly	For example, when a person extends a hand to radius lies parallel to ulna
10.	Pronation	Rotating the forearm and hand medially so that palm faces	For example, patting a child on the head faces posteriorly. Radius crosses ulna diagonally
11.	Protrusion	Moving anteriorly	Sticking the chin out
12.	Retrusion	Moving posteriorly	Tucking the chin retraction
13.	Elevation	To lift	Elevation of eyeball to look upwards
14.	Depression	To lower	Depression of eyeball to look at the feet

Commonly used anatomical and clinical abbreviations

A,aa   Artery, arteries
ANS   Autonomic nervous system
A-V   Atrioventricular
C1-C17(C8)   First to seventh cervical vertebrae or 1st to 8th spinal nerves cancer, carcinoma
Ca   Cancer, carcinoma

CAD	Coronary artery disease
CAT or CT	Computerized axial tomography
CN	Cranial nerve
CNS	Central nervous system
CSF	Cerebrospinal fluid
ECG	Electrocardiogram
EEG	Electroencephalogram/graphy Greek
G;GK	Greek
GI/GIT	Gastrointestinal/Gastrointestinal tract interphalangeal
IP	Interphalangeal
IV	Interventricular or intervertebral
IV	Intravenous
IVC	Inferior vena cava
IVF	In vitro fertilization
Jt	Joint
L1-L5	1st to 5th lumbar nerves/vertebrae
LA	Left atrium
LICS	Left intercostal space
Lig	Ligament
LP	Lumbar puncture
LV	Left ventricle
m, mm	Muscle, muscles
MCP	Metacarpophalangeal
MI	Myocardial infarction
MRI	Magnetic resonance imaging
MTP	Medical termination of pregnancy
MV	Mitral valve
N, nn	Nerve, nerves
PA	Posteroanterior
PNS	Peripheral nervous system, paranasal sinuses
RA	Right atrium
RV	Right ventricle
S1-S5	First to fifth sacral vertebrae/nerves
SA	Sinuatrial/Sinoatrial
SVC	Superior vena cava
T1-T12	1st to 12th thoracic vertebrae/nerves
TIA	Transient ischemic attack
TMJ	Temporomandibular joint
V,VV	Vein/veins

STRUCTURE OF CELL, CELL ORGANELLES AND THEIR FUNCTIONS

Introduction

- The cell was discovered by English scientist Robert Hook in the year 1665.
- Human cells are the smallest functional and structural unit of the body.
- They are connected together to form the tissues. These tissues are grouped together to form different type of organs, such as stomach, kidney, heart, brain, and lungs. These organs are grouped together to form a particular system, each of which performs a particular function.

Example: The digestive system is responsible for digesting and absorbing of food.

- Our body develops from a single cell called zygote, which is result from the fertilization of ovum and sperm.
- Human cell consists of a plasma membrane, cytoplasm and its organelles and a nucleus, which includes mitochondria, ribosome, endoplasmic reticulum, Golgi apparatus, lysosomes and the centrosomes, microtubules, microfilaments and vacuoles.

CELL STRUCTURE (FIG. 1.3)

- Cell visible by a microscope. It is unable to seen by naked eyes.
- The size and the shape of the cell range from millimeter to microns, which are generally based on the type of function. A cell generally varies in their shape and sizes.
- **Human cell shape:** Spherical, oval and rectangular, etc.

The cell is divided in the three parts these are as follows:
1. Cell membrane
2. Cytoplasm and its organelles
3. Nucleus

Cell Membrane

It is also called as plasma membrane. The cell membrane is present outside the cell and providing outer protective covering and contains the cytoplasm.

- The cell membrane consists of two layers of phospholipids with proteins and carbohydrates.
- The lipid molecules on the outer and inner part (lipid bilayer) allow it to selectively transport substances in and out of the cell.

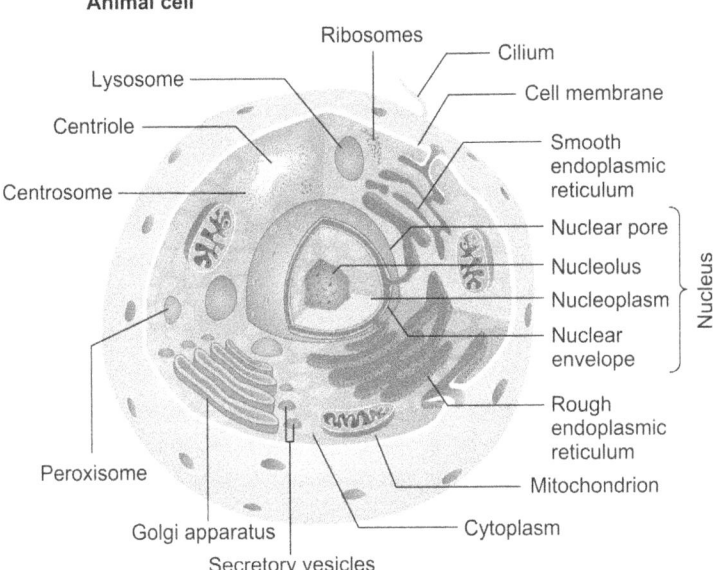

Fig. 1.3: Cell structure.

- Phospholipids make up the basic structure of a cell membrane.
- A single phospholipids molecule has two different ends—head and tail.
- The head end contains a phosphate group and is hydrophilic. This means that it is like to attract with water molecules.
- Tail end is made up of two strings of hydrogen and carbon atom called fatty acid chains. These chains are hydrophobic, mean do not like to attract with water molecules.

Functions of the Cell Membrane

- It acts as a physical barrier.
- It acts as receptors for hormones and other chemical messengers.
- It regulates exchange of materials with its surrounding.
- Some are enzymes transmembrane proteins form channels that are filled with water and allow very small, water-soluble ions to cross the membrane.
- To maintain the physical integrity of the cell.
- To control the movement of particles, e.g., ions or molecules.

Cytoplasm and its Organelles (Fig. 1.4)

- Cytoplasm is the fluid substance that fills the space between the cell membrane and the cellular organelles.

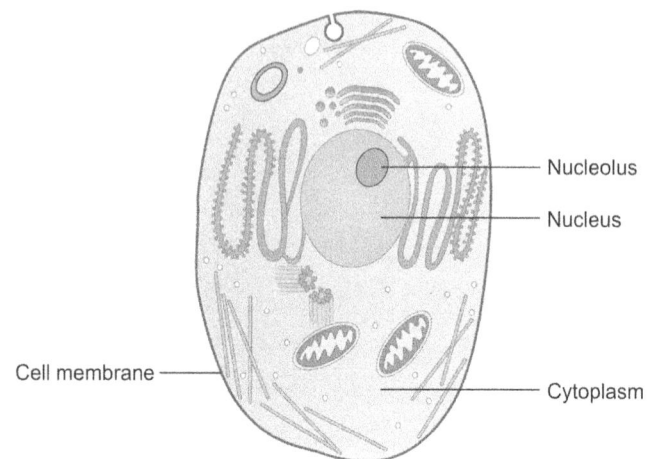

Fig. 1.4: Cytoplasm.

- The physical nature of cytoplasm is colloidal. It has a high percentage of water and particles of various shapes and sizes are suspended in it.
- Chemically cytoplasm contains water (60-90%) and 10% include a mixture of organic and inorganic compounds in various proportions. An organic component includes glucose, maltose, sucrose and inorganic components include phosphate, sodium, potassium and chloride.
- Cytoplasm is responsible for giving a cell its shape. It helps to fill out the cell and keep organelles in their place. Without cytoplasm the cell would be deflated and materials would not be able to pass easily from one organelle to another.

Mitochondria (Fig. 1.5)

- Mitochondria were first discovered in year 1886 by Robert Altman.
- Mitochondria are known as the powerhouse of the cell because they are responsible for the release of energy during cellular respiration.
- Energy is released in the form of ATP. While the cells release 2 ATP. Mitochondria release 34 ATP which adds up to 36 ATP. Since major portion of the ATP is released by mitochondria.
- The most active cell types have the greatest number of mitochondria, e.g., liver, muscles and spermatozoa.
- Mitochondria are shaped perfectly to maximize their productivity. They are made of two membranes.

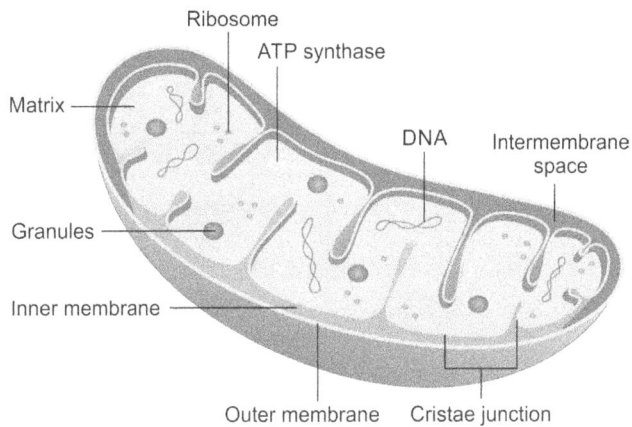

Fig. 1.5: Mitochondria.

- The outer membrane covers the organelle and contains it like a skin.
- The inner membrane folds over many times and creates layered structure called cristae.

Functions of Mitochondria

- The main function of mitochondria is the production of ATP.
- Contribution to synthesizing certain hormones, e.g., estrogen and testosterone.
- Cholesterol metabolism.
- Neurotransmitter metabolism.
- Detoxification of ammonia in the urea cycle.

Ribosome (Fig. 1.6)

- Ribosomes are the small structure and it is composed of RNA and protein. They synthesize proteins from amino acids, using RNA.
- They present in the cytoplasm in the form of small clusters.
- Ribosomes are originates on the surface of nuclear envelope and endoplasmic reticulum, where they produce protein for export from the cell. This is also called as protein factory or cell engine.

Endoplasmic Reticulum (ER)

Endoplasmic reticulum is a broad series of interconnecting membranous channels in the cytoplasm. They are two types of ER—smooth and rough.

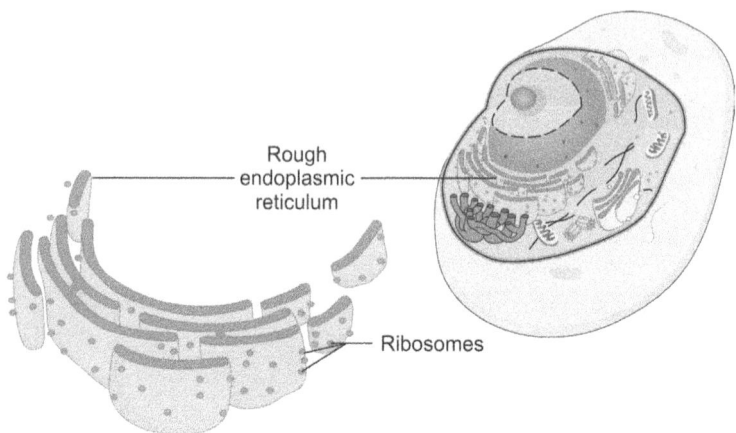

Fig. 1.6: Ribosome.

Smooth ER	Rough ER
SER does not bear ribosomes over the surface of its membranes.	RER possess ribosomes attached to its membranes.
It is mainly formed of vesicles and tubules.	It is mainly formed of cisternae and a few tubules.
It is engaged in the synthesis of glycogen, lipids and steroids.	The reticulum text part in the synthesis of proteins and enzymes.
SER gives rise to spherosomes.	It help in the information of lysosomes through the agency of Golgi apparatus.
Pores are absent so that materials synthesized by SER do not pass into its channels.	RER possesses narrow pores below its ribosomes for the passage of synthesized polypeptides into ER channels.
SER is often peripheral. It may be connected with plasma membrane.	It is often internal and connected with nuclear envelope.
Ribophorins (transmembrane glycoproteins) are absent.	RER contains ribophorins for providing attachment to ribosomes.
It may develop from RER	It develop from nuclear envelope.
It has enzymes for detoxification.	The same are absent.

Golgi Apparatus (Fig. 1.7)

❖ These are the group of closely folded flattened membranous sacs. It presents in all cells but is larger in those that synthesis and export proteins.

❖ The Golgi apparatus receives proteins and lipid from the rough endoplasmic reticulum. It modifies some of them and sorts, concentrates and packs them into sealed droplets called vesicles.

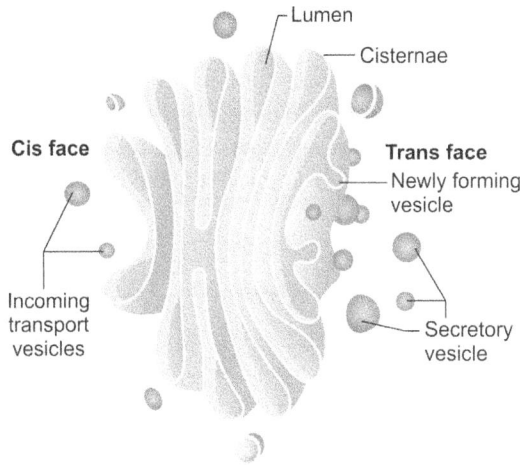

Fig. 1.7: Golgi apparatus.

- The vesicles are stored and when needed, they move to the plasma membrane and combine with plasma. These contents are secreted from the cell by the process of exocytosis.

Lysosomes (Fig. 1.8)

- Lysosomes are tiny sacs filled with fluid containing enzymes. Which enable the cell to process its nutrients and are also responsible for breaking down fragments of organelles and large molecules, such as RNA, DNA, carbohydrates, proteins inside the cell into smaller

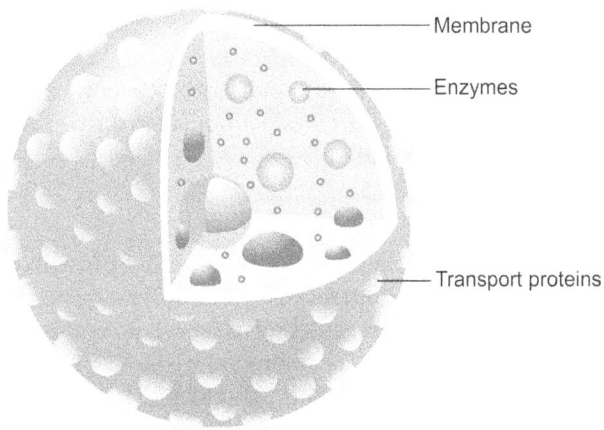

Fig. 1.8: Lysosome.

particles that are either recycled or extruded from the cell as waste material
- Lysosomes in white blood cells contain enzymes that digest foreign material, such as microbes. In case of disturbance of their cellular metabolism, they digest their own cell by releasing own enzyme that is why the lysosomes are called suicidal bags.

Functions of Lysosomes

- Intracellular digestion
- Autolysis
- Phagocytosis
- Osteogenesis

Centrosomes

Centrosomes consist of pair of centrioles. The centrioles are tiny cluster of microtubules.

Functions of Centrosomes

- It plays an important role in cell division.
- It maintains the equal distribution of chromosomes in daughter cell during cell division.

Microtubules

These are larger contractile protein fibers that are helpful in movement of cell extensions and cell and cell division.

Microfilaments

These are the smallest protein fibers. They provide shape, support and structural of the cell.

Vacuoles

Vacuoles are storage that bubbles found in cells. Vacuoles might store food of nutrients. They can store waste products so the rest of the cell is protected from contamination.

Nucleus (Fig. 1.9)

- All the cells have a nucleus but in RBCs, it is not present. Skeletal muscle fibers and some other cell contain several nuclei.
- The nucleus is the larger organelle of the cell. It is contained within the nuclear envelope, a nuclear membrane is similar to the plasma membrane but with tiny pores through which some substances can pass between it and the cytoplasm.

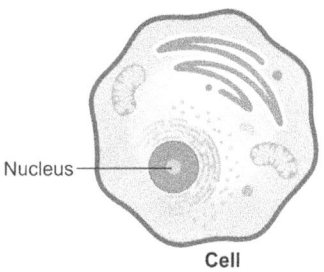

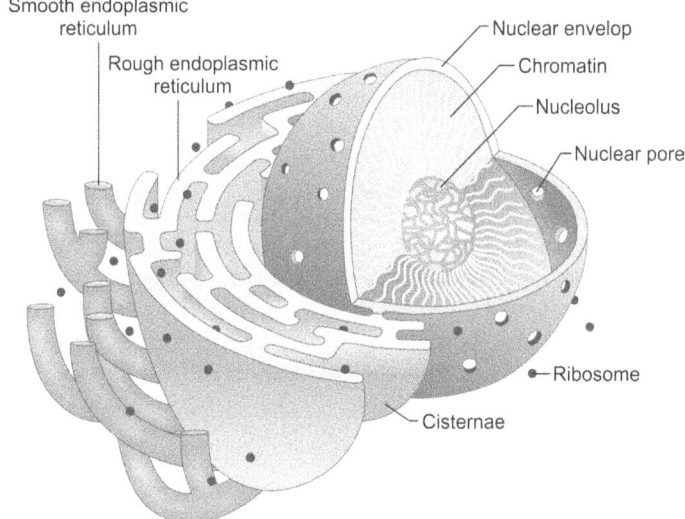

Fig. 1.9: Nucleus.

- Nucleus contains the body's genetic material which is called DNA. This directs all its metabolic activities.
- It is a non-dividing cell DNA which is present as a fine network of threads called chromatin. The cell prepares to divided the chromatin are called chromosomes. Substance like RNA is also found in the nucleus but all not found in nucleus.
- Nucleus is a spherical shape structure called the nucleolus. This is involved in synthesis of ribosomes.

CELL CYCLE (FIG. 1.10)

- Cell cycle described by Howard and Pelc (1953) first time. The sequence of events which occur during cell growth and cell division are collectively called cell cycle.

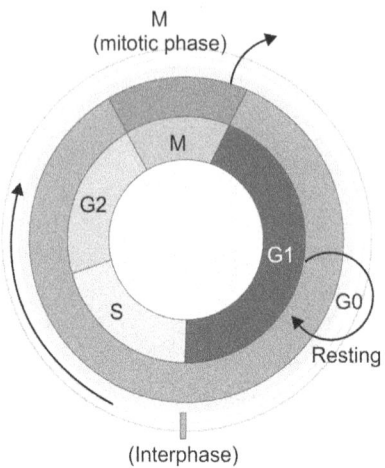

Fig. 1.10: Cell cycle.

- Cell division is the process by which a parent cell divides and gives rise to two or more daughter cells. It is a means of reproduction for single-cell organism.
- In multicellular organism cell division contributes to growth, development, repair and the generation of reproductive cells (sperms and eggs).

Mitosis and Meiosis (Fig. 1.11)

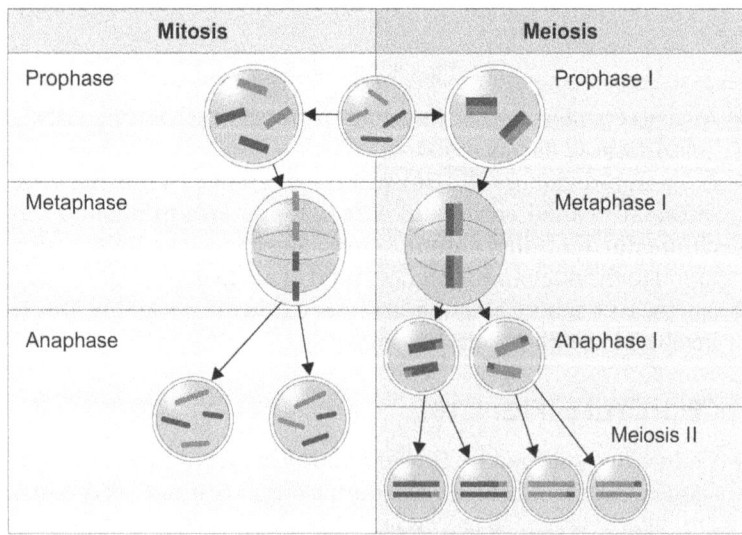

Fig. 1.11: Mitosis and meiosis.

Sl. No.	Characters	Mitosis	Meiosis
General			
1.	Site of occurrence	Somatic cells and during the multiplicative phase of gametogenesis in germ cells.	Reproductive germ cells of gonads.
2.	Period of occurrence	Throughout life.	During sexual reproduction.
3.	Nature of cells	Haploid or diploid	Always diploid
4.	Number of divisions	Parental cell divides once	Parental cell divides twice.
5.	Number of daughter cells	Two	Four
6.	Nature of daughter cells	Genetically similar to parental cell. Amount of DNA and chromosome number is same as in parental cell.	Genetically different from parental cell. Amount of DNA and chromosome number is half to that of parent cell.
II. Prophase			
7.	Duration	Shorter (of a few hours) and simple.	Prophase-I is very long (may be in days or month or years) and complex.
8.	Subphases	Formed of 3 subphases: Early-prophase, mid-prophase and late-prophase.	Prophase-I is formed of 5 subphases: leptotene, zygotene, pachytene, diplotene and diakinesis.
9.	Bouquet stage	Absent	Present in leptotene stage.
10.	Synapsis	Absent	Pairing of homologous chromosomes in zygotene stage.
11.	Chiasma formation and crossing over	Absent	Occurs during pachytene stage of prophase-I
12.	Disappearance of nucleolus and nuclear membrane	Comparatively in earlier part.	Comparatively in later part of prophase-I
13.	Nature of coiling	Plectonemic	Paranemic

Contd...

Contd...

Sl. No.	Characters	Mitosis	Meiosis
III. Metaphase			
14.	Metaphase plates	Only one equatorial plate	Two plate in metaphase-I but one plate in metaphase-II
15.	Position of centromeres	Lie at the equator. Arms are generally directed towards the poles.	Lies between equator and towards poles in metaphase-I and lies at the equator in metaphase-II
16.	Number of chromosomal fibers Two chromosomal fibers joint at centromere.		Single in metaphase-I while two metaphase-II
IV. Anaphase			
17.	Nature of separating chromosomes	Daughter chromosomes (chromatids with independent centromeres) separate.	Homologous chromosomes separate in anaphase-I while chromatids separate in anaphase in anaphase-II.
18.	Splitting of separating chromosomes	Occurs in anaphase.	No splitting of centromeres. Interzonal fibers are developed in metaphase-I
V. Telophase			
19.	Occurrence	Always occurs	Telophase-I may be absent but telophase-II is always present.
VI. Cytokinesis			
20.	Occurrence	Always occurs	Cytokinesis-I may be absent but cytokinesis-II is always present
21.	Nature of daughter cells	2N amount of DNA than 4N amount of DNA in parental cell.	1N amount of DNA than 4 N amount of DNA in parental cell.
22.	Fate of daughter cells	Divide again after interphase.	Do not divide and act as gametes.
VII. Significance			
23.	Functions	Helps in growth, healing, repair and multiplication of somatic cells. Occurs in both asexually and sexually reproducing organism.	Produces gametes which help in sexual reproduction.

Contd...

Contd...

Sl. No.	Characters	Mitosis	Meiosis
24.	Variations	Variations are not produced as it keeps quality and quantity of genes same.	Produces variations due to crossing over and chance arrangement of bivalents at metaphase-I
25.	In evolution	No role in evolution	It plays an important role in speciation and evolution.

HUMAN TISSUES, TYPES, STRUCTURE AND FUNCTION

Four groups of tissue in the body are known as the elementary tissues. These are epithelial tissue, muscular tissue, nervous tissue and connective tissue.

Epithelial Tissue (Fig. 1.12)

All epithelial cells lie on and are held together by a homogenous substance called a basement membrane. It is covering the body and lining cavities, hollow organs and tubes. Epithelial tissue consists of:
❖ Simple epithelium
❖ Stratified epithelium

Simple Epithelium

This consists of a single layer of cells and is divided into four types:
1. **Squamous epithelium:** It is composed of a single layer of flattened cells. These cells formed the alveoli of the lungs. They are found

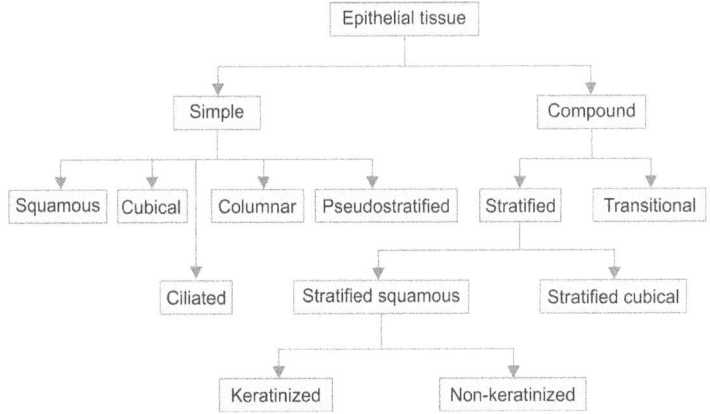

Fig. 1.12: Classification of epithelial tissue.

whenever a very smooth surface is essential as in the lining of the head, lining of blood vessels and lymphatics.
2. **Cuboidal epithelium:** These are the cube-shaped cells. It forms the kidney tubules and is found in some glands.
3. **Columnar epithelium:** This forms a single layer of cells which line the ducts of most glands, the gallbladder nearly the whole of the digestive tract in which goblet cells are interspersed and parts of the genitourinary tract (GIT).
4. **Ciliated epithelium:** It is found lining the air-passages and their ramifications, such as the frontal and maxillary sinuses. It also lines the uterine tubes and part of the uterus and ventricles of the brain. Ciliated cells are like columnar cells in shape but they have in addition fine hair like processes attached to their free edge. These processes are called cilia.

Stratified Epithelium

It consists of several layers of cells of various shapes. The superficial layers grow up from below. Basement membranes are usually absent. There are two main types—stratified squamous and transitional.
1. **Stratified squamous epithelium:** This is composed of a number of layers of cells of different shapes representing newly formed and mature cells. There are two types:
   i. *Non-keratinized stratified epithelium* (**Fig. 1.13**)*:* This is found on wet surfaces subjected to wear and tear but are protected

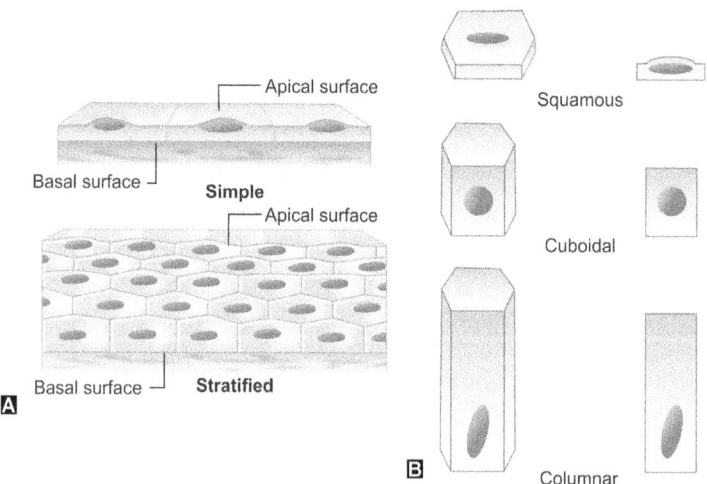

Fig. 1.13: Classification of epithelium: (A) Classification based on number of cell layers; (B) Classification based on cell shape..

from dying. For example, the lining of the mouth, the pharynx, the esophagus and the vagina.

  ii. *Keratinized stratified epithelium:* This is found on dry surfaces subjected to wear and tear in skin, hair and nails.
2. **Transitional epithelium:** This consists of several layers of pea-shaped cells. It is found in lining the urinary bladder and allows for stretching as the bladder fills.

Connective Tissue

Connective tissue provides the framework of the body. There are several types of connective tissue. This consists of loosely woven tissue which is distributed widely throughout the body. It is placed immediately beneath the skin and mucous surfaces forming the subcutaneous and submucous tissue and it also forms the sheaths of fascia which support and bind and connect together muscles, nerves, blood and other organs.

- **Adipose tissue:** It consists of fat cells, containing large fat globules in a matrix of areolar tissue. There are two types—white and brown:
  1. *White adipose tissue:* This makes up 20-25% of body weight in well-nourished adults. It is found supporting the kidney and the eyes, between muscle fiber and under the skin, where it acts as a thermal insulator and energy store.
  2. *Brown adipose tissue:* This is present in the newborn. It has a more extensive capillary network than white adipose tissue. In some adults, it is present in small amounts.
- **Dense connective tissue:** This contains more fibers and fewer cells than loose connective tissue.
- **Fibrous tissue:** This tissue is made up of closely packed bundles of collagen fibers with very little matrix. Fibrous tissue is found:
  - Forming ligaments
  - Act as an outer protecting covering for bone
  - Act as an outer protecting covering for some organs, e.g., the kidneys, lymph nodes and the brain
  - Forming muscle sheaths.
- **Elastic tissue:** It is found in organs where stretching or alteration of shape is required, e.g., in large blood vessel walls, the trachea and bronchi and the lungs.

Blood

It is a fluid connective tissue.

Lymphoid Tissue

This tissue, also known as reticular tissue has as semisolid matrix with fine branching reticulin fibers. It contains reticular cells and white blood cells (WBCs). Lymphoid tissue is found in lymph nodes and all organs of the lymphatic system.

Cartilage

It is firm but less firm than other connective tissue and clear blue-white substance. It is found principally at joints and between bones. There are three types—hyaline cartilage, fibrocartilage and elastic fibrocartilage.
1. **Hyaline cartilage:** It consists of collagen fibers embedded in a clear, glassy, tough ground substance or matrix. It is firm and elastic and is found covering the ends of the long bones as articular cartilage, in the costal cartilages in the nose, larynx, trachea and bronchial tubes where it keeps open the orifices.
2. **Fibrocartilage:** This consists of dense masses of white collagen fibers in a matrix similar to that of hyaline cartilage with the cells widely dispersed. It is a tough, slightly flexible supporting tissue found:
   - As pads between the bodies of the vertebrae, the intervertebral discs
   - Between the articulating surfaces of the bones of the knee joint
   - On the rim of the bony sockets of the hip and the shoulder joints depending the cavities without restricting movement
   - As ligaments joining bones.
3. **Elastic fibrocartilage:** This flexible tissue consists of yellow elastic fibers lying in a solid matrix. It provides support and maintains shape of pinna or lobe of the ear, the epiglottis and part of the tunica media of blood vessel walls.

Muscular Tissue (Fig. 1.14)

It is able to contract and relax providing movement within the body and of the body itself. Muscle contraction requires an adequate blood supply to provide sufficient oxygen, calcium and nutrients and to remove waste products. There are three types of muscle tissue, i.e., skeletal muscle, smooth muscle, and cardiac muscle.
1. **Skeletal muscle tissue:** This type is described as skeletal because it forms those muscles that move the bones, striated because striations can be seen in microscopic examination and voluntary as it is under conscious control.

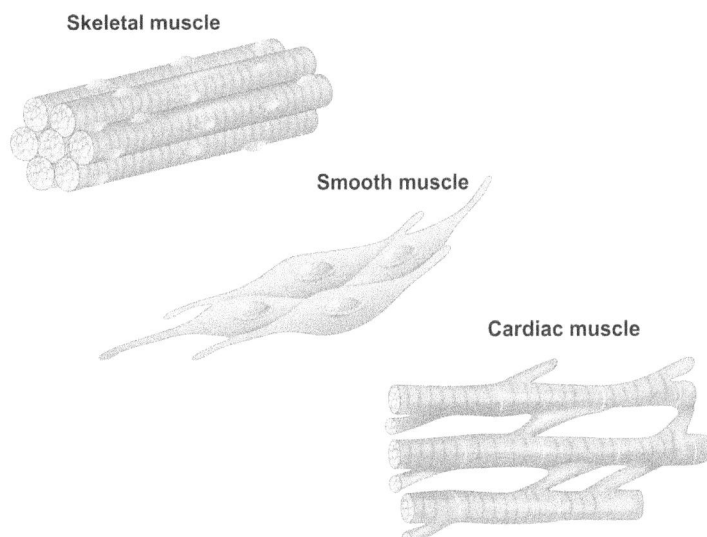

Fig. 1.14: Types of muscle tissue.

2. **Smooth muscle tissue:** Smooth muscle may also be described as non-striated or involuntary. Smooth muscle has the intrinsic ability to contract and relax. Contraction of smooth muscle is slower and more sustained than skeletal muscle. It is found in the walls of hollow organs.
    - Regulating the calamities of blood vessels and parts of the respiratory tract
    - Propelling contents of the ureters, ducts of glands and alimentary tract
    - Expelling contents of the urinary bladder and uterus.
3. **Cardiac muscle tissue:** This type of muscle tissue is found only in the heart wall. It is not under conscious control. The ends of the cells and their branches are in very close contact with the ends and branches of adjacent cells. The end-to-end continuity of cardiac muscle cells has significance in relation to the way the heart contracts. A wave of contraction spreads from cell to cell across the intercalated discs, which means that cells do not need to be stimulated individually.

Nervous Tissue

Two types of tissue are found in the nervous system:
1. **Excitable cells:** These are called neurons and they initiate, receive and transmit information.

2. **Non-excitable cells:** It is also known as great cells, these support the neurons.

■ OSTEOLOGY: SKELETAL SYSTEM (FIG. 1.15)

The skeletal system in an adult body is made up of 206 individual bones. These bones are arranged into two major divisions: The *axial skeleton* and the *appendicular skeleton*. The axial skeleton runs along the body's midline axis and is made up of 80 bones in the following regions:
- Skull
- Hyoid
- Auditory ossicles
- Ribs
- Sternum
- Vertebral column

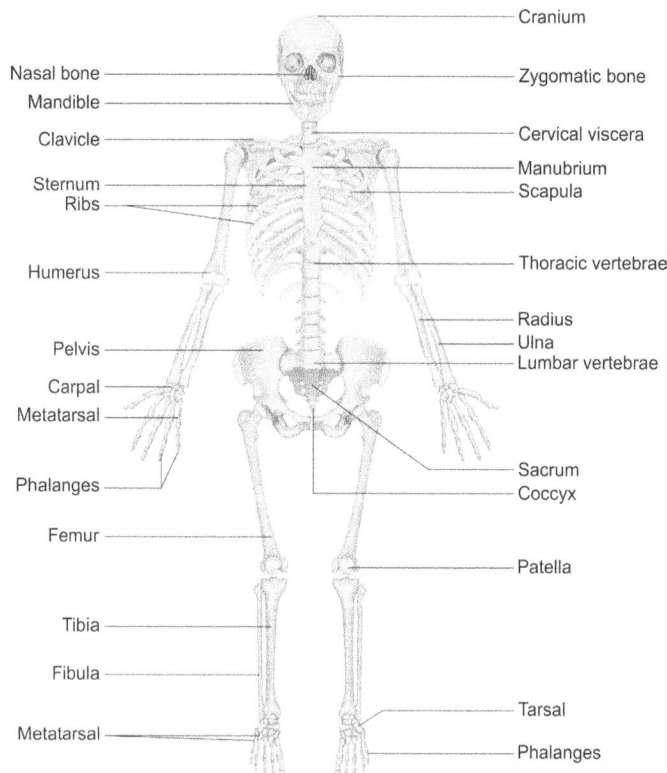

Fig. 1.15: The skeletal system.

The appendicular skeleton is made up of 126 bones in the following regions:
* Upper limbs
* Lower limbs
* Pelvic girdle
* Pectoral (shoulder) girdle.

Skull

The **skull** is composed of 22 bones that are fused together except for the mandible. These 21 fused bones are separate in children to allow the skull and brain to grow, but fuse to give added strength and protection as an adult. The **mandible** remains as a movable jaw bone and forms the only movable joint in the skull with the **temporal bone**. The bones of the superior portion of the skull are known as the **cranium** and protect the brain from damage. The bones of the inferior and anterior portion of the skull are known as **facial bones** and support eyes, nose, and mouth.

Hyoid and Auditory Ossicles

The **hyoid** is a small, U-shaped bone found just inferior to the mandible. The hyoid is the only bone in the body that does not form a joint with any other bone—it is a floating bone. The hyoid's function is to help to hold the **trachea** open and to form a bony connection for the **tongue muscles**.

The malleus, incus, and stapes—known collectively as the **auditory ossicles** are the smallest bones in the body, found in a small cavity inside of the temporal bone, they serve to transmit and amplify sound from the eardrum to the inner ear.

Vertebrae

Twenty-six vertebrae form the **vertebral column** of the human body. They are named by region:
* **Cervical** (neck)—7 vertebrae
* **Thoracic** (chest)—12 vertebrae
* **Lumbar** (lower back)—5 vertebrae
* **Sacrum**—1 vertebra
* **Coccyx** (tailbone)—1 vertebra.

With the exception of the singular sacrum and coccyx, each vertebra is named for the first letter of its region and its position along the superior-inferior axis. For example, the most superior thoracic vertebra is called T1 and the most inferior is called T12.

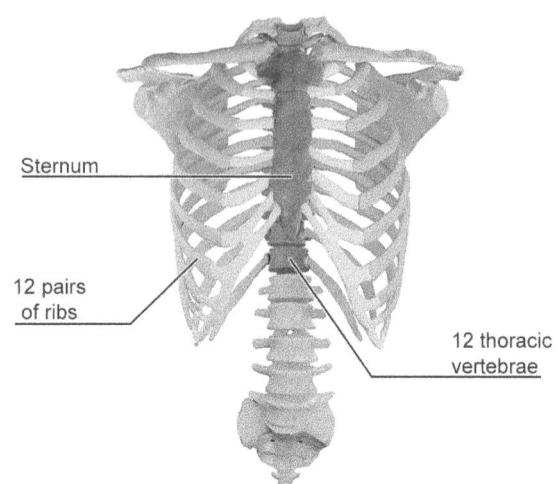

Fig 1.16: Ribs and sternum.

■ RIBS AND STERNUM (FIG. 1.16)

The sternum, or breastbone, is a thin, knife-shaped bone located along the midline of the anterior side of the **thoracic region of the skeleton**. The sternum connects to the ribs by thin bands of cartilage called the **costal cartilage**.

There are 12 pairs of ribs that together with the sternum form the ribcage of the thoracic region. The first seven ribs are known as **true ribs** because they connect to the thoracic vertebrae directly to the sternum through their own band of costal cartilage. Ribs 8, 9, and 10 all connect to the sternum through cartilage that is connected to the cartilage of the seventh rib, so we consider these to be **false ribs**. Ribs 11 and 12 are also false ribs, but are also considered to be **floating ribs** because they do not have any cartilage attachment to the sternum at all.

■ PECTORAL GIRDLE AND UPPER LIMB (FIG. 1.17)

The pectoral girdle connects the **upper limb (arm) bones** to the axial skeleton and consists of left and right clavicles and left and right scapulae.

The humerus is the bone of the upper arm. It forms the **ball and socket joint of the shoulder** with the scapula and forms the **elbow joint** with the lower arm bones. The radius and ulna are the two bones of the forearm. The ulna is on the medial side of the forearm and forms

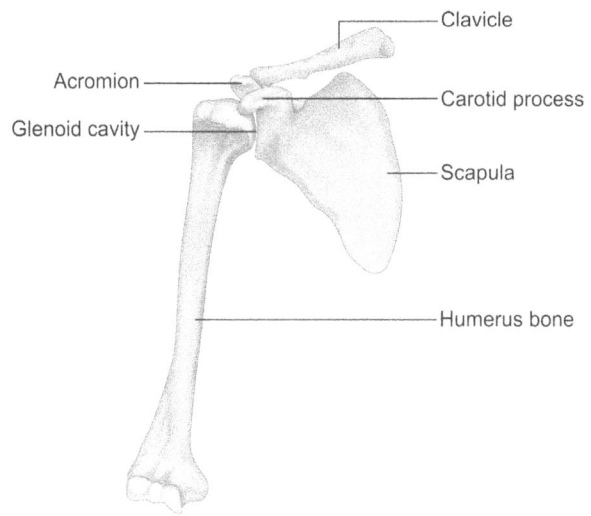

Fig. 1.17: Pectoral girdle.

a **hinge joint** with the humerus at the elbow. The radius allows the forearm and hand to turn over at the wrist joint.

The lower arm form the wrist joint with the carpals, a group of eight small bones that give added flexibility to the wrist. The carpals are connected to the five metacarpals that form the **bones of the hand** and connect to each of the fingers. Each finger has three bones known as phalanges, except for the thumb, which only has two phalanges.

PELVIC GIRDLE AND LOWER LIMB (FIG. 1.18)

Formed by the left and right hip bones, the pelvic girdle connects the **lower limb (leg) bones** to the axial skeleton.

The **femur** is the largest bone in the body and the only bone of the thigh (femoral) region. The femur forms the **ball and socket hip joint** with the hip bone and forms the **knee joint** with the tibia and patella. Commonly called the kneecap, the patella is special because it is one of the few bones that are not present at birth. The patella forms in early childhood to support the knee for walking and crawling.

The tibia and fibula are the bones of the lower leg. The tibia is much larger than the fibula and bears almost all of the body's weight. The fibula is mainly a muscle attachment point and is used to help maintain balance. The tibia and fibula form the ankle joint with the talus, one of the seven tarsal bones in the **foot**.

The tarsals are a group of seven small bones that forms the posterior end of the foot and heel. The tarsals form joints with the five long

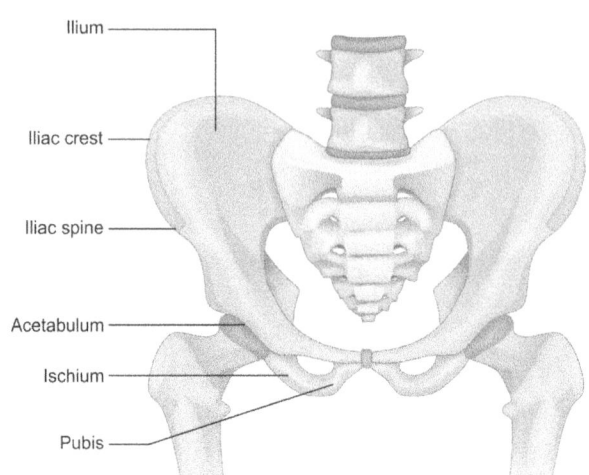

Fig. 1.18: Pelvic girdle.

metatarsals of the foot. Then, each of the metatarsals forms a joint with one of the set of phalanges in the toes. Each toe has three phalanges, except for the big toe, which only has two phalanges.

Microscopic Structure of Bones

The skeleton makes up about 30-40% of an adult's body mass. The skeleton's mass is made up of nonliving bone matrix and many tiny bone cells. Roughly half of the bone matrix's mass is **water**, while the other half is collagen protein and solid crystals of calcium carbonate and calcium phosphate.

Living bone cells are found on the edges of bones and in small cavities inside of the bone matrix. Although, these cells make up very little of the total bone mass, they have several very important roles in the functions of the skeletal system. The bone cells allow bones to:
❖ Grow and develop
❖ Repaired following an injury or daily wear
❖ Broken down to release their stored minerals.

■ TYPES OF BONES (FIG. 1.19)

All the bones of the body can be broken down into five types:
1. **Long:** Long bones are longer than they are wide and are the major bones of the limbs. They grow more than the other classes of bone throughout childhood and so are responsible for the bulk of our height as adults. A hollow medullary cavity is found in the center of

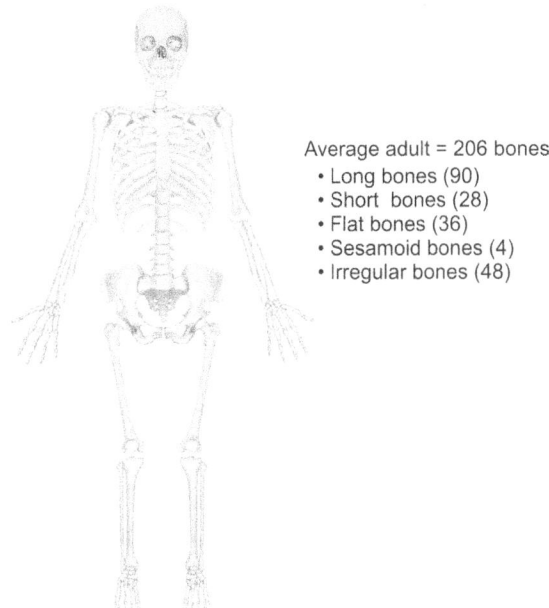

Average adult = 206 bones
- Long bones (90)
- Short bones (28)
- Flat bones (36)
- Sesamoid bones (4)
- Irregular bones (48)

Fig. 1.19: Types of bones.

long bones and serves as a storage area for bone marrow. Examples of long bones include the femur, tibia, fibula, metatarsals, and phalanges.

2. **Short:** Short bones are about as long as they are wide and are often cubed or round in shape. The carpal bones of the wrist and the tarsal bones of the foot are examples of short bones.
3. **Flat:** Flat bones vary greatly in size and shape, but have common feature of being very thin in one direction. Because they are thin, flat bones do not have a medullary cavity like the long bones. The frontal, parietal, and occipital bones of the cranium—along with the ribs and hip bones—are all examples of flat bones.
4. **Irregular:** Irregular bones have a shape that does not fit the pattern of the long, short, or flat bones. The vertebrae, sacrum, and coccyx of the spine—as well as the sphenoid, ethmoid, and zygomatic bones of the skull—are all irregular bones.
5. **Sesamoid:** The sesamoid bones are formed after birth inside of tendons that run across the joints. Sesamoid bones grow to protect the tendon from stresses and strains at the joint and can help to give a mechanical advantage to muscles pulling on the tendon. The patella and the pisiform bone of the carpals are the only sesamoid

bones that are counted as part of the 206 bones of the body. Other sesamoid bones can form in the joints of the hands and feet, but are not present in all people.

Parts of Bones

The long bones of the body contain many distinct regions due to the way in which they develop. At birth, each long bone is made of three individual bones, separated by hyaline cartilage. Each end bone is called an **epiphysis** (epi=on; physis=to grow) while the middle bone is called a **diaphysis** (dia=passing through). The epiphysis and diaphysis grow towards one another and eventually fuse into one bone. The region of growth and eventual fusion in between the epiphysis and diaphysis is called the **metaphysis** (meta=after). Once the long bone parts have fused together, the only hyaline cartilage left in the bone is found as articular cartilage on the ends of the bone that form joints with other bones. The **articular cartilage** acts as a shock absorber and gliding surface between the bones to facilitate movement at the joint.

Looking at a bone in cross section, there are several distinct layered regions that make up a bone. The outside of a bone is covered in a thin layer of dense irregular connective tissue called the **periosteum**. The periosteum contains many strong collagen fibers that are used to firmly anchor the tendons and muscles to the bone for movement. Stem cells and osteoblast cells in the periosteum are involved in the growth and repair of the outside of the bone due to stress and injury. Blood vessels present in the periosteum provide energy to the cells on the surface of the bone and penetrate into the bone itself to nourish the cells inside of the bone. The periosteum also contains nervous tissue and many nerve endings to give bone its sensitivity to pain when injured.

Deep to the periosteum is the compact bone that makes up the hard, mineralized portion of the bone. **Compact bone** is made of a matrix of hard mineral salts reinforced with tough collagen fibers. Many tiny cells called **osteocytes** live in small spaces in the matrix and help to maintain the strength and integrity of the compact bone. Deep to the compact bone layer is a region of spongy bone where the bone tissue grows in thin columns called **trabeculae** with spaces for red bone marrow in between. The trabeculae grow in a specific pattern to resist outside stresses with the least amount of mass possible, keeping bones light but strong. Long bones have a spongy bone on their ends but have a hollow medullary cavity in the middle of the diaphysis. The medullary cavity contains red bone marrow during childhood, eventually turning into yellow bone marrow after puberty.

Articulations

An articulation, or joint, is a point of contact between bones, between a bone and cartilage, or between a bone and a tooth. Synovial joints are the most common type of articulation and feature a small gap between the bones. This gap allows a free range of motion and space for synovial fluid to lubricate the joint. Fibrous joints exist where bones are very tightly joined and offer little to no movement between the bones. Fibrous joints also hold **teeth** in their bony sockets. Finally, cartilaginous joints are formed where bone meets cartilage or where there is a layer of cartilage between two bones. These joints provide a small amount of flexibility in the joint due to the gel-like consistency of cartilage.

Support and Protection

The skeletal system's primary function is to form a solid framework that supports and protects the body's organs and anchors the skeletal muscles. The bones of the axial skeleton act as a hard shell to protect the internal organs—such as the **brain** and the **heart**—from damage caused by external forces. The bones of the appendicular skeleton provide support and flexibility at the joints and anchor the muscles that move the limbs.

Movement

The bones of the skeletal system act as attachment points for the skeletal muscles of the body. Almost every skeletal muscle works by pulling two or more bones either closer together or further apart. Joints act as pivot points for the movement of the bones. The regions of each bone where muscles attach to the bone grow larger and stronger to support the additional force of the muscle. In addition, the overall mass and thickness of a bone increase when it is under a lot of stress from lifting weights or supporting body weight.

Hematopoiesis

Red bone marrow produces red and white blood cells (RBCs and WBCs) in a process known as hematopoiesis. Red bone marrow is found in the hollow space inside of bones known as the **medullary cavity**. Children tend to have more red bone marrow compared to their body size than adults do, due to their body's constant growth and development. The amount of red bone marrow drops off at the end of puberty, replaced by yellow bone marrow.

Storage

The skeletal system stores many different types of essential substances to facilitate growth and repair of the body. The skeletal system's cell matrix acts as our calcium bank by storing and releasing calcium ions into the blood as needed. Proper levels of calcium ions in the blood are essential to the proper function of the nervous and muscular systems. Bone cells also release osteocalcin, a hormone that helps to regulate blood sugar and fat deposition. The yellow bone marrow inside of our hollow long bones is used to store energy in the form of lipids. Finally, red bone marrow stores some iron in the form of the molecule ferritin and uses this iron to form hemoglobin in RBCs.

Growth and Development

The skeleton begins to form early in fetal development as a flexible skeleton made of hyaline cartilage and dense irregular fibrous connective tissue. These tissues act as a soft, growing framework and placeholder for the bony skeleton that will replace them. As development progresses, blood vessels begin to grow into the soft fetal skeleton, bringing stem cells and nutrients for bone growth. Osseous tissue slowly replaces the cartilage and fibrous tissue in a process called **calcification**. The calcified areas spread out from their blood vessels replacing the old tissues until they reach the border of another bony area. At birth, the skeleton of a newborn has more than 300 bones; as a person ages, these bones grow together and fuse into larger bones, leaving adults with only 206 bones.

Flat bones follow the process of intramembranous ossification where the young bones grow from a primary ossification center in fibrous membranes and leave a small region of fibrous tissue in between each other. In the skull, these soft spots are known as **fontanels**, and give the skull flexibility and room for the bones to grow. Bone slowly replaces the fontanels until the individual bones of the skull fuse together to form a rigid adult skull.

Long bones follow the process of endochondral ossification where the diaphysis grows inside of cartilage from a primary ossification center until it forms most of the bone. The epiphyses then grow from secondary ossification centers on the ends of the bone. A small band of hyaline cartilage remains in between the bones as a growth plate. As we grow through childhood, the growth plates grow under the influence of growth and sex hormones, slowly separating the bones. At the same time, the bones grow larger by growing back into the growth plates. This process continues until the end of puberty, when the growth plate stops growing and the bones fuse permanently into a single bone. The vast difference in height and limb length between birth and adulthood are mainly the result of endochondral ossification in the long bones.

ARTHROLOGY JOINTS: TYPES, BASIC STRUCTURE

The term arthrology is applied to the study of joints. There are three main classes—fibrous, cartilaginous and synovial joints.

- **Fibrous joints:** These joints are immovable or fixed joints in which no movement between the bones is possible, e.g., joints of the flat skull bones.
- **Cartilaginous joints:** These are slightly movable joints in which the joints surfaces are separated by some intervening substance and slight movement is only possible, e.g., the pubic symphysis and the intervertebral joints.
- **Synovial joints:** These are freely movable joints, e.g., the joints of the carpus and the tarsus.
- **Joints of the vertebral arches:** These are cartilaginous joints formed by pads of fibrocartilage placed between each two vertebrae, strengthened by ligaments running in front and behind the vertebral bodies throughout the entire length of the column. Masses of muscle on each side materially aid in the stability of the spine. The intervertebral discs are three pads of fibrocartilage between the bodies of the movable vertebrae.
- **Temporomandibular joint:** The mandible forms the lower jaw. It is the only movable bone in the skull apart from the ossicles of the ear. It consists of a body which is the central curved horizontal part containing the lower teeth and forming the chain and two upright portions called rami, one at each side which joins the body at the angle of the jaw.

The ramus terminates above processes, the coronoid process in front and the condyle of the jaw or as it sometimes called the head of the mandible which lies behind. This mandibular head or condyle articulates with the temporal bone to form the temporomandibular joint.

- **Joints of the upper extremity (Fig. 1.20):**
  - *The sternoclavicular joint:* It is a gliding joint formed by the large sternal extremity of the clavicle, articulating with the clavicular fact on the sternum.
  - *The acromioclavicular joint:* It is formed by the outer end of the clavicle articulating with the acromion process of the scapula.
  - *The shoulder joint (humeroscapular joint):* It is a synovial joint of the ball and socket variety. The head of the humerus forming

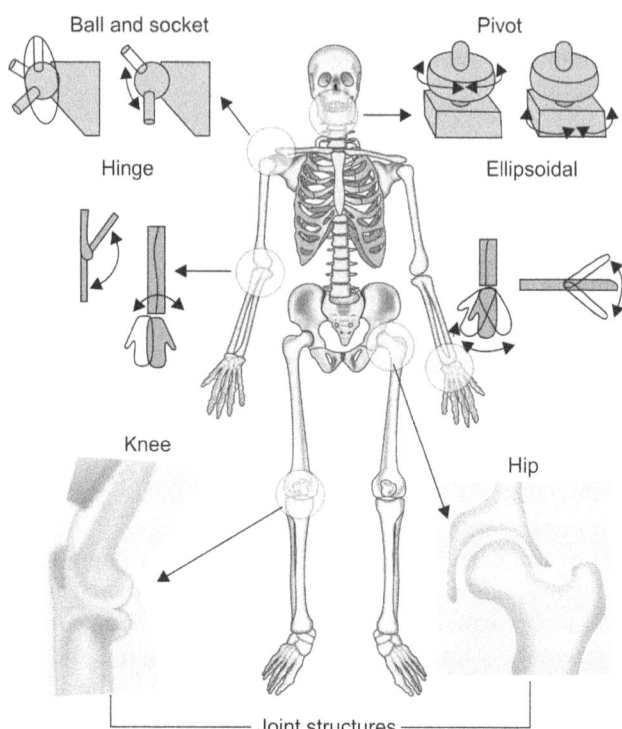

Fig. 1.20: Various joints present in the skeleton.

one-third of a space articulates within the glenoid cavity of the scapula.

- *The elbow joint:* It is a hinge joint between the trochlear surface on the lower extremity of the humerus and the trochlear notch of the ulna. This forms the principle part of the joint, the humeroulnar joint. The head of the radius articulates with the capitulum of the humerus forming the humeroradial joint.
- *The radioulnar joints:* These are two movable joints between the radius and the ulna, the superior and inferior radioulnar joints. The interosseous membrane forms a third joint—the middle radioulnar joint. This membrane also separates the muscles on the front from those on the back of the forearm.
- *The wrist joint:* The wrist joint or radiocarpal joint is a condyle joint between the lower end of the radius and the articular disc below the head of the ulna which together form a concave surface for the reception of the upper aspects of the scaphoid, lunate and triquetral bones.

- **Joints of hand and fingers:**
  - *The carpal joints:* The articulating surfaces between the carpal bones are flat and smooth. These flat surfaces move easily on each other, forming gliding joints between the different bones. The carpal bones are placed closely together so that only limited movements are possible but are fairly considerable amount of movement occurs when the bones move together.
  - *The carpometacarpal joints:* These are gliding joints formed between the distal aspect of the lower row of carpal bones and the superior articulating surfaces on each of the five metacarpal bones. The carpometacarpal found of thumb saddle joint which is formed between the base of the first metacarpal and the trapezium. Intermetacarpal joints are formed between the bases of the metacarpal bones, the lateral articulating surface form plane or gliding joints between these bones.
  - *The metacarpophalangeal joints:* These are joints of the condyloid type. The heads of the five metacarpal bones are received into articulating surfaces on the bases of the proximal phalanges.
  - *The interphalangeal joints:* These are hinge joints. These joints are formed by the heads of the proximal phalanges being received into articulating surfaces on the bases of the distal phalanges.
- **Joints of the lower extremity:**
  - *The hip joint:* It is a synovial joint of the ball and socket variety. The head of the femur is received into the acetabulum of the innominate bone. The acetabulum is depended by the attachment of the acetabular labrum to its circumference. This ligament is in the native of a rim of fibrocartilage which deepens and increases the adaptability of the surface formed by the acetabulum for the reception of the head of the femur.
  The capsular ligament of the hip joint is thick and string and limits the movement of the joint in all directions. The ligament is also especially strengthened by bands of fibers in several parts. One of the most important of these bands lies in front of the joint, the iliofemoral ligament. This ligament limits extension at the joint and so helps to maintain the crest position in standing.
  - *The knee joint:* It is a modified hinge joint formed by the condyles of the femur articulating with the superior surfaces of the condyles of the tibia. The patella lies on the smooth patellae surface of the femur over which it glides during the movements of the joint. It lies infront of the main articular parts of the joint but does not enter into the formation of the knee joint.

- *The tibiofibular joints:* These joints are formed between the upper and lower extremities of the two bones of the leg, the shafts of the bones being united by an interosseous ligament which forms a third joint between these bones as in the malleolus of the tibia which together forms a socket to receive the body of the talus. The capsule of the joint is strengthened by additional important ligaments.
- *Joints of the foot:* The joints between the tarsal bones are gliding joints. The bones are united by dorsal, plantar and interosseous ligaments.

  The interosseous ligament placed between the under surface of the talus and the upper surface of the calcaneus is thick and strong, and grooves the joint surfaces of both these bones.

MYOLOGY

It is the term which is used to describe the study of muscles

Muscles of the Face (Fig. 1.21)

There are many muscles involved in changing the facial expression and with movement of the lower jaw during chewing and speaking.

- **Occipitofrontalis (Unpaired):** This consists of a posterior muscular part over the occipital bone, an anterior part over the frontal bone and an extensive flat tendon that stretches over the dome of the skull and joins the two muscular parts.
- **Levator palpebrae superioris:** This muscle extends from the posterior part of the orbital cavity to the upper eyelid.
- **Orbicularis oculi:** This muscle surrounds the eye, eyelid and orbital cavity. It closes the eye and when strongly contracted 'screws up' the eyes.
- **Buccinator:** This flat muscle of the cheek draws the cheeks towards the teeth in chewing and in forcible expulsion of arc from the mouth.
- **Orbicularis oris (Unpaired):** It surrounds the mouth and blends with the muscles of the cheeks. It closes the lips and strongly contracted the shapes of mouth for whistling.
- **Masseter:** This is a broad muscle extending from the zygomatic arch to the angle of the jaw.
- **Temporalis:** This muscle covers the squamous part of the temporal bone. It passes behind zygomatic arch to be inserted into the coronoid process of the mandible. It closes the mouth and assists with chewing.
- **Pterygoid:** This muscle extends from the sphenoid bone to the mandible. It closes the mouth and parts of the lower jaw forward.

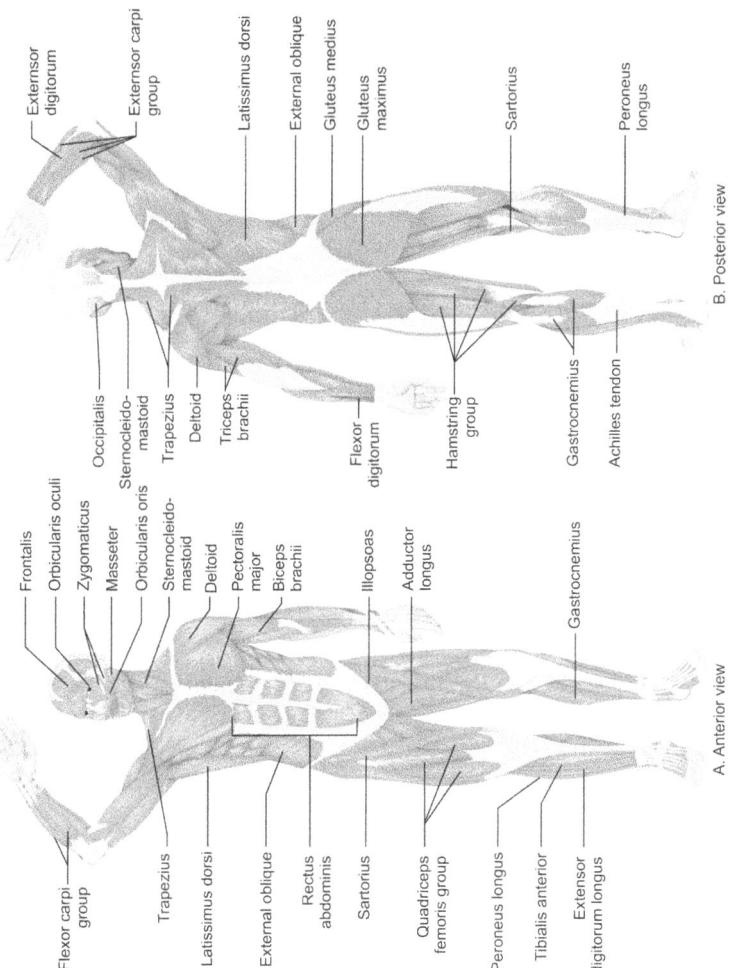

Fig. 1.21: Various muscles present in the body.

Muscles of the Neck

The region of the neck is divided into two main triangles—anterior and posterior by the sternomastoid muscle which running obliquely from the mastoid process of the temporal bone to the front of the clavicle which is palpable in its entire length.

The posterior of the neck is bounded infront by the sternomastoid muscle and behind by the anterior border of trapezius; it contains portions of the cervical and brachial plexuses of nerves—a chain of lymphatic glands which lie posterior to the sternomastoid and nerves and blood vessels. At the base of this, lies the first rib cover in which the subclavian artery passes. It is here that digital pressure can be applied to the subclavian artery.

Muscles of the Pelvic Floor

- **Levator ani:** This is a part of broad flat muscles, forming the anterior part of the pelvic floor.
- **Coccygeus:** This is a paired triangular sheet of muscle and tendinous fibers situated behind the levator ani.

Muscles of the Shoulder and Upper Limb

These muscles stabilize the association between the appendicular and axial skeletons at the pectoral girdle and stabilize and allow movement of the shoulders and upper arms.

- **Deltoid:** These muscles fiber originate from the clavicle, acromion process and spine of scapula and radiate over the shoulder joint to be inserted into the deltoid tuberosity of the humerus.
- **Pectoralis major:** This lies on the anterior thoracic wall. The fibers originate from the middle third of the clavicle and from the sternum and are inserted into the lip of the intertubercular groove of the humerus.
- **Coracobrachialis:** This lies on the upper medial aspect of the arm.

Muscles of the Thorax

The main muscles used in normal breathing are the intercostal and the diaphragm.

- **Intercostal muscles:** There are 11 pairs of intercostal muscles that occupy the spaces between the 12 pairs of ribs. They are arranged in two layer—the external and internal intercostal muscles.
    - *The external intercostal muscle fibers:* These extent downwards and forwards from the lower border of the rib above to the upper border of the rib below.
    - *The internal intercostal muscle fibers:* These extend downwards and backwards from the lower border of the rib above to the upper border of the rib below, crossing the external intercostal muscle fibers and right angles.
- **Diaphragm:** The diaphragm is dome-shaped muscular structure separating the thoracic and abdominal cavities. It forms the floor of the thoracic cavity and the roof the abdominal cavity and consists of a central tendon from which muscle fibers radiate to be attached to the lower ribs and sternum and to the vertebral column by two crura.

Muscles of the Trunk

These muscles stabilize the association between the appendicular and axial skeletons at the pectoral girdle and stabilize and allow movement of the shoulders upper arms.

Muscles of the Back (Fig. 1.22)

The arrangement of these muscles is the same on each side of the vertebral column.

- ❖ **Trapezius:** This muscle covers the shoulder and the back of the neck.
- ❖ **Latissimus dorsi:** This arises from the posterior part of the iliac crest and the spinous processes of the lumbar and the lower thoracic vertebrae.
- ❖ **Teres major:** This originates from the inferior angle of the scapula and is inserted into the humerus just below the shoulder joint.
- ❖ **Quadratus lumborum:** This muscle originates from the iliac crest, and then it passes upwards, parallel and close to the vertebral column and it is inserted into the 12th rib.
- ❖ **Sacrospinalis:** This is a group of muscles lying between the spinous and transverse processes of the vertebrae. They originate from the sacrum and are finally inserted into the occipital bone.

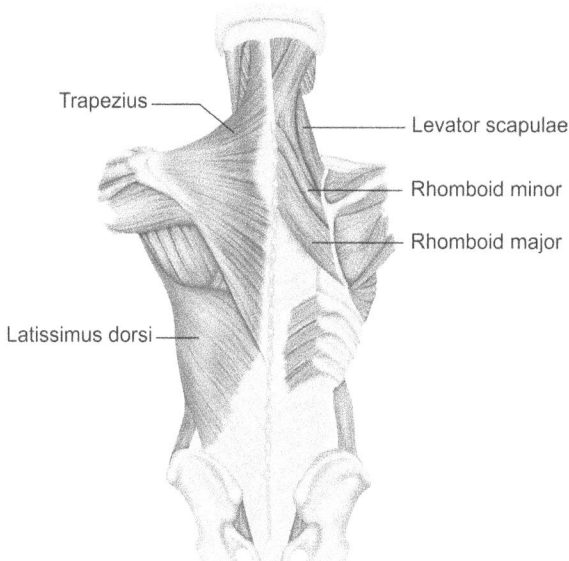

Fig. 1.22: Muscles of the back.

Muscles of the Abdominal Wall (Fig. 1.23)

Four parts of muscles from the abdominal wall are:
1. **Rectus abdominis:** It is the most superficial muscle. It originating from the transverse part of pubic bone then passing upwards to be inserted into the lower ribs and the xiphoid process of the sternum.
2. **Transverse abdominis:** The fiber arise from the iliac crest and the lumbar vertebrae and pass across the abdominal wall to be inserted into the linea alba by an aponeurosis. This is the deepest muscle of the abdominal wall.
3. **External oblique:** This muscle extends from the lower ribs downwards and forward to be inserted into the iliac crest.
4. **Internal oblique:** This muscle lies deep to the external oblique. Its fibers arise from the iliac crest and by a broadband of fascia from the spinous processes of the lumbar vertebrae.

Muscles of Arm

❖ **Biceps:** This lies on the anterior aspect of the upper arm. At its proximal end, it is divided into two parts each of which has its own tendon. The short head rises from the coracoid process of the scapula and passes in front of the shoulder joint to the arm.
❖ **Brachialis:** This lies on the anterior aspect of the upper arm deep to the biceps. It originates from the shaft of the humerus, extends across the elbow joint.
❖ **Triceps:** This lies on the posterior aspect of the humerus. It arises from three heads, one from the scapula and two from the posterior surface of the humerus.

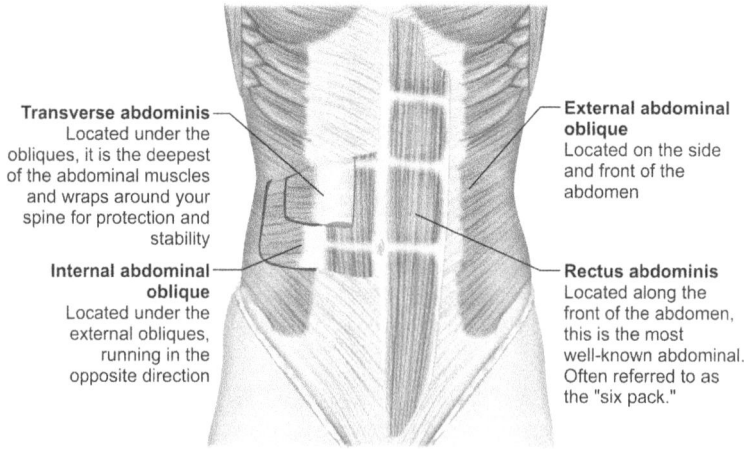

Fig. 1.23: Muscles of abdominal wall.

- **Brachioradialis:** The brachioradialis spans the elbow joint, originating on the distal end of the humerus and inserts on the lateral epicondyle of the radius.
- **Pronator quadratus:** This square-shaped muscle is the main muscle causing pronation of the hand and has attachments on the lower sections of both the radius and the ulna.
- **Pronator teres:** This lies obliquely across the upper third of the front of the forearm. It arises from the medial epicondyle of the humerus and the coronoid process of the ulna and passes obliquely across forearm which to be inserted into the lateral surface of the shaft of the radius.
- **Supinator:** This lies obliquely across the posterior and lateral aspects of the forearm.
- **Flexor carpi radialis:** This lies on the medial aspect of the forearm.
- **Extensor carpi radialis longus and brevis:** These lies on the posterior aspect of the forearm. The fibers originate from the lateral epicondyle of the humerus and are inserted by a long tendon into the second and third metacarpal bones.
- **Extensor carpi ulnaris:** This lies on the posterior surface of the forearm. It originates from the lateral epicondyle of the humerus and is inserted into the fifth metacarpal bone.
- **Palmaris longus:** This muscle resists shearing forces that might pull the skin and fascia of the palm away from the underlying structures, flexes and wrist.
- **Extensor digitorum:** This muscle originates on the lateral epicondyle of the humerus and spans both the elbow and wrist joints; in the wrist, it divides into four tendons, one for each finger.

Muscle that Control Finger Movements

Large muscles in the forearm that extend to the hand give power to the hand and fingers but not to the delicacy of movement needed for fine and dextrons finger control.

Muscles of the Hip and Lower Limb

- **Psoas:** The upper part of the psoas lies behind the diaphragm in the lower part of the media sternum. It also lies in relation to the quadratus lumborum. The lumbar plexus lies in the substance of this muscle and the abdominal aorta, the inferior vena cava and the receptaculum chyli and many lymphatic glands lie infront of it.
- **Iliacus:** This lies in the iliac fossa of the innominate bone. It originates from the iliac crest passes over the iliac fossa and joins

the tendon of the psoas muscle, to be inserted into the lesser trochanter of the femur.
- **Quadriceps femoris:** This is a group of four muscles lying in the front and sides of the thigh. They are rectus femoris and three vastus—lateralis, medialis and intermedius.
- **Obturators:** These are the deep muscles of the buttock, have their origins in the rim of the obturator foramen of the pelvis and insert into the proximal femur.
- **Gluteals:** These consist of the gluteus maximus, medius and minimus which together form the flesh part of the buttock.
- **Sartorius:** This is the longest muscle in the body and crosses both the hip and knee joints.
- **Adductor group:** This lies on the medial aspect of the thigh. They originate from the pubic bone and are inserted into the linea aspera of the femur.
- **Hamstrings:** These lie on the posterior aspect of the thigh. They originate from the ischium and are inserted into the upper end of the tibia.
- **Gastrocnemius:** This forms the bulk of the calf of the leg. It arises by two heads, one from each condyle of the femur and passes down behind the tibia to be inserted into the calcaneus by the calcaneal tendon.
- **Anterior tibialis:** This originates from the upper end of the tibia, lies on the anterior surface of the leg and is inserted into the middle uniform bone by a long tendon.
- **Soleus:** This is one of the main muscles of the calf of the leg, lying immediately deep to the gastrocnemius.

ANATOMICAL SPACES

- **The axilla:** It is a pyramidal-shaped space between the arm and the wall of the chest. It is bounded medially by the chest wall and the structures upon it laterally by the humerus and the muscles attached to it anteriorly by the pectoral muscles and posteriorly by the muscles attached to the axillary border of the scapula.
- **The cubital fossa:** It is a space at the bend of the elbow. It is bounded above by an imaginary line drawn transversely across the lower end of the anterior surface of the arm medially by the pronator teres muscle and laterally by the brachioradialis. The floor of this cavity is formed by the brachialis muscle.

- **The ischiorectal fossa:** It is placed immediately below the inguinal ligament which forms the base of the triangles; it is then bounded laterally by the adductors of the thigh. The floor is formed by the deep muscles of the thigh.
- **The subsartorial canal:** It is a passage running along the front and medial aspect of the thigh to reach the back.
- **The popliteal space:** It lies at the back of the knee joint, the posterior surface of which forms the floor of the space. It is a diamond shape space bounded above by the medial and lateral hamstring muscles and below by the medial and lateral heads of gastrocnemius.

HISTOLOGY SKIN AND APPENDAGES

The skin is the largest organ of the body, covering an area of approximately 2 m². The skin is composed of the cutis (including the dermis and epidermis), subcutaneous tissue, and skin appendages. The epidermis, which is derived from ectoderm, is the outermost layer of the skin and is mainly composed of keratinocytes. The dermis, which is derived from mesoderm, is located underneath the epidermis and is mainly, composed of elastic fibers, type I collagen, and connective tissue. It is formed by the papillary dermis and the reticular dermis. The subcutaneous tissue, which is derived from the mesoderm, is the innermost layer of the skin and is mainly composed of fat and connective tissue. Skin appendages are derived from the skin and include hair, nails, and glands. The main functions of the skin are protection (barrier against ultraviolet radiation, microorganisms, and water loss), the synthesis of vitamin D, detection of sensation (e.g., touch, temperature, pain), and the regulation of body temperature.

Structure of the Skin
See **Figure 1.24**.

Hair Follicles
Definition: Invaginations of the epidermis into the deep dermis, forming a cavity where the hair grows and develops.
- **Composition:** Hair
- A skin appendage that grows from follicles in the dermis
- Contains medulla, cortex, and cuticle
- Functions include conservation of body heat, sensation, and protection of the skin
- Most prominent on the scalp, pubis, axilla, extremities, and face

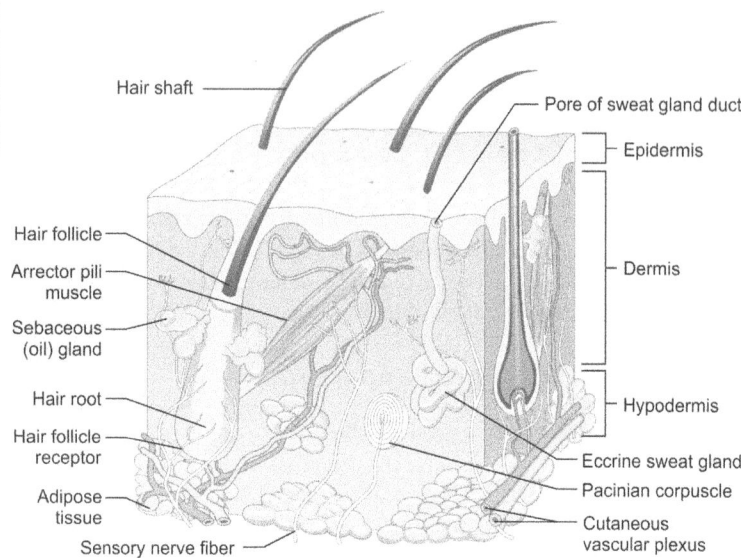

Fig. 1.24: Structure of skin.

- **See also "Phases of hair growth":** Hair shaft
- Extends above the epidermis
- **Connects to the hair root in the deep dermis:** Hair bulb
- Root of the hair follicle; located deep in the dermal papilla
- **Receives blood and nutrients from a capillary network of vessels to sustain hair growth:** Arrector pili muscle
- **Description:** obliquely directed smooth muscle fibers that attach to the dermal sheath surrounding hair follicles
- **Function:**
  - Contraction, which is responsible for piloerection (goosebumps)
  - Conservation of body heat
- Innervated by the sympathetic autonomic nervous system
- **Types:** Vellus hair follicle
- Extends into the reticular dermis
- Found throughout the body
- **During puberty, vellus hairs in the axillae and the genital area become terminal hairs:** Terminal hair follicle
- Extends into subcutaneous fat
- Found on the scalp, eyebrows, and eyelashes

Functions of the Skin

The main functions of the skin include:
- Barrier and protection against the external environment

- Thermoregulation (e.g., perspiration, regulation of blood circulation)
- **Sensory function:** Sensations of pressure, vibration, touch, pain, and temperature
- Hormone synthesis of vitamin D
- **Melanin synthesis:** Provides protection against ultraviolet (UV) radiation and determines the color of the skin and iris.

ALIMENTARY SYSTEM: GIT

The human digestive system (**Fig. 1.25**) consists of the *GIT* plus the accessory organs of digestion (its *tongue, salivary glands, pancreas, liver,* and *gallbladder*). In this system, the process of *digestion* has many stages, the first of which starts in the *mouth* (oral cavity). Digestion involves the breakdown of food into smaller and smaller components, until they can be absorbed and assimilated into the body. The secretion of *saliva* helps to produce a *bolus* which can be swallowed to pass down the *esophagus* and into the *stomach*.

Saliva also contains a *catalytic enzyme* called *amylase* which starts to act on food in the mouth. Another *digestive enzyme* called *lingual lipase* is secreted by some of the *lingual papillae* on the tongue and also from *serous glands* in the main salivary glands. Digestion is helped by the *mastication* of food by the *teeth* and also by the *muscular actions* of *peristalsis* and *segmentation contractions*. *Gastric juice* in the stomach is essential for the continuation of digestion as is the production of *mucus* in the stomach.

Liver

The liver is the largest gland in the body, weighing between 1 and 2-3 kg is situated in the upper part of the abdominal cavity occupying the greater part of the right hypochondriac region, part of the epigastric region and extending into the left hypochondriac region.

The liver has four lobes. The two most obvious are the large right lobe and the smaller, wedge-shaped left lobe. The other two, the caudate and quadrate lobes.

Structure

The lobes of the liver are made up of tiny functional units called *lobules*. Liver lobules are hexagonal in outline and are formed by cells called *hepatocytes*, arranged in pairs of columns radiating from a central vein between two pairs of columns of cells are sinusoids containing a mixture of blood from the tiny branches of the portal

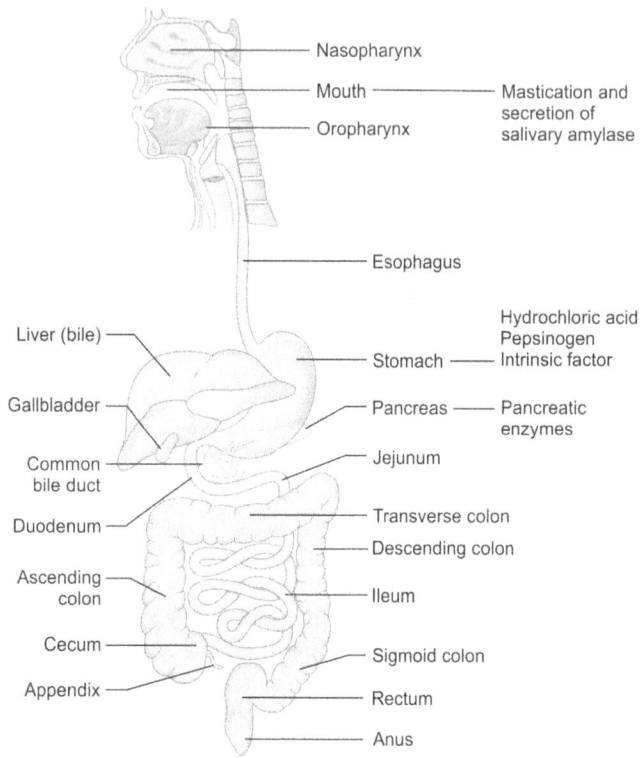

Fig. 1.25: Human digestive system.

vein and hepatic artery. This arrangement allows the arterial blood and portal venous blood to mix and come into close in contact with the liver cells.

Blood drains from the sinusoids into central or centrilobular veins. These then join with veins from other lobules, forming large veins, until eventually they become the hepatic veins which leave the liver and empty into the inferior vena cava.

Functions of Liver
- Carbohydrate metabolism
- Fat metabolism
- Protein metabolism
- Breakdown of erythrocytes and defense against microbes
- Detoxification of drugs and noxious substance
- Inactivation of hormones
- Production of heat
- Secretion of bile.

Stomach

The stomach is a J-shaped dilated portion of the alimentary tract situated in the epigastric, umbilical and left hypochondriac regions of the abdominal cavity.

Organs associated with the stomach are:
- Anteriorly—left lobe of liver and anterior abdominal wall
- Posteriorly—abdominal aorta, pancreas, spleen, left kidney and adrenal gland
- Superiorly—diaphragm, esophagus and left lobe of liver
- Inferiorly—transverse colon and small intestine
- To the left—diaphragm and spleen
- To the right—liver and duodenum.

Structure of the Stomach (Fig. 1.26)

The stomach is continuous with the esophagus at the cardiac sphincter and with the duodenum at the pyloric sphincter. It has two curvatures—*the lesser and greater curvature*. The lesser curvature is short lies on the posterior surface of the stomach and is the downward continuation of the posterior wall of the esophagus. Just before the pyloric sphincter, it curves upward to complete the J-shape where the esophagus joins the stomach. The anterior region angles acutely upwards, curves downwards forming the greater curvature and the slightly upwards towards the pyloric sphincter.

Parts of the Stomach

The stomach is divided into three parts:
1. **Fundus:** The fundus of the stomach is the dilated portion to the left and superior to the cardiac orifice. This is the most superior part of the stomach.
2. **Body of the stomach:** It is the major portion of the stomach. It lies between the fundus and the pyloric antrum.
3. **Pyloric antrum:** Antrum is continued as the narrow canal which is called pyloric canal or pyloric end. Pyloric canal opens into first part of small intestine called duodenum. The opening of pyloric canal is guarded by a sphincter called pyloric sphincter.

Walls of the Stomach

- The four layers of tissue that comprise the basic structure of the alimentary canal are found in the stomach bud with some modifications.

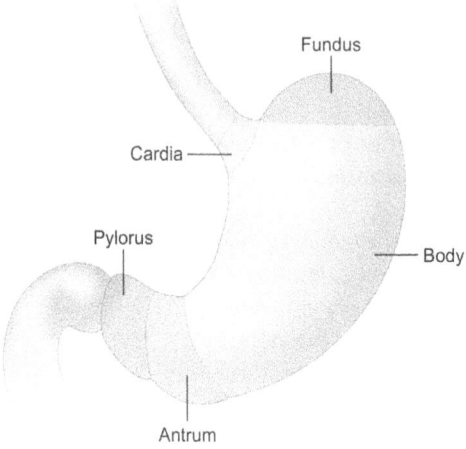

Fig. 1.26: Parts of the stomach.

- **Muscle layer:** This consist of three layers of smooth muscle:
  1. An outer layer is longitudinal fiber
  2. Middle layer is circular fibers
  3. Inner layer is oblique fibers
- **Mucosa layer:** When the stomach is empty the mucous membrane lining is thrown into longitudinal folds or rugae. Numerous gastric glands are situated below the surface in the mucous membrane. They consist of specialized cell that secrete juice into the stomach.
- **Blood supply:** Arterial blood to the stomach is by the left gastric artery, the right gastric artery and the gastro epiploic arteries.
- **Venous drainage:** Right and left gastric veins and in the portal vein; short gastric and left gastroepiploic vein drains into the superior mesenteric vein.

Functions of the Stomach

- It acts as a reservoir of food.
- By its peristaltic activity, it makes the food particles smaller and softer and mixes the food thoroughly with gastric juice.
- The gastric enzymes produced by gastric glands have an important role in digestion.
- The hypochondriac acid secreted by gastric glands destroys many organisms present in food and drinks.

❖ Stomach secretes the intrinsic factors necessary for the absorption of vitamin B_{12}.
❖ Some substances are absorbed in the stomach, e.g., some drugs, alcohol, glucose, etc.

The Gallbladder (Fig. 1.27)

The gallbladder is a pear-shaped musculomembranous bag lying in a fossa on the under surface of the liver and reaching to the front margin of that organ. It is about 8–10 cm in length. It is divided into a fundus, body, and neck, consists of three coats:
1. An outer serous peritoneal coat
2. A middle unstriped muscular tissue
3. An inner mucous membrane, which is continuous with that lining the bile ducts.

The cystic duct is about 4 cm in length. It passes from the neck of the gallbladder and forms the hepatic duct, there by forming the common bile duct which conveys the bile to the duodenum.

Functions

❖ Reservoir for bile.
❖ Concentration of the bile by up to 10 or 15 fold by absorption of water through the walls of the gallbladder.
❖ Release of stored bile.

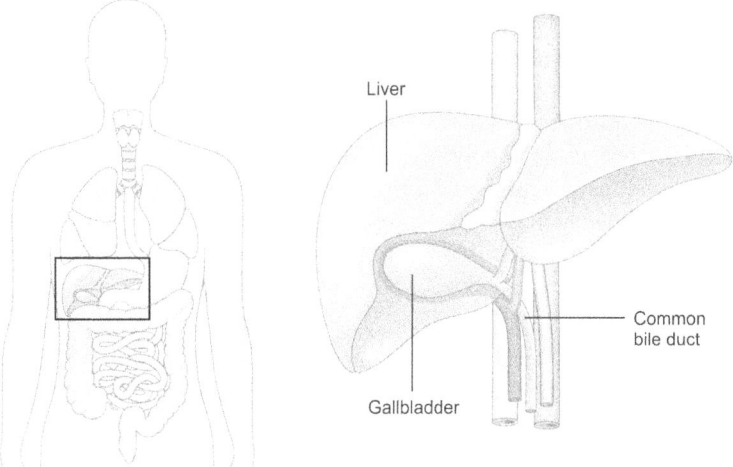

Fig. 1.27: Gallbladder.

PROCESS OF FOOD INGESTION, DIGESTION, ABSORPTION AND DEFECATION

Obtaining nutrition and energy from food is a multi-step process. For true animals, the first step is ingestion, the act of taking in food. This is followed by digestion, absorption, and elimination. In the following sections, each of these steps will be discussed in detail.

Ingestion

The large molecules found in intact food cannot pass through the cell membranes. Food needs to be broken into smaller particles so that animals can harness the nutrients and organic molecules. The first step in this process is ingestion. Ingestion is the process of taking in food through the mouth. In vertebrates, the teeth, saliva, and tongue play important roles in mastication (preparing the food into bolus). While the food is being mechanically broken down, the enzymes in saliva begin to chemically process the food as well. The combined action of these processes modifies the food from large particles to a soft mass that can be swallowed and can travel the length of the esophagus.

Digestion and Absorption

Digestion is the mechanical and chemical break down of food into small organic fragments. It is important to break down macromolecules into smaller fragments that are of suitable size for absorption across the digestive epithelium. Large, complex molecules of proteins, polysaccharides, and lipids must be reduced to simpler particles, such as simple sugar before they can be absorbed by the digestive epithelial cells. Different organs play specific roles in the digestive process. The animal diet needs carbohydrates, protein, and fat, as well as vitamins and inorganic components for nutritional balance. How each of these components is digested is discussed in the following sections.

Carbohydrates

The digestion of carbohydrates begins in the mouth. The salivary enzyme amylase begins the breakdown of food starches into maltose, a disaccharide. As the bolus of food travels through the esophagus to the stomach, no significant digestion of carbohydrates takes place. The esophagus produces no digestive enzymes but does produce mucous for lubrication. The acidic environment in the stomach stops the action of the amylase enzyme.

The next step of carbohydrate digestion takes place in the duodenum. Recall that the chyme from the stomach enters the duodenum and mixes with the digestive secretion from the pancreas, liver, and gallbladder. Pancreatic juices also contain amylase, which continues the breakdown of starch and glycogen into maltose, a disaccharide. The disaccharides are broken down into monosaccharides by enzymes called maltases, sucrases, and lactases, which are also present in the brush border of the small intestinal wall. Maltase breaks down maltose into glucose. Other disaccharides, such as sucrose and lactose are broken down by sucrase and lactase, respectively. Sucrase breaks down sucrose (or "table sugar") into glucose and fructose, and lactase breaks down lactose (or "milk sugar") into glucose and galactose. The monosaccharides (glucose) thus produced are absorbed and then can be used in metabolic pathways to harness energy. The monosaccharides are transported across the intestinal epithelium into the bloodstream to be transported to the different cells in the body. The steps in carbohydrate digestion are summarized in **Figure 1.28** and **Table 1.1**.

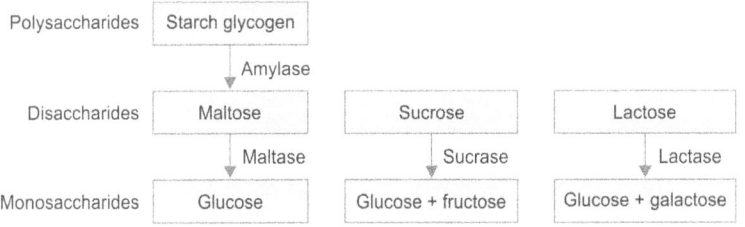

Fig. 1.28: Digestion of carbohydrates is performed by several enzymes. Starch and glycogen are broken down into glucose by amylase and maltase. Sucrose (table sugar) and lactose (milk sugar) are broken down by sucrase and lactase, respectively.

Table 1.1: Digestion of carbohydrates.

Enzyme	Produced by	Site of action	Substrate acting on	End products
Salivary amylase	Salivary glands	Mouth	Polysaccharides (Starch)	Disaccharides (maltose), oligosaccharides
Pancreatic amylase	Pancreas	Small intestine	Polysaccharides (starch)	Disaccharides (maltose), monosaccharides
Oligosaccharidases	Lining of the intestine; brush border membrane	Small intestine	Disaccharides	Monosaccharides (e.g., glucose, fructose, galactose)

Protein (Table 1.2)

A large part of protein digestion takes place in the stomach. The enzyme pepsin plays an important role in the digestion of proteins by breaking down the intact protein to peptides, which are short chains of four to nine amino acids. In the duodenum, other enzymes—trypsin, elastase, and chymotrypsin—act on the peptides reducing them to smaller peptides. Trypsin elastase, carboxypeptidase, and chymotrypsin are produced by the pancreas and released into the duodenum where they act on the chyme. Further breakdown of peptides to single amino acids is aided by enzymes called peptidases (those that break down peptides). Specifically, carboxypeptidase, dipeptidase, and aminopeptidase play important roles in reducing the peptides to free amino acids. The amino acids are absorbed into the bloodstream through the small intestines.

Table 1.2: Digestion of protein.

Enzyme	Produced by	Site of action	Substrate acting on	End products
Pepsin	Stomach chief cells	Stomach	Proteins	Peptides
Trypsin Elastase Chymotrypsin	Pancreas	Small intestine	Proteins	Peptides
Carboxypeptidase	Pancreas	Small intestine	Peptides	Amino acids and peptides
Aminopeptidase Dipeptidase	Lining of intestine	Small intestine	Peptides	Amino acids

Lipids

Lipid digestion begins in the stomach with the aid of lingual lipase and gastric lipase. However, the bulk of lipid digestion occurs in the small intestine due to pancreatic lipase. When chyme enters the duodenum, the hormonal responses trigger the release of bile, which is produced in the liver and stored in the gallbladder. Bile aids in the digestion of lipids, primarily triglycerides by emulsification. Emulsification is a process in which large lipid globules are broken down into several small lipid globules. These small globules are more widely distributed in the chyme rather than forming large aggregates. Lipids are hydrophobic substances—in the presence of water, they will aggregate to form globules to minimize exposure to water. Bile contains bile salts, which are amphipathic, meaning they contain hydrophobic and hydrophilic parts. Thus, the bile salts hydrophilic side can interface with water on one side and the hydrophobic side interfaces with lipids on the other. By doing so, bile salts emulsify large lipid globules into small lipid globules.

Pancreatic juices contain enzymes called lipases (enzymes that break down lipids). If the lipid in the chyme aggregates into large globules, very little surface area of the lipids is available for the lipases to act on, leaving lipid digestion incomplete. By forming an emulsion, bile salts increase the available surface area of the lipids many fold. The pancreatic lipases can then act on the lipids more efficiently and digest them. Lipases break down the lipids into fatty acids and glycerides. These molecules can pass through the plasma membrane of the cell and enter the epithelial cells of the intestinal lining. The bile salts surround long-chain fatty acids and monoglycerides forming tiny spheres called micelles. The micelles move into the brush border of the small intestine absorptive cells where the long-chain fatty acids and monoglycerides diffuse out of the micelles into the absorptive cells leaving the micelles behind in the chyme. The long-chain fatty acids and monoglycerides recombine in the absorptive cells to form triglycerides, which aggregate into globules and become coated with proteins. These large spheres are called chylomicrons. Chylomicrons contain triglycerides, cholesterol, and other lipids and have proteins on their surface. The surface is also composed of the hydrophilic phosphate "heads" of phospholipids. Together, they enable the chylomicron to move in an aqueous environment without exposing the lipids to water. Chylomicrons leave the absorptive cells via exocytosis. Chylomicrons enter the lymphatic vessels, and then enter the blood in the subclavian vein.

Vitamins

Vitamins can be either water-soluble or lipid-soluble. Fat-soluble vitamins are absorbed in the same manner as lipids. It is important to consume some amount of dietary lipid to aid the absorption of lipid-soluble vitamins. Water-soluble vitamins can be directly absorbed into the bloodstream from the intestine.

Elimination

The final step in digestion is the elimination of undigested food content and waste products. The undigested food material enters the colon, where most of the water is reabsorbed. Recall that the colon is also home to the microflora called "intestinal flora" that aid in the digestion process. The semi-solid waste is moved through the colon by peristaltic movements of the muscle and is stored in the rectum. As the rectum expands in response to storage of fecal matter, it triggers the neural signals required to set up the urge to eliminate. The solid waste is eliminated through the anus using peristaltic movements of the rectum.

Common Problems with Elimination

Diarrhea and constipation are some of the most common health concerns that affect digestion. Constipation is a condition where the feces are hardened because of excess water removal in the colon. In contrast, if enough water is not removed from the feces, it results in diarrhea. Many bacteria, including the ones that cause cholera, affect the proteins involved in water reabsorption in the colon and result in excessive diarrhea.

Emesis

Emesis, or vomiting, is elimination of food by forceful expulsion through the mouth. It is often in response to an irritant that affects the digestive tract, including but not limited to viruses, bacteria, emotions, sights, and food poisoning. This forceful expulsion of the food is due to the strong contractions produced by the stomach muscles. The process of emesis is regulated by the medulla.

Summary

Digestion begins with ingestion, where the food is taken in the mouth. Digestion and absorption take place in a series of steps with special enzymes playing important roles in digesting carbohydrates, proteins, and lipids. Elimination describes removal of undigested food contents and waste products from the body. While most absorption occurs in the small intestines, the large intestine is responsible for the final removal of water that remains after the absorptive process of the small intestines. The cells that line the large intestine absorb some vitamins as well as any leftover salts and water. The large intestine (colon) is also where feces is formed.

■ RESPIRATORY SYSTEM (FIG. 1.29)

The respiratory system (also referred to as the ventilator system) is a complex biological system comprised of several organs that facilitate the inhalation and exhalation of oxygen and carbon dioxide in living organisms (or, in other words, breathing).

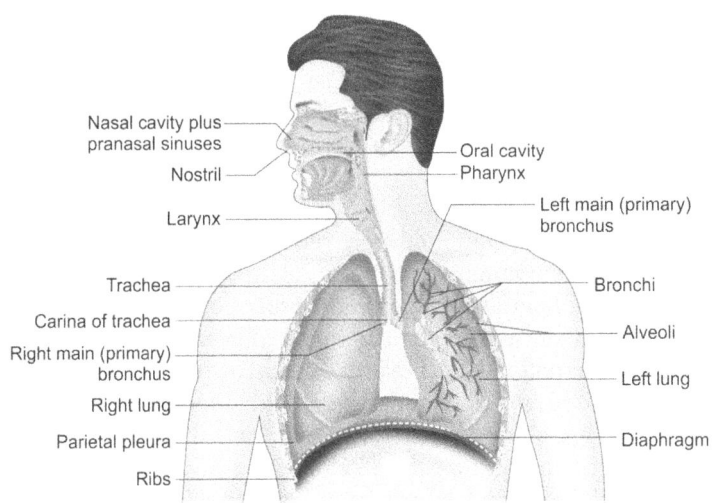

Fig. 1.29: Anatomy of respiratory system.

For all air-breathing vertebrates, respiration is handled by the lungs, but these are far from the only components of the respiratory system. In fact, the system is composed of the following biological structures—nose and nasal cavity, mouth, pharynx, larynx, trachea, bronchi and bronchioles, lungs and the muscles of respiration.

A properly functioning respiratory system is a vital part of our good health. Respiratory infections can be acute and sometimes life-threatening. They can also be chronic, in which case they place tremendous long-term stress on the immune system, endocrine system, *HPA (Hypothalamus-pituitary gland-adrenal gland) axis*, and much more.

Anatomical Components

Nose and Nasal Cavity

The nose and nasal cavity constitute the main external opening of the respiratory system. They represent the entryway to the respiratory tract—a passage through the body which air uses for travel in order to reach the lungs. The nose is made out of bone, muscle, cartilage and skin, while the nasal cavity is, more or less, hollow space. Although, the nose is typically credited as being the main external breathing apparatus, its role is actually to provide support and protection to the nasal cavity. The cavity is lined with mucous membranes and little hairs that can filter the air before it goes into the respiratory tract. They can trap all harmful particles, such as dust, mold and pollen and prevent them from reaching any of the internal components. At the same time, the cold outside air is warmed up and moisturized before going through the respiratory tract. During exhalation, the warm air that is eliminated returns the heat and moisture back to the nasal cavity, so this forms a continuous process.

Oral Cavity

The oral cavity, more commonly referred to as the mouth, is the only other external component that is a part of the respiratory system. In truth, it does not perform any additional functions compared to the nasal cavity, but it can supplement the air inhaled through the nose or act as an alternative when breathing through the nasal cavity is not possible or exceedingly difficult. Normally, breathing through nose is preferable to breathing through the mouth. Not only does the mouth not possess the ability to warm and moisturize the air coming in, but it also lacks the hairs and mucous membranes to filter out unwanted contaminants. On the plus side, the pathway leading from the mouth is shorter and the diameter is wider, which means that more air can enter in the body at the same speed.

Pharynx

The pharynx is the next component of the respiratory tract, even though most people refer to it simply as the throat. It resembles a funnel made out of muscles that acts as an intermediary between the nasal cavity and the larynx and esophagus. It is divided into three separate sections—nasopharynx, oropharynx and laryngopharynx. The nasopharynx is the upper region of the structure, which begins at the posterior of the nasal cavity and simply allows air to travel through it and reach the lower sections. The oropharynx does something similar, except it is located at the posterior of the oral cavity. Once the air reaches the laryngopharynx, something called the epiglottis will divert it to the larynx. The *epiglottis* is a flap that performs a vital task by switching access between the esophagus and trachea. This ensures that air will travel through the trachea, but that food which is swallowed and travels through the pharynx is diverted to the esophagus.

Larynx (Fig. 1.30)

The larynx is the next component, but represents only a small section of the respiratory tract that connects the laryngopharynx to the trachea. It is commonly referred to as the voice box, and it is located near the anterior section of the neck, just below the hyoid bone. The aforementioned epiglottis is a part of the larynx, as are the thyroid

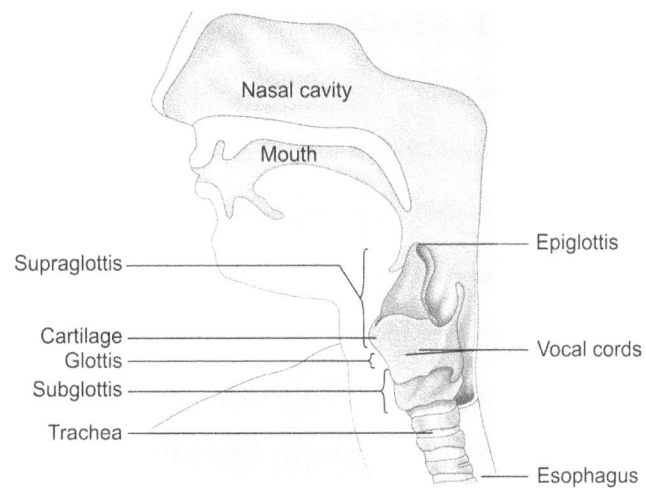

Fig. 1.30: Larynx.

cartilage, the cricoid cartilage and the vocal folds. Both cartilages offer support and protection to other components, such as the vocal folds and the larynx itself. The thyroid cartilage also goes by a more common name—the Adam's apple—although, contrary to popular belief, it is present in both men and women. It is typically more pronounced in adult males. The vocal folds are mucous membranes that tense up and vibrate in order to create sound, hence, the term *voice box*. The pitch and volume of these sounds can be controlled by modifying the tension and speed of the vocal folds.

Trachea (Fig. 1.31)

The trachea is a longer section of the respiratory tract, shaped like a tube and approximately 5 inches in length. It has several C-shaped hyaline cartilage rings which are lined with pseudostratified ciliated columnar epithelium. These rings keep the trachea open for air all the time. They are C-shaped in order to allow the open end to face the esophagus. This allows the esophagus to expand into the area normally occupied by the trachea in order to permit larger chunks of food to pass through. The trachea, more commonly referred to as the windpipe, connects the larynx to the bronchi and also has the role of filtering the air prior to it entering the lungs. The epithelium which lines the cartilage rings produces mucus which traps harmful particles. The cilia then move the mucus upward towards the pharynx, where it is redirected towards the gastrointestinal tract (GIT) in order for it to be digested.

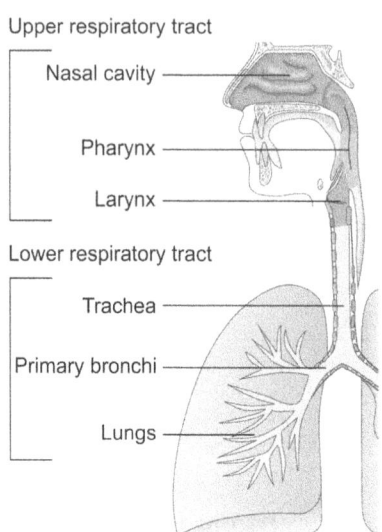

Fig. 1.31: Trachea.

Bronchi

The lower end of the trachea splits the respiratory tract into two branches that are named the primary bronchi. These first run into each of the lungs before further branching off into smaller bronchi. These secondary bronchi continue carrying the air to the lobes of the lungs, then further split into tertiary bronchi. The tertiary bronchi then split into even smaller sections that are spread out throughout the lungs called *bronchioles*. Each one of these bronchioles continues to split into even smaller parts called *terminal bronchioles*. At this stage, these tiny bronchioles number in the millions, are less than a millimeter in length, and work to conduct the air to the lungs' alveoli. The larger bronchi contain C-shaped cartilage rings similar to the ones used in the trachea to keep the airway open. As the bronchi get smaller, so do the rings that become progressively more widely spaced. The tiny bronchioles do not have any kind of cartilage and instead rely on muscles and elastin.

This system creates a tree-like pattern, with smaller branches growing from the bigger ones. At the same time, it also ensures that air from the trachea reaches all the regions of the lungs. Besides simply carrying the air, the bronchi and bronchioles also possess mucus and cilia that further refine the air and get rid of any leftover environmental contaminants. The walls of the bronchi and bronchioles are also lined with muscle tissue, which can control the flow of air going into the lungs. In certain instances, such as during physical activity, the muscles relax and allow more air to go into the lungs.

Lungs (Fig. 1.32)

The lungs are two organs located inside the thorax on the left and right sides. They are surrounded by a membrane that provides them with enough space to expand when they fill up with air. Because the left lung is located lateral to the heart, the organs are not identical—the left lung is smaller and has only two lobes while the right lung has three. Inside, the lungs resemble a sponge made of millions and millions of small sacs that are named *alveoli*. These alveoli are found at the ends of terminal bronchioles and are surrounded by capillaries through which blood passes. Thanks to an epithelium layer which covering the alveoli, the air that goes inside them is free to exchange gases with the blood that goes through the capillaries.

Muscles of Respiration

The last component of the respiratory system is a muscle structure known as the *muscles of respiration*. These muscles surround the lungs and allow the inhalation and exhalation of air. The main muscle in this system is known as the *diaphragm*, a thin sheet of muscle that constitutes the bottom of the thorax. It pulls in air into the lungs by contracting several inches with each breath. In addition to the diaphragm, multiple intercostal muscles are located between the ribs and they also help in compress and expand the lungs.

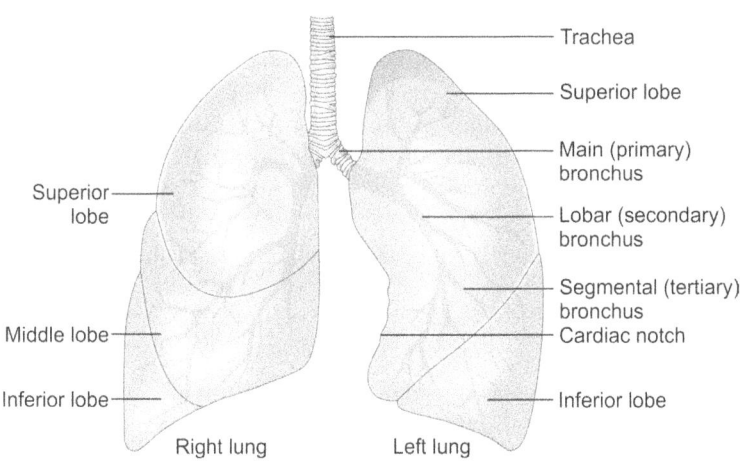

Fig. 1.32: Lungs.

BREATHING MECHANISM, DIFFERENT RESPIRATORY VOLUMES

The air that we breathe in and out of the lungs varies in its pressure. So basically when there is a fall in air pressure the alveolar spaces fall and the air enters the lungs (inspiration) and as the pressure of the alveoli within exceeds the atmospheric pressure, the air is blown from the lungs (expiration). The flow rate of air is in proportion to the magnitude of the pressure difference.

The breathing mechanism involves two processes:
1. Inspiration
2. Expiration

Inspiration

In the process of inspiration, there would be a contraction of muscles attached to the ribs on the outer side which pulls out the ribs and results in the expansion of the chest cavity.

Later, the diaphragm, contracts, moves downwards and expands the chest cavity resulting in the contraction of the abdominal muscles.

The expansion of the chest cavity produces a partial vacuum which sucks air into the lungs and fills the expanded alveoli.

Mechanism of Inspiration

- ❖ The process of intake of atmospheric air is known as inspiration. It is an active process.
- ❖ When the volume of the thoracic cavity increases and the air pressure decreases, inspiration takes place.
- ❖ Contraction of external intercostal muscles increases the volume of the thoracic cavity.
- ❖ Contraction of the diaphragm further increases the size of the thoracic activity. Simultaneously, the lungs expand.
- ❖ With the expansion of the lungs, the air pressure inside the lungs decreases.
- ❖ The pressure equalizes and the atmospheric air rushes inside the lungs.

Expiration

The expiration process is considered once after the gaseous exchange occurs in the lungs and the air is expelled. This expulsion of air is called expiration.

During this process, muscles attached to the ribs contract, the muscles of the diaphragm and the abdomen relax which leads to a decrease in the volume of the chest cavity and increases the pressure of the lungs, causing the air in the lungs to be pushed out through the nose.

Mechanism of Expiration

- ❖ The process of exhaling carbon dioxide is called expiration. It is a passive process.
- ❖ It occurs when the size of the thoracic activity decreases and the air pressure outside increases.
- ❖ Now the external intercostal muscles relax and the internal intercostal muscles contract.
- ❖ As a result, the ribs are pulled inwards and the size of the thoracic cavity is reduced.
- ❖ The diaphragm is relaxed and the lungs get compressed.
- ❖ Consequently, the pressure increases and the air is forced outside.

Mechanism of Respiration (Fig. 1.33)

Mechanism of respiration involves the breathing mechanism and exchange of gases.

The gaseous exchange occurs by diffusion in the alveoli. It depends upon the pressure differences between blood and tissues, or atmospheric air and blood. The **exchange of gases** takes place at the surface of the alveolus.

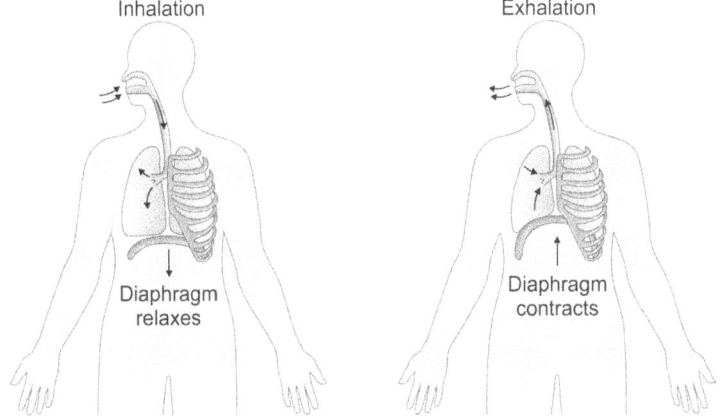

Fig: 1.33: Respiration.

The mechanism of breathing has already been explained above. Let us have a look at the steps involved in the exchange of gases.

Exchange of Gases

The exchange of gases takes place in the following manner:

Transport of Oxygen

- Oxygen in the blood is carried to the tissue in two forms—oxyhemoglobin—chemical composition of oxygen with hemoglobin, and solution of oxygen in the blood plasma.
- The oxygen in the blood combines with hemoglobin when the concentration of oxygen is high in the blood.
- Oxyhemoglobin, being unstable, dissociates to release oxygen. Low oxygen, low pH and high temperatures stimulate the dissociation process.

Internal Respiration

The gaseous exchange taking place in the tissues is called internal respiration. Here, the oxygen carried in the form of oxyhemoglobin gets dissociated to release oxygen.

This oxygen breaks down glucose to release carbon dioxide, water, and energy. The energy is utilized by the body, while the carbon dioxide is diffused from the tissues.

Transport of Carbon Dioxide from Tissues to Lungs

Carbon dioxide is transported by four mechanisms:
1. Some carbon dioxide dissolves in the water of plasma to form carbonic acid.
2. Carbonic acid ionizes to form bicarbonate ions. The hydrogen ions are catalyzed by the enzyme carbonic anhydrase. Bicarbonate ions combine with sodium and potassium to form sodium bicarbonate and potassium bicarbonate.
3. Some carbon dioxide combines with hemoglobin for the formation of carbaminohemoglobin.
4. It is finally carried from the lungs and released out of the body through expiration.

Intrapleural Breathing

Intrapleural breathing is used to refer to the pressure that is present in the space between the pleura and the lungs. This space is referred to as the pleural cavity. The pressure in this region is normally less than the atmospheric pressure. This is the reason why pleural pressure is termed as negative pressure.

The lung movement is governed by the pressure gradient, the transpulmonary pressure, which exists between the pleura and the lungs. The difference in the pressures between intrapulmonary and intrapleural pressures is known as transpulmonary pressure.

The pressure in the pleural cavity while breathing turns negative while there is an increase in the transpulmonary pressure causing the lungs to expand. While expiration, the lungs recoil as a result of an increase in the pleural pressure.

The competing forces inside the thorax results in the formation of negative intrapleural pressure, one of these forces is associated with the lung's elasticity. The lungs have elastic tissues which cause it to be pulled inwards off the thoracic wall. An inward pull of the lung tissue is also generated by the surface tension of the alveolar fluid. The inward tension generated from the lungs is opposed by forces from the thoracic wall and the pleural fluid.

Respiratory Gas Transport

After the gases have scattered in the lungs, causing the blood to become oxygenated, leaving carbon dioxide, the next phase of transportation of oxygen-rich blood to the tissues takes place. Meanwhile, the next round of deoxygenated blood needs to be brought to the lungs for the cycle to continue.

In the bloodstream, the transportation of gases occurs all through the body which is contributed to the cardiovascular system comprising the blood vessels and the heart. The blood carrying oxygen leaves the lungs to flow into the heart through the pulmonary veins, which are pumped to the rest of the body from the left ventricle through the aorta and its corresponding branches.

RESPIRATORY VOLUME (FIG. 1.34)

Lung volumes are also known as respiratory volumes. It refers to the volume of gas in the lungs at a given time during the respiratory cycle. Lung capacities are derived from a summation of different lung volumes. The average total lung capacity of an adult human male is about 6 liters of air. Lung volumes measurement is an integral part of pulmonary function test. These volumes tend to vary, depending on the depth of respiration, ethnicity, gender, age, body composition and in certain respiratory diseases. A number of the lung volumes can be measured by Spirometry—tidal volume, inspiratory reserve volume, and expiratory reserve volume. However, measurement of residual volume, functional residual capacity, and total lung capacity

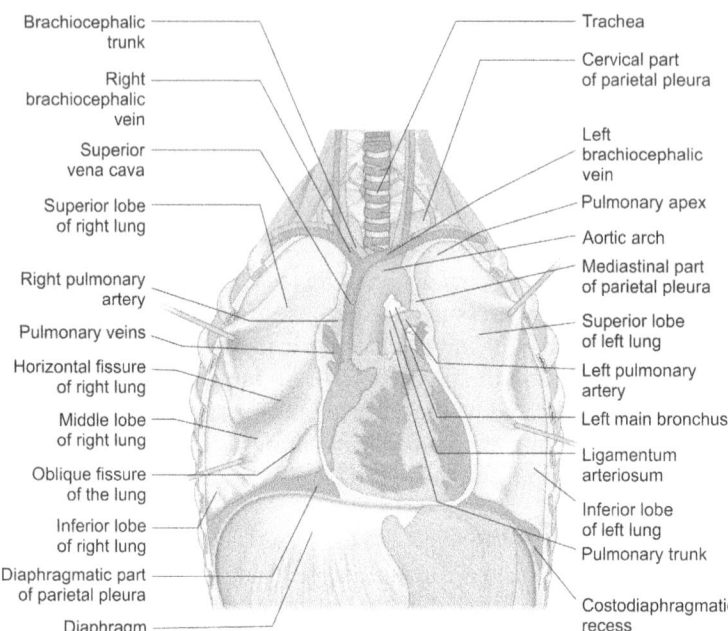

Fig. 1.34: Respiratory volume.

is through body plethysmography, nitrogen washout and helium dilution technique.

Lung Volume

- **Tidal volume (TV):** It is the amount of air that can be inhaled or exhaled during one respiratory cycle. This depicts the functions of the respiratory centers, respiratory muscles and the mechanics of the lung and chest wall.
  The normal adult value is 10% of vital capacity (VC), approximately 300–500 mL (6–8 mL/kg); but can increase up to 50% of VC on exercise.
- **Inspiratory reserve volume (IRV):** It is the amount of air that can be forcibly inhaled after a normal tidal volume. IRV is usually kept in reserve, but is used during deep breathing. The normal adult value is 1900–3300 mL.
- **Expiratory reserve volume (ERV):** It is the volume of air that can be exhaled forcibly after exhalation of normal tidal volume. The normal adult value is 700–1200 mL. ERV is reduced with obesity, ascites or after upper abdominal surgery.

❖ **Residual volume (RV):** It is the volume of air remaining in the lungs after maximal exhalation. Normal adult value is averaged at 1200 mL (20-25 mL/kg). It is indirectly measured from summation of FRC and ERV and cannot be measured by spirometry.
In obstructive lung diseases with features of incomplete emptying of the lungs and air trapping, RV may be significantly high. The RV can also be expressed as a percentage of total lung capacity and values in excess of 140% significantly increase the risks of barotrauma, pneumothorax, infection and reduced venous return due to high intrathoracic pressures as noticed in patients with high RV who require surgery and mechanical ventilation thus needs high perioperative inflation pressures.

LUNG CAPACITIES

❖ **Inspiratory capacity (IC):** It is the maximum volume of air that can be inhaled following a resting state. It is calculated from the sum of inspiratory reserve volume and tidal volume. IC = IRV+TV
❖ **Total lung capacity (TLC):** It is the maximum volume of air the lungs can accommodate or sum of all volume compartments or volume of air in lungs after maximum inspiration. The normal value is about 6,000 mL (4-6 L). TLC is calculated by summation of the four primary lung volumes (TV, IRV, ERV, RV).
TLC may be increased in patients with obstructive defects, such as emphysema and decreased in patients with restrictive abnormalities including chest wall abnormalities and kyphoscoliosis.
❖ **Vital capacity (VC):** It is the total amount of air exhaled after maximal inhalation. The value is about 4800 mL and it varies according to age and body size. It is calculated by summing tidal volume, inspiratory reserve volume, and expiratory reserve volume. VC = TV + IRV + ERV.
VC indicates ability to breathe deeply and cough, reflecting inspiratory and expiratory muscle strength. VC should be 3 times greater than TV for effective cough. VC is sometimes reduced in obstructive disorders and always in restrictive disorders.
❖ **Function residual capacity (FRC):** It is the amount of air remaining in the lungs at the end of a normal exhalation. It is calculated by adding together residual and expiratory reserve volumes. The normal value is about 1800-2200 mL. FRC = RV + ERV.
FRC does not rely on effort and highlights the resting position when inner and outer elastic recoils are balanced. FRC is reduced in restrictive disorders. The ratio of FRC to TLC is an index of hyperinflation. In COPD, FRC is up to 80% of TLC.

URINARY SYSTEM (FIG. 1.35)

Ureters

Ureters are the tubes that convey urine from the kidneys to the urinary bladder. They are about 25 cm long. It is continuous with the funnel-shaped renal pelvis. It passes downwards through the abdominal cavity behind the peritoneum in front of the psoas muscle into the pelvic cavity and passes through the posterior wall of the bladder.

Structure

Ureters consist of three layers of tissue:
1. An outer covering of fibrous tissue
2. A middle muscular layer consisting of interlacing smooth muscle fibers.
3. An inner layer, the mucosa composed of transitional epithelium.

Functions

❖ The ureter propel urine from the kidneys into the bladder by peristaltic contraction of the smooth muscle layer.
❖ Peristaltic waves occur several times per minute increasing in frequency with the volume of urine produced and send little spurts of urine into the bladder.

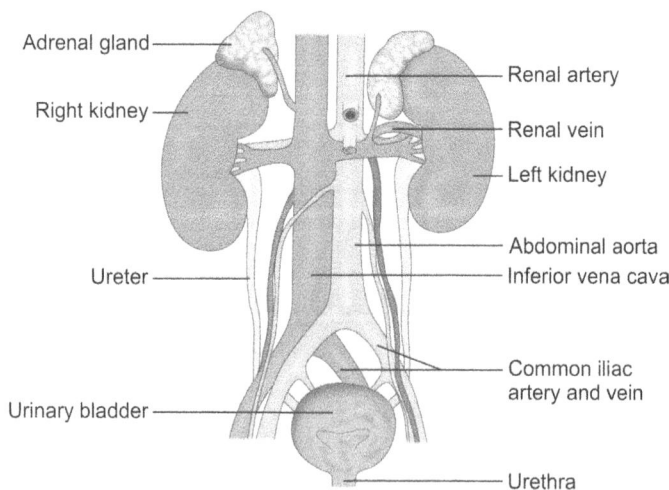

Fig. 1.35: Urinary system.

Urinary Bladder

The bladder acts as a reservoir for urine; it is a pear-shaped organ. It lies in the true pelvis in front of the other contents and the behind the symphysis pubis. The bladder consists of:
* An outermost serous coat
* A muscular coat
* A submucous coat and mucus using, of transitional epithelium.

Structure

The bladder wall is composed of three layers:
1. The outer layer of loose connective tissue, containing blood and lymphatic vessels and nerves covered on the upper surface by the peritoneum.
2. The middle layer consisting of a mass of interlaying smooth muscle fibers and elastic tissue, are loosely arranged in three layers.
3. The mucosa, composed of transitional epithelium.

The total capacity of the bladder is rarely more than about 600 mL. The three orifices in the bladder wall form a triangle or trigone. The upper two orifices on the posterior wall are the openings of the ureters. The lower orifice is the opening into the urethra.

Kidneys

The kidneys are a pair of excretory organs situated on the posterior abdominal wall, behind the peritoneum and below the diaphragms. The left kidney is slightly at a higher level than the right kidney, because of the considerable space occupied by the liver.

Shape and Size

Each kidney is bean-shaped and measures 7.5–10 cm long, 6 cm wide and 3 cm thick. Each kidney weighs 150 g.

Organs Associated with the Kidneys

Right Kidney

Superiorly: The right adrenal gland
Anteriorly: The right lobe of the liver, the duodenum and the hepatic flexure of the colon
Posteriorly: The diaphragm and muscles of the posterior abdominal wall.

Left Kidney

Superiorly: The left adrenal gland

Anteriorly: The spleen, stomach, pancreas, jejunum and splenic flexure of the colon
Posteriorly: The diaphragm and muscles of the posterior abdominal wall.

Structure of the Kidney

- An outer fibrous capsule, surrounding the kidney.
- The cortex, a reddish brown layer of tissue.
- The medulla, the innermost layer, consisting of pale conical-shaped striations, the renal pyramids.

The hilum is the concave medial border of the kidney where the renal blood and lymph vessels, the ureter and nerves enter. The renal pelvis is the funnel-shaped structure that act as a receptacle for the urine formed by the kidney. It has a number of distal branches called *calyces*, each of which surrounds the apex of the renal pyramid. Urine formed in the kidney passes through a *papilla* at the apex of the pyramid into a minor calyx, then into a major calyx before passing through the pelvis into the ureter.

Microscopic Structure of the Kidney

The kidney is composed of about 1 million functional units, the nephrons and a smaller number of collecting ducts.

Nephron

The nephron consists of a twisted tubule closed at one end and the other end opening into a collecting tubule. The closed end is to form the cup-shaped glomerular capsule or Bowman's capsule, the reminder of nephron is about 3 cm long and is described in three parts.
1. Proximal convoluted tubule
2. Medullary loop (loop of Henle)
3. Distal convoluted tubule, leading into a collecting ducts.

The collecting ducts unit, forming larger ducts that empty into the minor calyces after entering the kidney at the hilum. The renal artery divides into the smaller arteries and arterioles. In the cortex as arteriole, the afferent arteriole enters into each glomerular capsule and then subdivides into a cluster of capillaries, forming the glomerulus.

The blood vessels leading away from the glomerulus is the afferent arteriole. It breaks up into a second capillary network, and exchange across capillary walls. Regulates the composition of the blood and supplies local tissues with oxygen and a nutrients.

The walls of the glomerulus and the glomerular capsule consists of a single layer of flattened epithelial cells. The remained of the

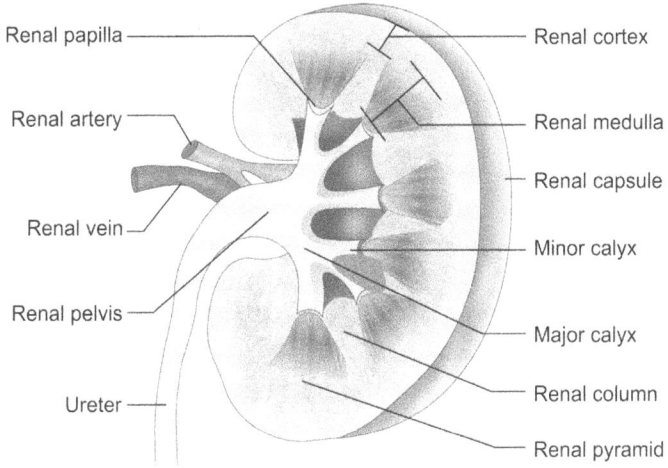

Fig. 1.36: Cross section of kidney.

nephron and the collecting tubule are formed by a single layer of highly specialized cells.

The blood vessels of kidney are supplied by both sympathetic and parasympathetic nerves.

Functions of the Kidney (Fig. 1.36)

- Formation and secretion of urine.
- Excretion of metabolic waste product and many drugs.
- Regulation of body fluid volume by excreting either dilute or concentrated urine.
- Regulation of concentration of electrolytes and various ions.
- Regulation of acid-base balance by excreting either excess of acid and/or base.
- Regulation of arterial blood pressure by adjusting sodium and water excretion.
- Secretion and the protection of some hormones, such as erythropoietin and renin, etc.
- Metabolism of various hormones, such as insulin, glucagon, parathyroid hormone.

PROCESS OF URINE FORMATION

Waste is excreted from the human body, mainly in the form of urine. Our kidneys play a major role in the process of excretion. Constituents of normal human urine include 95% water and 5% solid wastes. It is produced in the nephron, which is the structural and functional

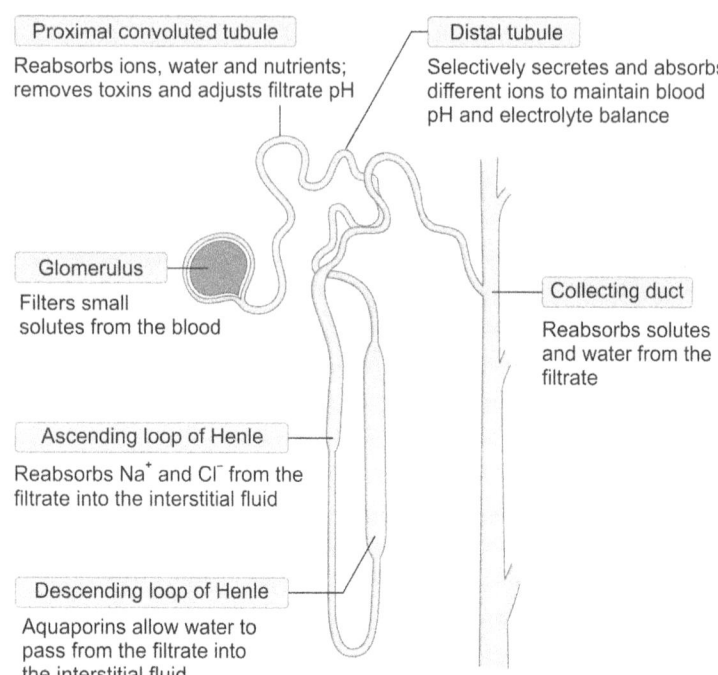

Fig. 1.37: Formation of urine.

unit of the kidney. Urine formation in our body is mainly carried out in three phases, namely **(Fig. 1.37)**:
1. Glomerular filtration
2. Reabsorption
3. Secretion

Glomerular Filtration

Glomerular filtration occurs in the glomerulus where blood is filtered. This process occurs across the three layers—the epithelium of Bowman's capsule, the endothelium of glomerular blood vessels, and a membrane between these two layers.

Blood is filtered in such a way that all the constituents of the plasma reach the Bowman's capsule, except proteins. Therefore, this process is known as ultrafiltration.

Reabsorption

Around 99% of the filtrate obtained is reabsorbed by the renal tubules. This is known as reabsorption. This is achieved by active and passive transport.

Secretion

The next step in urine formation is tubular secretion. Here, tubular cells secrete substances, such as hydrogen ions, potassium ions, etc. into the filtrate. Through this process, the ionic, acid-base and the balance of other body fluids are maintained. The secreted ions combine with the filtrate and form urine. The urine passes out of the nephron tubule into a collecting duct.

Urine

The urine produced is 95% water and 5% nitrogenous wastes. Wastes, such as urea, ammonia, and creatinine are excreted in the urine. Apart from these, the potassium, sodium and calcium ions are also excreted.

Osmoregulation

Osmoregulation is the process of regulating body fluids and their compositions. It maintains the osmotic pressure of the blood and helps in homeostasis. This is why, it is recommended to consume more water about 2-3 liters, which helps in the proper functioning of our kidneys. For example, we consume lots of water during summers, but still, we urinate fewer times in summers than in winters and the concentration of the urine is also more. The reason is that we lose lots of water from our body in summer through sweating. Thus, to maintain the fluid balance in the body our kidneys reabsorb more water.

Key points on urine formation and osmoregulation:

- ❖ Urine is formed in three main steps-glomerular filtration, reabsorption and secretion.
- ❖ It comprises 95% water and 5% wastes, such as ions of sodium, potassium and calcium, and nitrogenous wastes, such as creatinine, urea and ammonia.
- ❖ Osmoregulation is the process of maintaining homeostasis of the body.
- ❖ It facilitates the diffusion of solutes and water across the semi-permeable membrane thereby maintaining osmotic balance.
- ❖ The kidney regulates the osmotic pressure of blood through filtration and purification by a process known as osmoregulation.

REPRODUCTIVE SYSTEM

Male Reproductive System (Fig. 1.38)

The male reproductive system organs are:

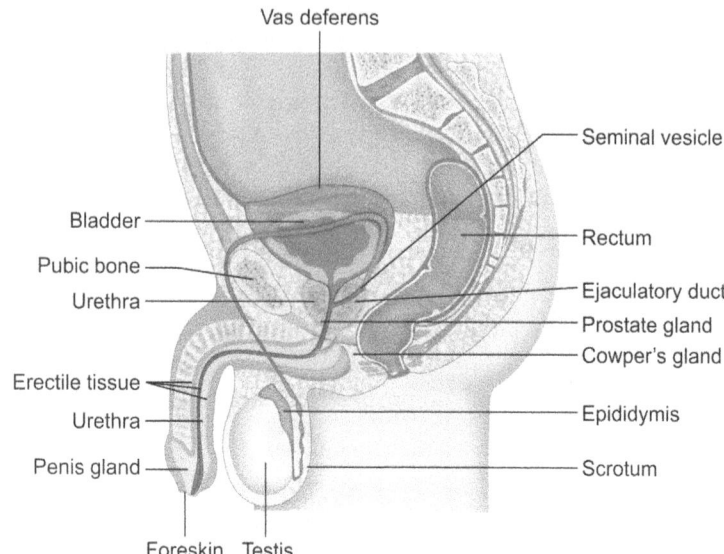

Fig. 1.38: Male reproductive system.

Scrotum

The scrotum is a pouch of deeply pigmented skin, fibrous and connective tissue and smooth muscle. It is divided into two compartments each of which contains one testis, one epididymis and the testicles end of a spermatic cord. It lies below the symphysis pubis, in front of the upper part of the thighs and behind the penis.

Testes

The testes are the reproductive glands of the male and are equivalent of the ovaries in the female. They are about 4.5 cm long, 2.5 cm width and 3 cm thick and are suspended in the scrotum by the spermatic cords. They are surrounded by three layers of tissue.

Tunica Vaginalis

This is a double membrane, forming the outer covering of the testes, and is a downgrowth of the abdominal and pelvic peritoneum. During early fetal life, the testes develop in the lumbar region of the abdominal cavity just below the kidneys. They then descend into the scrotum, taking with them coverings of peritoneum. Descent of the testes into the scrotum should be complete by the 8th month of fetal life.

Tunica Albuginea

This is a fibrous covering beneath the tunica vaginalis that surrounds the testes.

Tunica Vasculosa

This consists of a network of capillaries supported by delicate connective tissue.

Structure of the Testes

In each testes, there are 200 to 300 lobules, and within each lobule are 1 to 4 convoluted loops composed of germinal epithelial cells, called seminiferous tubules. Between the tubules, are groups of interstitial cells (of Leydig) that secrete the hormone testosterone after puberty. At the upper pole of the testis, the tubules combine to form a single tubule. This tubule, about 6 in its full length, is repeatedly folded and tightly packed into a mass called the epididymis. It leaves the scrotum as the deferent duct in the spermatic cord. Blood and lymph vessels pass to the testes in the spermatic cord.

Functions

Spermatozoa (sperm) are produced in the seminiferous tubules of the testes, and mature as they pass through the long and convoluted epididymis where they are stored. The hormone controlling sperm production is FSH from the anterior pituitary. A mature sperm has a head, a body and a tail used for motility. The head is almost filled by the nucleus, containing its deoxyribonucleic acid (DNA). It also contains the enzymes required to penetrate the outer layers of the ovum to reach, and fuse with its nucleus. The body of the sperm is packed with mitochondria to fuel the propelling action of the tail that powers the sperm along with female reproductive tract.

Spermatic Cords

The spermatic cords suspend the lists in the scrotum. Each cord contains a testiculer artery, testicular veins, lymphatics, a deferent duct and testicular nerves which come together to form the cord from their various origins in the abdomen. The cord, which is covered in a sheath of smooth muscle of connective and fibrous tissues, extends through the inguinal canal and is attached to the testes on the posterior wall.

Penis

The penis has a root and a body. The root has in the perineum and the body surrounds the urethra. It is formed by three cylindrical masses of erectile tissue and smooth muscle.

The two lateral columns are called the corpora cavernosa and the column between them, containing the urethra, is the corpus spongiosum. At its tip, expanded into a triangular structure known as the glans penis. Just above the glans, the skin is folded upon itself and forms a movable double layer, the foreskin or prepuce. Arterial blood is supplied by deep, dorsal and bulbar arteries. The series of veins drain blood into the internal pudendal or and internal iliac veins.

■ FEMALE REPRODUCTIVE SYSTEM (FIG. 1.39)

The female reproductive organs are divided into external and internal organs.

External Genitalia (Vulva)

External genitalia consist of the labia majora and labia minora, the clitoris, the vaginal orifice, the vestibule, the hymen and the vestibular glands (Bartholin's glands).

- ❖ **Labia majora:** These are the two large folds forming the boundary of the vulva. They are composed of skin fibrous tissue and fat and large numbers of sebaceous glands.

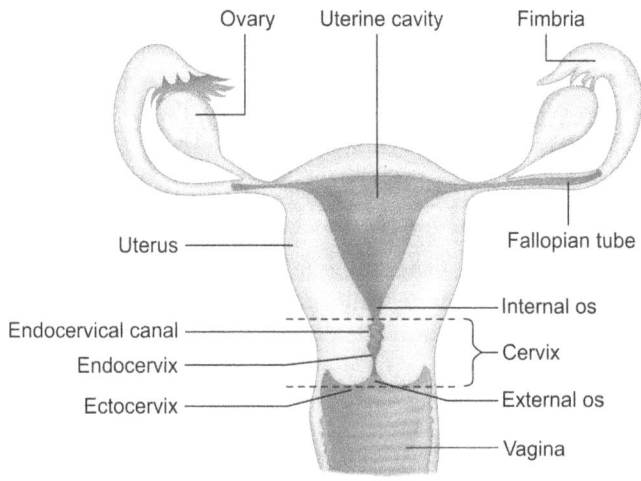

Fig. 1.39: Female reproductive system.

- **Labia minora:** These are two smaller folds of skin between the labia majora containing numerous sebaceous glands.
- **Vestibule:** The cleft between the labia minora is the vestibule. The vagina, urethra and elutes of the greater vestibular glands open into the vestibule.
- **Clitoris:** The clitoris corresponds to the penis in the male and contains sensory nerve endings and erectile tissue, but it has no reproductive significance.
- **Hymen:** The hymen is the layer of mucous membrane which partially occludes the opening of the vagina.
- **Vestibular glands (Bartholin's glands):** These are situated one on each side near the vaginal opening. They secrete mucus that keeps the vulva moist.
- **Arterial supply:** This is by branches from the internal pudendal arteries that branch from the internal iliac arteries and by external pudendal arteries that branch from the femoral arteries.

Venous Drainage

This forms a large plexus which eventually drains into the internal iliac veins.

Lymph Drainage

This is through the superficial inguinal lymph nodes.

Nerve Supply

This is by branches from pudendal nerves.

Internal Genitalia

Its lies in the pelvic cavity and consist of the vagina, uterus, two uterine tubes and two ovaries.

Vagina

The vagina is a fibromuscular tube used with stratified squamous epithelium, connecting the external and internal organs of reproduction. It runs obliquely upwards and backwards at an angle of about 45° between the bladder in front and rectum and anus behind. In the adult, the anterior wall is about 7.5 cm long and the posterior wall about 9 cm long.

Structure of the Vagina

The vagina has three layers—an outer covering of areolar tissue, a middle layer of smooth muscle and an inner lining of stratified squamous epithelium that forms ridges or rugae. It has no secretory glands but the surface is kept moist by cervical secretions.

Uterine Tubes (Fallopian Tubes)

The uterine tubes are about 10 cm long and extend from the sides of the uterus between the fundus. The end of each tube has finger like projections called fimbriae. The longest of these is the ovarian fimbriae, which is in close association with the ovary.

Structure

The wall of uterine tube is made up of mucous membrane, surrounded by a muscle coat which is covered externally by peritoneum.

The mucous membrane shows numerous branching folds which almost fill in the lumen of the tube. These folds are most conspicuous in the ampulla. Each fold has a highly cellular core of connective tissue. It is lined by columnar epithelium, that rests on a basement membrane. Some of the lining cells are ciliated; ciliary action helps to move ova towards the uterus. Other cells are secretory.

The muscle coat has an inner circular layer and an outer longitudinal layer of smooth muscle.

Functions

The uterine tubes move the ovum from the ovary to the uterus by peristalsis is and ciliary movement. The mucus secreted by the mucosa provides ideal conditions for movement of ovum and spermatozoa. Fertilization of the ovum usually takes place in the uterine tube and the zygote is propelled into the uterus for implantation.

Ovaries

The right and left ovaries are the female gonads. Female gametes called ova (singular ovum) are produced in them. The ovary also produces female sex hormones. Each ovary is shaped like an almond. It is approximately 3 cm in length, 1.5 cm in width, and 1 cm in thickness. It is covered by a germinal epithelium that is continuous with the peritoneum. The broad ligament stretches from the side of the uterus to the lateral wall and floor of the pelvis. The ovary is attached to the posterosuperior aspect of the broad ligament by a fold of peritoneum called the mesovarium. The part of the broad ligament between the attachment of the mesovarium and lateral wall of the pelvis is called the *suspensory ligament of the ovary*. The lateral surface of the ovary lies in contact with the peritoneum covering the lateral wall of the pelvis. It lies in a depression called the ovarian fossa. The free surface of the ovary is lined by a single layer of cuboidal cells (germinal epithelium). The substance of the ovary is linked into a thick cortex and a much smaller medulla. Immediately, deep to the terminal epithelium the cortex is covered by a condensation of connective tissue called the tunica albugines.

Functions of the Ovaries

Maturation of the follicle stimulated peritoneum follicle stimulating hormone from the anterior pituitary and estrogen secreted by the follicle lining cells. Ovulation is triggered by a surge of luteinizing hormone from the anterior pituitary, which occurs a few hours before ovulation.

After ovulation, the follicle lining cells develop into the corpus indium, under the influence of LH from the anterior pituitary. The corpus luteum produces the hormone progesterone and some estrogen if the ovum is fertilized, it embeds itself in the wall of the uterus where it grows and develops and produces the hormone Human Chorionic Gonadotropin (HCG) which stimulates the corpus luteum to continue secreting progesterone and estrogen for the first 3 months of pregnancy, after which function is continued by the placenta. If the ovum is not the corpus luteum degenerates and a new cycle begins with menstruation.

Uterus

The uterus is a hollow muscular pear-shaped organ, flattened anteroposteriorly. It lies in the pelvic cavity between the urinary bladder and the rectum when the body is the uterus lies in an horizontal position. It is about 7.5 long, 5 cm wide, its walls are about 2.5 cm thick. Its weight from 30–40 g. The parts of the uterus are:
- ❖ **Fundus:** This is the dome-shaped part of uterus above the opening of the uterine tubes.
- ❖ **Body:** This is the main part. It is narrowest inferiorly at the internal where it is continuous with the cervix.
- ❖ **Cervix ('neck' of the uterus):** This protrudes to the anterior wall of the vagina, opening into it at the external.

Structure

The walls of the uterus are composed of three layers of tissue—perimetrium, myometrium and endometrium.
1. **Perimetrium:** Anteriorly over the fundus and the body where it is folded on to the upper surface of the urinary bladder. This folded peritoneum forms the vesicouterine pouch.

Posteriorly, the peritoneum extends over the fundus, the body and the cervix, then it continues on the rectum to form the rectouterine pouch. Laterally, it lies only the fundus is covered because the peritoneum forms a double fold with the uterine tubes in the upper free borders. This double fold is the broad ligament.

2. **Myometrium:** This is the thickest layer of tissue in the uterine wall. It is a mass of smooth muscle fibers interlaced with areolar tissue, blood vessels and nerves.
3. **Endometrium:** This consists of columnar epithelium containing a large number of mucus secreting tubular glands. It is divided functionally into two layers:
   i. *Functional layer:* It is the upper layer and it thickens and becomes rich in blood vessels in the first half of menstrual cycle. If the ovum is not fertilized and does not implant, this layer is shed during menstruation.
   ii. *Basal layer:* It lies next to the myometrium, and is not lost during menstruation. It is the layer from which the fresh functional layer is regenerated during each cycle.

The function of uterus is to accept the fertilized ovum which will turn into a fetus and hold each in during development.
- It also helps to support the fetus during gestational period.
- Once the egg is unplanned, the uterus provides nutrition to the fetus that is embedded in the endometrium through blood vessels that are develop specifically for this purpose.
- The fertilize ovum becomes embryo attaches to a wall of the uterus, creates a placenta and develops into a fetus until birth.

Blood supply

Arterial supply: This is by the uterine arteries branches of internal iliac arteries.
Venous drainage: It is drain into the internal iliac veins.

Functions of the uterus
- It is the site of menstrual bleeding.
- It is the site for embryo development.

■ ENDOCRINE SYSTEM (FIG. 1.40)

The endocrine system is made up of glands body that produce and secrete hormones, chemical substance produced in the body that regulate the activity of cells or organs. These hormones regulate the body's growth, metabolism and sexual development and function.

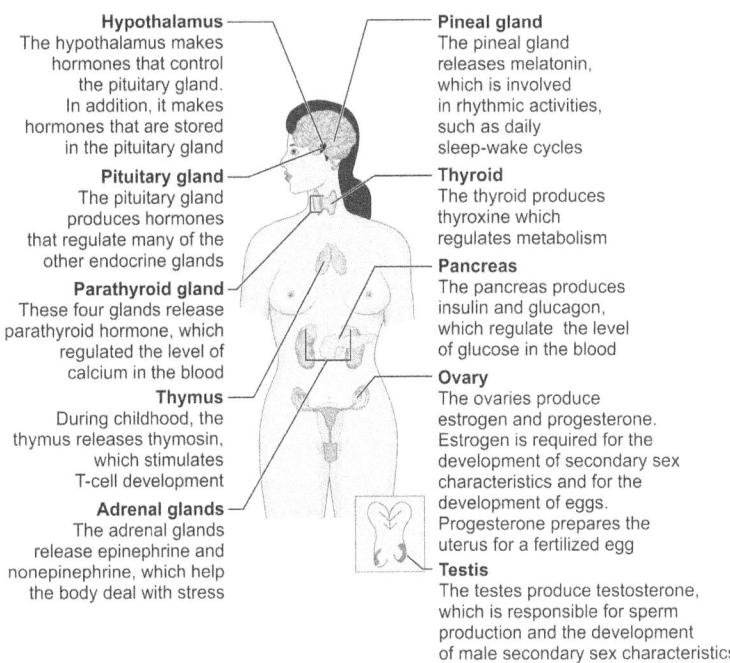

Fig. 1.40: Organs of the endocrine system and other organs containing tissues that secrete hormones.

The hormones are released into the bloodstream and may affect one or several organs throughout the body.

The major glands of the endocrine system are the hypothalamus, pituitary, thyroid, parathyroid, adrenals, pineal body and the reproductive organs (ovaries and testes). The pancreas is also a part of the system; it has a role in hormone production as well as in digestion.

Hypothalamus

The hypothalamus is located in the lower central part of the brain. This part of the brain is important in regulation of satiety metabolism and body temperature. It secretes hormones that stimulate or suppress the release of hormones in the pituitary gland. Many of these hormones are releasing hormones which are secreted into an artery that carries them directly to the pituitary gland. In the pituitary gland, these releasing hormones send signal for the secretions of stimulating hormones. The hypothalamus also secretes a hormone called somatostatin, which causes the pituitary gland to stop the release of growth hormone.

Pituitary Gland

The pituitary gland is located at the base of the skull in the pituitary fossa of the sphenoid. It consists of three lobes—anterior and posterior and an intermediate part or the pars intermedia. For the purpose of the study of its own functions, it is considered in two parts—the anterior and posterior lobes.

The Anterior Lobe

The anterior lobe of the pituitary produces a number of hormones which are instrumental in controlling the production of the secretion of all the other endocrine organs.
- The growth hormone controls the growth of the body.
- The thyrotropic hormone controls the activity of the thyroid gland in the production of thyroxine.
- The adrenocorticotropic hormone (ACTH) controls the activity of the adrenal glands in the production of cortisol from the cortex of the gland.
- The gonadotropic hormones are the follicle-stimulating hormone (FSH) which stimulates the development of graafian follicles in the ovary and the formation of spermatozoa in the testes.
- The luteinizing hormone controls the secretion of the estrogens and progesterone in the ovary and testosterone in the tests.
- Luteotropin or prolactin (PRL) controls the secretion of milk and maintains the existence of the corpus luteum during pregnancy.

Posterior Lobe Secretions

The posterior lobe of the pituitary secretes two hormones—*antidiuretic hormone (ADH)* which regulates the amount of water passed by the kidneys and the oxytocin hormone stimulating the contraction of the uterus during the birth of a baby and the release of milk during breastfeeding.

Thyroid Gland

The thyroid gland consists of two lobes, placed one on each side of the trachea and connected together by a strip of thyroid tissue called the *isthmus of the thyroid* which lies across in front of the trachea.

Structure

The thyroid gland is composed of numbers of vesicles lined with the cubical epithelium, abundantly supplied with blood and held together by connective tissue. These cells secrete a sticky fluid, the colloid of the thyroid which contains an iodine compound; the active principle of this compound is a thyroxine hormone. This secretion fills the vesicles and from here, passes to the bloodstream either directly or through the lymphatics.

Function

The secretion of the thyroid is regulated by a hormone of the anterior lobe of the pituitary gland, the thyrotropic hormone. The thyroid gland is intimately concerned with the metabolic activities regulating the chemistry of the tissues and is instrumental in stimulating oxidation and consequently the output of carbon dioxide (CO_2).

Hyposecretion

Deficiency of the secretion of the gland at birth produces a condition known as cretinism in which mental and physical growth are retarded. In adults, deficiency of the secretion produces myxedema—the general metabolic processes slowdown, there is a tendency to gain weight, movements are lethargic, there is slowness of mind and speech, the skin becomes thickened and dry and the hair falls out or gets thin.

Hypersecretion

In enlargement of the gland and increased secretion, hyperthyroidism occurs, the symptoms are the opposite of those of myxedema. The metabolic rate is raised and the body temperature may be higher than normal.

Parathyroid Glands

There are four small parathyroid glands, two embedded in the posterior surface of each lobe of the thyroid gland. They are surrounded by fine connective tissue capsules. The cells forming the glands are spherical in shape and are arranged in columns with channels containing blood between them.

Function

The parathyroid glands secrete parathyroid hormone (PTH). Secretion is regulated by the blood level of calcium. When this falls, secretion of PTH is increased and vice versa.

The main function of PTH is to increase the blood calcium level when it is slow.

Parathyroid hormone and calcitonin from the thyroid gland act in a complementary manner to maintain blood calcium levels within the normal range. This is needed for:
* Muscle contraction
* Blood clotting
* Nerve impulse transmission.

The Thymus Gland

The thymus gland lies in the thorax about the level of the bifurcation of the trachea. It is pinkish-gray in color and consists of two lobes. At birth, the gland is quite small, weighing about 10 grams or a little more; it increases in size and at puberty, weighs from 30-40 grams and then shrinks again.

The Adrenal Gland (Fig. 1.41)

The adrenal or suprarenal gland lies on the upper pole of each kidney. The adrenal gland consists of an outer yellowish part—the cortex which produces cortisol, a close relation of cortisone and an inner medullary portion both adrenaline and noradrenaline.

These substances are secreted under the control of the sympathetic nervous system. The secretion is increased in conditions of emotion, such as anger and fear and in states of asphyxia and starvation and an increased output raises the blood pressure in order to combat the shock produced by these emergencies.

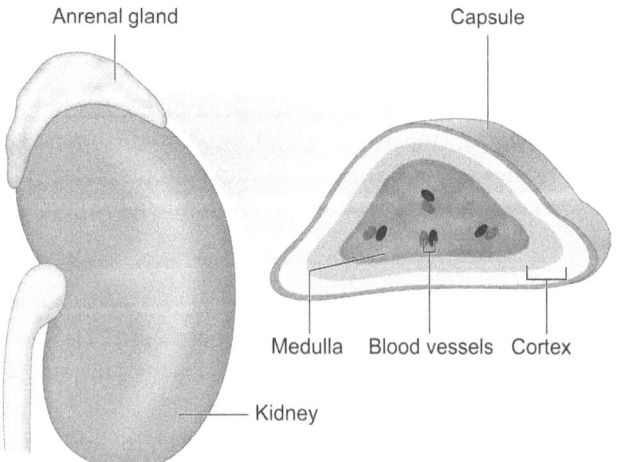

Fig. 1.41: Hormones of adrenal glands.

Noradrenaline gland raises the blood pressure by stimulating the muscular fibers in the walls of the blood vessels causing them to contract. *Adrenaline* aids carbohydrate metabolism by increasing the output of glucose from the liver.

The important hormones secreted by the adrenal cortex are hydrocortisone, aldosterone and corticosterone which are intimately concerned with metabolism, growth, renal function and muscle tone. These functions are essential of life.

Pancreatic Islets

The cells that make up the pancreatic islets are found in clusters, irregularly disturbed throughout the substance of the pancreas. Unlike exocrine pancreas, which produces pancreatic juice there are no ducts leading from the clusters of islet cells. Pancreatic hormones are secreted directly into the bloodstream and circulate throughout the body. There are three main types of cells in the pancreatic islets:
1. (Alpha) cells, which secrete glucagon
2. (Beta) cells, which secrete insulin
3. (Delta) cells, which secrete somatostatin

The normal blood glucose level is between 3.5 and 8 mmol/liter. Blood glucose levels are controlled mainly by the opposing actions of insulin and glucagon:
* Glucagon increases blood glucose levels
* Insulin reduces blood glucose levels

Pancreas (Fig. 1.42)

The pancreas is a compound racemose gland, very similar in structure to the salivary glands. It is about 23 cm long, extending from the duodenum to the following three parts of spleen and is described as consisting of the following three parts:
1. **The head of the pancreas:** The broadest part lies to the right of the abdominal cavity and in the curve of the duodenum which particularly encircles it.
2. **The body of the pancreas:** It is the main part of the organ; it is behind the stomach and in front of the first lumbar vertebra.
3. **The tail of the pancreas:** It is a narrow part to the left which actually touches the spleen.

The substance of the pancreas is composed of lobules which begin by the function of the small ducts of lobules situated in the tail of the pancreas and passing through the body from left to right, receiving ducts from other lobules and uniting to form the main duct—the duct of Wirsung.

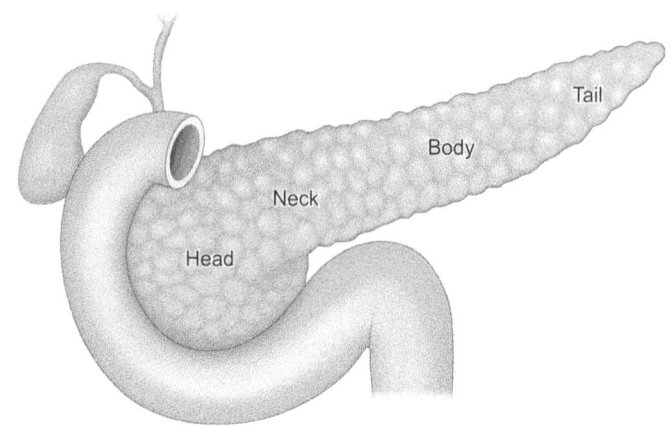

Fig. 1.42: Parts of pancreas.

Functions

The pancreas is both an exocrine and endocrine gland. The function of the exocrine pancreas is to produce pancreatic juice containing enzymes that digest carbohydrates, proteins and fats. The endocrine pancreas secretes the hormones; insulin and glucagon which are principally concerned with control of blood glucose levels.

NERVOUS SYSTEM: STRUCTURE OF BRAIN AND SPINAL CORD

The nervous system has two major parts: **The central nervous system (CNS) and the peripheral nervous system (PNS) (Fig. 1.43)**. The central system is the primary command center for the body, and is comprised of the brain and spinal cord. The peripheral nervous system consists of a network of nerves that connects the rest of the body to the CNS.

The two systems work together to collect information from inside the body and from the environment outside it. The systems process the collected information and then dispatch instructions to the rest of the body, facilitating an appropriate response.

In most cases, the brain is the final destination point for information gathered by the rest of the nervous system. Once data arrives, the brain sorts and files it before sending out any necessary commands.

The brain is divided into many different sections, including the cerebrum and brainstem. These parts handle pieces of the brain's overall workload, including storing and retrieving memory and

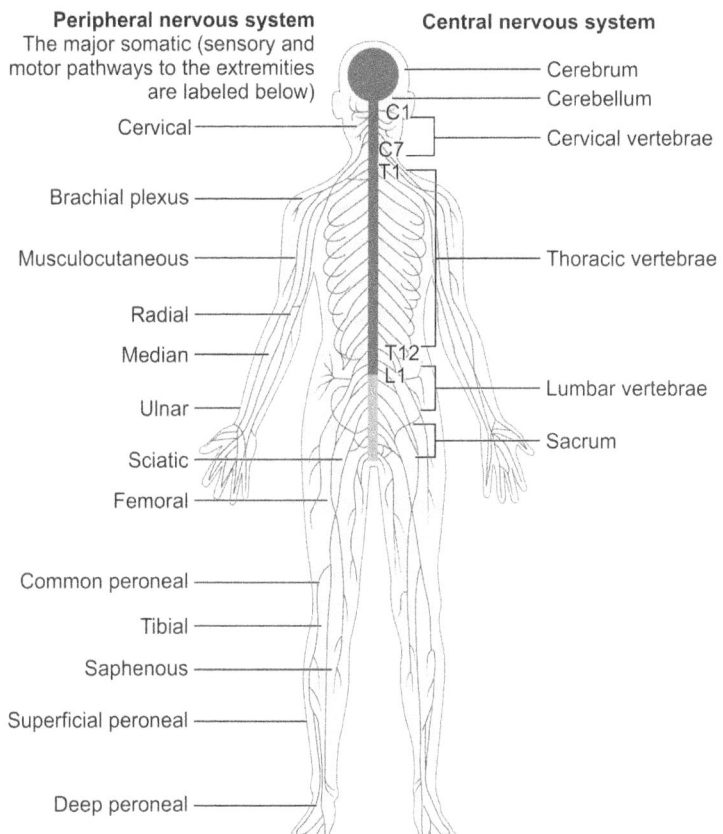

Fig. 1.43: The nervous system.

making body movement's smooth. Although the *brain* is the control center, its job would not be possible without the *spinal cord*, which is the major conduit for information traveling between brain and body. Peripheral system nerves branch from either the brainstem or the spinal cord. Each nerve is connected to a particular area of the torso or limbs and is responsible for communication to and from those regions.

The PNS can also be subdivided into smaller components—**the somatic and autonomic systems.** The somatic involves parts of the body a person can command at will, and the autonomic helps run involuntary functions, such as pumping blood.

Information conveyed through the nervous system moves along networks of cells called *neurons*. These neurons can only send information one way. Those transmitting to the brain are *sensory neurons*; those that transmit from the brain are known as *motor neurons*.

The nervous system can suffer from a number of afflictions, including cancer (e.g., brain tumors). Other problems include multiple sclerosis, in which damaged nerves prevent signals from traveling along them, and meningitis, which causes an inflammation of the membranes surrounding the brain and spinal cord.

The Meninges (Fig. 1.44)

Meninges have three membranes that envelop the *brain* and *spinal cord*. In mammals, the meninges are the *dura mater*, the *arachnoid mater*, and the *pia mater*. *Cerebrospinal fluid (CSF)* is located in the *subarachnoid space* between the arachnoid mater and the pia mater. The primary function of the meninges is to protect the CNS.

❖ **Dura mater:** The dura mater (*Latin: tough mother*) (also rarely called *meninx fibrosa* or *pachymeninx*) is a thick, durable membrane, closest to the skull and vertebrae. The dura mater, the outermost part, is a loosely arranged, fibroelastic layer of cells, characterized by multiple interdigitating cell processes, no extracellular collagen, and significant extracellular spaces. The middle region is a mostly fibrous portion. It consists of two layers—the *endosteal* layer, which lies closest to the *calvaria* (skullcap), and the inner meningeal layer, which lies closer to the brain. It contains larger blood vessels that split into the capillaries in the *pia mater*. It is composed of dense fibrous tissue, and its inner surface is covered by flattened cells, such as those present on the surfaces of the pia mater and arachnoid mater. The dura mater is a sac that envelops the arachnoid mater and surrounds and supports the large *dural sinuses* carrying blood from the brain toward the heart. The dura has four areas of infolding:

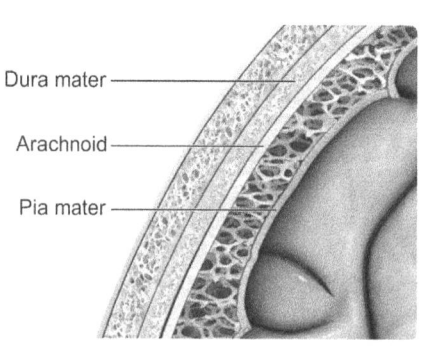
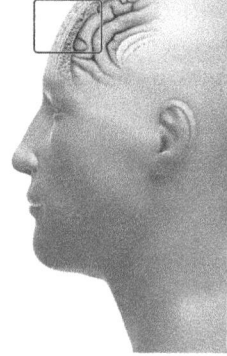

Fig. 1.44: Meninges.

- *Falx cerebri*, the largest, sickle-shaped; separates the *cerebral hemispheres*. Starts from the frontal crest of *frontal bone* and the *crista galli* running to the *internal occipital protuberance*.
- *Tentorium cerebelli*, the second largest, crescent-shaped; separates the *occipital lobes* from *cerebellum*. The falx cerebri attaches to it giving a tent-like appearance.
- *Falx cerebelli*, vertical infolding; lies inferior to the tentorium cerebelli, separating the *cerebellar hemispheres*.
- *Diaphragma sellae*, smallest infolding; covers the *pituitary gland* and *sella turcica*.

❖ **Arachnoid mater:** The middle element of the meninges is the arachnoid mater, so named because of its spider web-like appearance. It cushions the CNS. This thin, transparent membrane is composed of fibrous tissue and, like the pia mater, is covered by flat cells also thought to be impermeable to fluid.

The shape of the arachnoid does not follow the convolutions of the surface of the brain and so looks like a loosely fitting sac. In particular, in the region of the brain a large number of fine filaments called *arachnoid trabeculae* pass from the arachnoid through the subarachnoid space to blend with the tissue of the pia mater. The arachnoid is composed of an outermost portion (arachnoid barrier cell layer) with tightly packed cells and no extracellular collagen; that is why, it is considered to represent an effective morphological and physiological meningeal barrier between the CSF and subarachnoid space and the blood circulation in the dura. The arachnoid barrier layer is characterized by a distinct continuous basal lamina on its inner surface toward the innermost collagenous portion of the arachnoid reticular layer.

❖ **Pia mater:** The pia mater (*Latin: tender mother*) is a very delicate membrane. It is the meningeal envelope that firmly adheres to the surface of the brain and spinal cord, following all of the brain's contours (the *gyri* and *sulci*). It is a very thin membrane composed of fibrous tissue covered on its outer surface by a sheet of flat cells thought to be impermeable to fluid. The pia mater is pierced by blood vessels to the brain and spinal cord, and its *capillaries* nourish the brain.

❖ **Leptomeninges:** The *arachnoid* and *pia mater* together are sometimes called the *leptomeninges*, literally 'thin meninges'. The morphology of the brain in *meningococcal meningitis* is said to be covered by *exudate* on the surface of and within the leptomeninges. Because the arachnoid is connected to the pia by cob-web like strands, it is structurally continuous with the pia, hence, the name

pia-arachnoid or leptomeninges. They are responsible for the production of beta-trace.
- **Spaces:** The *subarachnoid space* is the space that normally exists between the *arachnoid* and the *pia mater*, which is filled with CSF. The *dura mater* is attached to the *skull*, whereas in the *spinal cord*, the dura mater is separated from the bone (vertebrae) by a space called the *epidural space*, which contain fat and blood vessels. The arachnoid is attached to the dura mater, while the pia mater is attached to the CNS tissue. When the dura mater and the arachnoid separate through injury or illness, the space between them is the *subdural space*. There is a *subpial space* underneath the pia mater that separates it from the *glia limitans*.

Brain (Fig. 1.45)

The brain is composed of the cerebrum, cerebellum, and brainstem
- The **cerebrum** is the largest part of the brain and is composed of right and left hemispheres. It performs higher functions, such as interpreting touch, vision and hearing, as well as speech, reasoning, emotions, learning, and fine control of movement.
- The **cerebellum** is located under the cerebrum. Its function is to coordinate muscle movements, maintain posture, and balance.
- The **brainstem** includes the midbrain, pons, and medulla. It acts as a relay center connecting the cerebrum and cerebellum to the spinal cord. It performs many automatic functions, such as breathing, heart rate, body temperature, wake and sleep cycles,

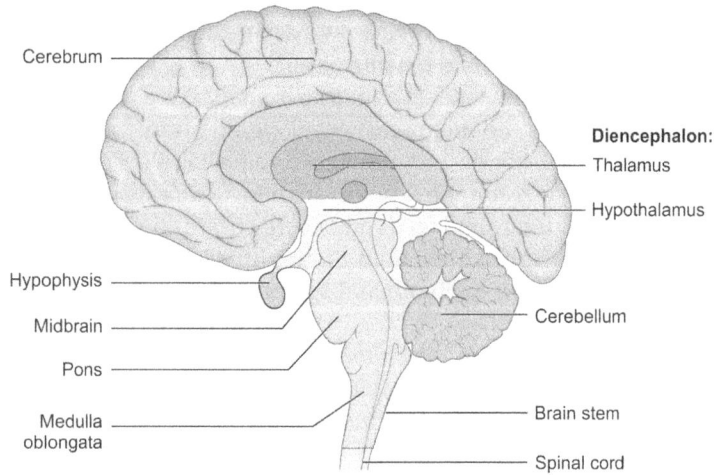

Fig. 1.45: Brain.

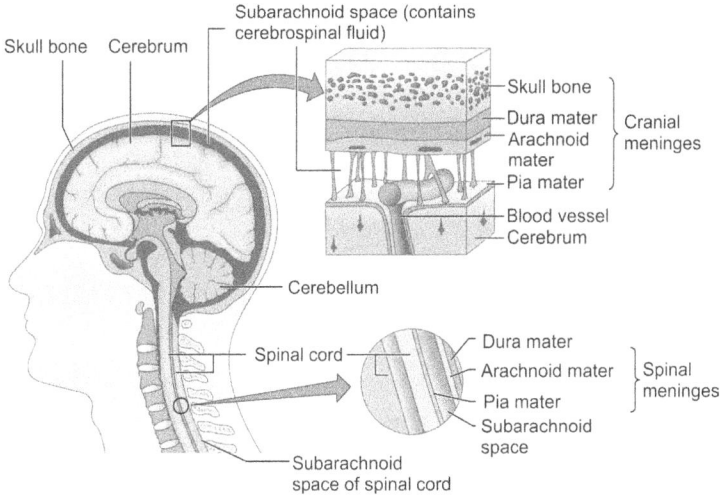

Fig. 1.46: Anatomy of brain and cross section of brain wall.

digestion, sneezing, coughing, vomiting, and swallowing. Ten of the twelve cranial nerves originate in the brainstem.

The surface of the cerebrum has a folded appearance called the *cortex*. The cortex contains about 70% of the 100 billion nerve cells. The nerve cell bodies color the cortex gray-brown and giving it its name—gray matter. Beneath the cortex are long connecting fibers between neurons, called *axons*, which make up the white matter.

The folding of the cortex increases the brain's surface area allowing more neurons to fit inside the skull and enabling higher functions. Each fold is called *a gyrus*, and each groove between folds is called a *sulcus*. There are names for the folds and grooves that help define specific brain regions **(Fig. 1.46)**.

Right Brain—Left Brain (Fig. 1.47)

The right and left hemispheres of the brain are joined by a bundle of fibers called the *corpus callosum* that delivers messages from one side to the other. Each hemisphere controls the opposite side of the body. If a brain tumor is located on the right side of the brain, your left arm or leg may be weak or paralyzed.

Not all functions of the hemispheres are shared. In general, the left hemisphere controls speech, comprehension, arithmetic, and writing. The right hemisphere controls creativity, spatial ability, artistic, and musical skills. The left hemisphere is dominant in hand use and language in about 92% of people.

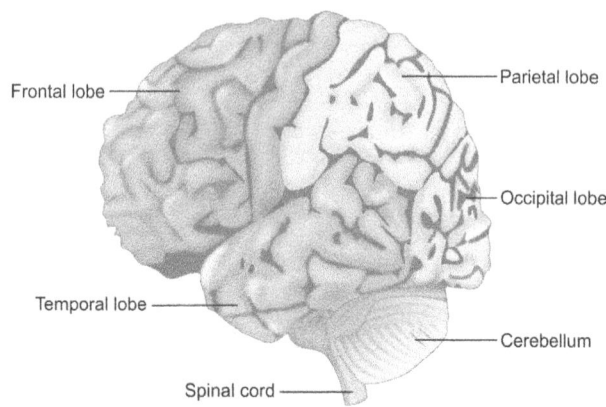

Fig. 1.47: Parts of the human brain.

Lobes of the Brain

The cerebral hemispheres have distinct fissures, which divide the brain into lobes. Each hemisphere has four lobes—frontal, temporal, parietal, and occipital. Each lobe may be divided, once again, into areas that serve very specific functions. It is important to understand that each lobe of the brain does not function alone. There are very complex relationships between the lobes of the brain and between the right and left hemispheres.

Frontal lobe
- Personality, behavior, emotions
- Judgment, planning, problem-solving
- **Speech:** Speaking and writing (Broca's area)
- Body movement (motor strip)
- Intelligence, concentration, self-awareness.

Parietal lobe
- Interprets language, words
- Sense of touch, pain, temperature (sensory strip)
- Interprets signals from vision, hearing, motor, sensory and memory
- Spatial and visual perception

Occipital lobe
Interprets vision (color, light, movement)

Temporal lobe
- Understanding language (Wernicke's area)
- Memory

❖ Hearing
❖ Sequencing and organization

Messages within the brain are carried along pathways. Messages can travel from one gyrus to another, from one lobe to another, from one side of the brain to the other, and to structures found deep in the brain (e.g., thalamus, hypothalamus).

Spinal Cord (Fig. 1.48)

The spinal cord is a long, fragile tube like structure that begins at the end of the brainstem and continues down almost to the bottom of the spine (spinal column). The spinal cord consists of nerves that carry incoming and outgoing messages between the brain and the rest of the body. It is also the center for reflexes, such as the knee jerk reflex.

Like the brain, the spinal cord is covered by three layers of tissue (meninges). The spinal cord and meninges are contained in the spinal canal, which runs through the center of the spine. In most adults, the spine is composed of 26 individual back bones (vertebrae). Just as the skull protects the brain, vertebrae protect the spinal cord. The vertebrae are separated by disks made of cartilage, which act as cushions, reducing the forces generated by movements, such as walking and jumping.

A column of bones called vertebrae make up the spine (spinal column). The vertebrae protect the spinal cord, a long, fragile structure contained in the spinal canal, which runs through the center of the spine.

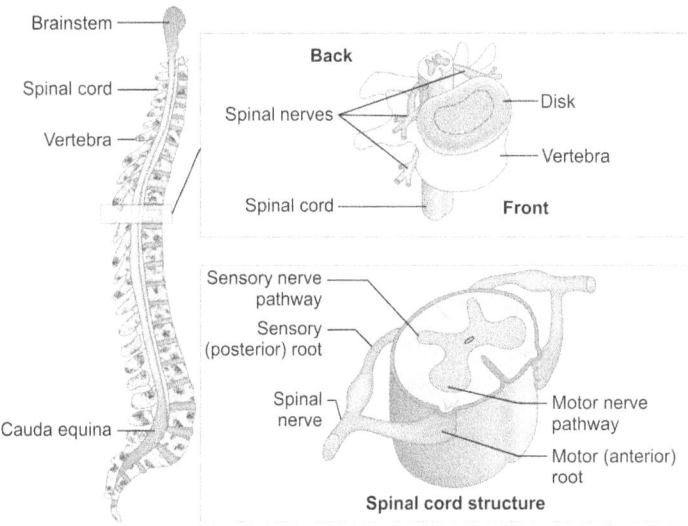

Fig. 1.48: Spinal cord.

Between the vertebrae are disks composed of cartilage, which help cushion the spine and give it some flexibility.

- **Spinal nerves:** Emerging from the spinal cord between the vertebrae are 31 pairs of spinal nerves. Each nerve emerges in two short branches (roots):
  1. One at the front (motor or anterior root) of the spinal cord
  2. One at the back (sensory or posterior root) of the spinal cord.

  The motor roots carry commands from the brain and spinal cord to other parts of the body, particularly to skeletal muscles.

  The sensory roots carry information to the brain from other parts of the body.

- **Cauda equina:** The spinal cord ends about three fourths of the way down the spine, but a bundle of nerves extends beyond the cord. This bundle is called the cauda equina because it resembles a horse's tail. The *cauda equina* carries nerve impulses to and from the legs.

Like the brain, the spinal cord consists of gray and white matter. The butterfly-shaped center of the cord consists of gray matter. The front 'wings' (called horns) contain motor nerve cells, which transmit information from the brain or spinal cord to muscles, stimulating movement. The back horns contain sensory nerve cells, which transmit sensory information from other parts of the body through the spinal cord to the brain. The surrounding white matter contains columns of nerve fibers that carry sensory information to the brain from the rest of the body (ascending tracts) and columns that carry impulses from the brain to the muscles (descending tracts).

BLOOD: COMPOSITION AND FUNCTIONS

It is a mobile, reddish-colored fluid that circulates in blood vessels in the human body and supplies nutrients and oxygen to all the living cells and removes waste products and carbon dioxide from them. It has two components—plasma and blood corpuscles. Blood corpuscles are of three types—red blood cells, white blood cells, and platelets. The blood that runs through the veins, arteries, and capillaries is known as whole blood, a mixture of about 55% plasma and 45% blood cells. About 7 to 8% of your total body weight is blood. An average-sized man has about 12 pints of blood in his body, and an average-sized woman has about 9 pints.

Functions of blood: Some of the important functions of the blood are as follows:
- Circulation of blood is responsible for transportation of soluble digested food from the small intestine to various parts of the body

where they are stored or assimilated. Blood also carries glucose from the liver to the muscles.
- ❖ Blood carries soluble excretory materials, such as urea to organs of excretion.
- ❖ Blood transports oxygen from the lungs to all the parts of the body. In blood, oxygen combines with hemoglobin to form oxyhemoglobin. When the blood reaches the tissue, oxygen from hemoglobin diffuses into the tissue cells.
- ❖ Circulations of blood help to maintain a constant body temperature by distributing the excess heat from the deeply seated organs.
- ❖ Blood carries carbon dioxide produced by the tissues to the lungs for breathing out.
- ❖ Blood carries hormones from the endocrine glands to target organs.
- ❖ Blood has a property of clotting which prevents excessive blood loss.
- ❖ The white blood cells act as soldiers of the body by killing the bacteria and other germs.
- ❖ The blood acts as a buffer and maintains a constant solute potential and pH.

The Components of Blood

Plasma

The liquid component of blood is called plasma. It is a mixture of water, sugar, fat, protein, and salts. The main job of the plasma is to transport blood cells throughout your body along with nutrients, waste products, antibodies, clotting proteins, chemical messengers, such as hormones, and proteins that help maintain the body's fluid balance.

Red Blood Cells

Red blood cells are the most abundant cell in the blood, accounting for about 40-45% of its volume. They are bright red color and are also called erythrocytes or RBCs. The shape of a red blood cell is a biconcave with a flattened center.

Production of red blood cells is controlled by erythropoietin, a hormone produced primarily by the kidneys. Red blood cells start as immature cells in the bone marrow and after approximately seven days of maturation are released into the bloodstream. Unlike many other cells, red blood cells have no nucleus and can easily change shape, helping them fit through the various blood vessels in your body. However, while the lack of a nucleus makes a red blood cell more flexible, it also limits the life of the cell as it travels through the smallest blood vessels, damaging the cell's membranes and depleting its energy supplies. The red blood cell survives on average only 120 days.

Red blood cells contain a special protein called hemoglobin, which helps in carrying oxygen from the lungs to the rest of the body and then returns carbon dioxide from the body to the lungs so it can be exhaled. Blood appears red because of the large number of red blood cells, which get their color from the hemoglobin. The percentage of whole blood volume that is made up of red blood cells is called the hematocrit and is a common measure of red blood cell levels.

White Blood Cells

White blood cells are also called leukocytes. White blood cells protect the body from infection. They are much fewer in number than red blood cells, accounting for about 1% of your blood.

The most common type of white blood cell is the neutrophil, and accounts for 55–70% of the total white blood cell count. Each neutrophil lives less than a day, so the bone marrow must constantly make new neutrophils to maintain protection against infection.

The other major type of white blood cell is a lymphocyte. There are two main populations of these cells:
1. T-Lymphocytes help to regulate the function of other immune cells and directly attack various infected cells and tumors.
2. B-Lymphocytes make antibodies, which are proteins that specifically target bacteria, viruses, and other foreign materials.

Platelets

Platelets are also called **thrombocytes**. Platelets are small fragments of cells. Platelets help the blood clotting process or coagulation by gathering at the site of an injury, sticking to the lining of the injured blood vessel, and forming a platform on which blood coagulation can occur.

Sometimes a higher than normal number of platelets can cause unnecessary clotting, which **can lead to strokes and heart attacks.**

Blood Clotting

Blood is a necessary component of the human body and the loss of this fluid may be life-threatening. Blood is generated via hematopoiesis and ultimately becomes the delivery method for oxygen to the tissues and cells. The human body protects against loss of blood through the clotting mechanism. Vascular mechanisms, platelets, coagulation factors, prostaglandins, enzymes, and proteins are the contributors to the clotting mechanism which act together to form clots and stop a loss of blood. Through vasoconstriction, adhesion, activation, and aggregation, the contributors form a transient plug to act as the cork to the leaking blood flow. Soon after, fibrin, the functioning form of fibrinogen, stabilizes this weak platelet plug. The scope of this article will highlight the physiological aspects of the clotting mechanism.

The cellular components of the clotting mechanism include platelets, endothelial cells, and a series of proteins, enzymes, and ions. The clotting mechanism involves the circulatory system which includes the lineage of blood cells and blood vessels.

The clotting mechanism is broken into 2 stages:
1. **Primary hemostasis:** Formation of a weak platelet plug
2. **Secondary hemostasis:** Stabilizing the weak platelet plug into a clot by the fibrin network.

Primary Hemostasis

Primary hemostasis is the formation of a weak platelet plug which is achieved in four phases—vasoconstriction, platelet adhesion, platelet activation, and platelet aggregation.

Vasoconstriction is the initial response whenever there is vessel injury. Vasospasm of the blood vessels occurs first in response to injury of the vasculature. This vasospasm, in turn, stimulates vasoconstriction. Vasoconstriction is primarily mediated by endothelin-1, a potent vasoconstrictor, which is synthesized by the damaged endothelium. Damaged endothelium exposes subendothelial collagen, von Willebrand factor (vWF), releases ATP, and inflammatory mediators. vWF is synthesized by megakaryocytes which later gets stored in a-granules of platelets. Weibel-Palade bodies of the endothelium also synthesize vWF. It is the combination of exposure of vWF, subendothelial collagen, ATP, and inflammatory mediators which provide the gateway into the second phase of primary hemostasis, platelet adhesion.

Platelet adhesion is the process by which platelets attach to the exposed subendothelial vWF. Post-vascular damage, platelets begin to roll along vessel walls and adhere to areas of exposed subendothelial collagen and vWF. Platelet membranes are rich in G protein (Gp) receptors located within the phospholipid bilayer. Specifically, it is Gp Ib-IX receptor on platelets that bind to vWF within the endothelium that creates the initial connection between the two. Once bound, a variety of events can occur in the third phase of primary hemostasis to activate the platelet.

Platelet activation consists of platelets undergoing two specific events once they have adhered to the exposed vWF (i.e., the damaged vessel site). First, platelets will undergo an irreversible change in shape from smooth discs to multi-pseudopodal plugs, which greatly increases their surface area. Second, platelets secrete their cytoplasmic granules.

Platelet activation is mediated via thrombin by two mechanisms. Thrombin directly activates platelets via proteolytic cleavage by binding the protease-activated receptor. Thrombin also stimulates platelet granule release which includes serotonin, platelet activating factor, and adenosine diphosphate (ADP). ADP is an important physiological agonist which is stored specifically in the dense granules of platelets. When ADP is released, it binds to P2Y1 and P2Y12 receptors on platelet membranes. P2Y1 induces the pseudopod shape change and aids in platelet aggregation. P2Y12 plays a major role in inducing the clotting cascade. When ADP binds to its receptors, it induces Gp IIb/IIIa complex expression at the platelet membrane surface. The Gp IIb/IIIa complex is a calcium-dependent collagen receptor which is necessary for platelet-to-endothelial adherence and platelet-to-platelet aggregation. Simultaneously, platelets synthesize Thromboxane A2 (TXA2). TXA2 further intensifies vasoconstriction and platelet aggregation (next step in the primary hemostasis process). The process of platelet activation readies the local environment for platelet aggregation.

Platelet aggregation begins once platelets have been activated. Once activated, the Gp IIb/IIIa receptors adhere to vWF and fibrinogen. Fibrinogen is found in the circulation and forms a connection between the Gp IIb/IIIa receptors of platelets to interconnect them with each other. This ultimately forms the weak platelet plug.

Ultimately, primary hemostasis allows the culmination of a weak platelet plug to temporarily protect from hemorrhage until further stabilization of fibrinogen to fibrin via thrombin occurs in secondary hemostasis.

Secondary Hemostasis

Secondary hemostasis involves the clotting factors acting in a cascade to ultimately stabilize the weak platelet plug. This is accomplished by completing three tasks: (1) triggering activation of clotting factors, (2) conversion of prothrombin to thrombin, and (3) conversion of fibrinogen to fibrin. These tasks are accomplished initially by 1 of 2 pathways; the extrinsic and intrinsic pathway, which converge at the activation of factor X and then complete their tasks via the common pathway. Please note that calcium ions are required for the entire process of secondary hemostasis.

The extrinsic pathway includes tissue factor (TF) and factor VII (FVII). It is initiated when TF binds to FVII, activating FVII to factor VIIa (FVIIa), forming a TF-FVIIa complex. This complex, in turn, activates factor X (FX). Note, the TF-FVIIa complex can also activate factor IX of the intrinsic pathway, which is called the alternate pathway. Once factor X is activated to FXa by TF-FVIIa complex, the cascade continues down the common pathway.

The intrinsic pathway includes Hageman factor (FXII), factor I (FXI), factor IX (FIX), and factor VIII (FVIII). The process is initiated when FXII comes into contact with exposed subendothelial collagen and becomes activated to FXIIa. Subsequently, FXIIa activates FXI to FXIa, and FXIa activates FIX to FIXa. FIXa works in combination with activated factor VIII (FVIIIa) to activate factor X. Once Factor X is activated by FIXa-FVIIIa complex, the cascade continues down the common pathway.

The common pathway is initiated via the activation of factor Xa. Factor Xa combines with factor Va and calcium on phospholipid surfaces to create a prothrombinase complex ultimately activating prothrombin (aka factor II) into thrombin. This activation of thrombin occurs via serine protease cleaving of prothrombin. Now, thrombin activates factor XIIIa (FXIIIa). FXIIIa crosslinks with fibrin forming the stabilized clot.

PATHOPHYSIOLOGY

Thrombosis is the process of blood clot (thrombus) formation in a blood vessel. Virchow triad is an important concept that highlights the primary abnormalities in pathology that can lead to the clotting mechanism proceeding to thrombosis. The triad is composed of stasis or turbulent blood flow, endothelial injury, and hypercoagulability of the blood.

- ❖ Abnormal (stasis) or turbulent blood flow can lead to thrombosis. Normal blood flow is laminar. Turbulent blood flow leads to endothelial injury thus promoting the formation of a thrombus. An example of turbulent blood flow is in the aneurysm of weakened vessels. Another aspect of abnormal blood flow, venous stasis, such as in postoperative bed rest, long distance traveling in a car or plane, or immobility due to obesity can lead to endothelial injury thus promoting thrombosis.
- ❖ Endothelial Injury leads to platelet activation and the formation of a thrombus. This may be a result of inflammation of the endothelial surface of the vasculature. Hypercholesterolemia is an example of a

chronic inflammatory condition which progresses into endothelial injury.
- Hypercoagulability (thrombophilia) is any disorder of the blood that predisposes a person to thrombosis. This may be a result of inherited clotting disorders, such as a factor V Leiden mutation or an acquired clotting disorder, such as disseminated intravascular coagulation.

Hemorrhage occurs when blood escapes from its vessel walls.

Platelet dysfunction, or clotting factor dysfunction, can be further broken down into which part of the clotting mechanism physiology is affected.

Disorders of Primary Hemostasis: vWF, Platelet Defects, or Receptor Interference

- Von Willebrand factor disease
- Bernard-Soulier disease
- Glanzmann thrombasthenia
- Medication-induced

Disorders of Secondary Hemostasis: Clotting Factor Defects

- Factor V Leiden
- Vitamin K deficiency
- Hemophilia
- Anti-phospholipid antibody syndrome
- Disseminated intravascular coagulation
- Liver disease
- Medication-induced

Defects in Small Vessels

- Trauma
- Aneurysm rupture
- Vasculitides

■ CLINICAL SIGNIFICANCE

In addition to the pathophysiology, a few ideas to keep in mind when you have a patient with clotting mechanism disorders:

Patients with:
- Primary hemostasis defects typically present with small bleeds in the skin or mucosal membranes. This includes petechiae and/or purpura.

1. Damaged blood vessel wall

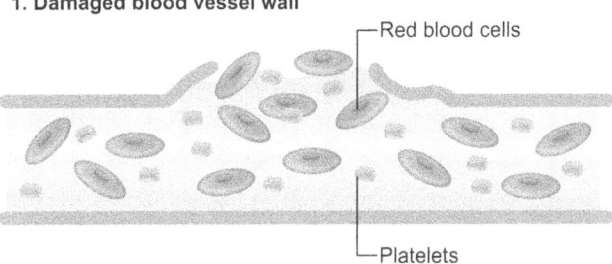

1. Repaired vessel wall

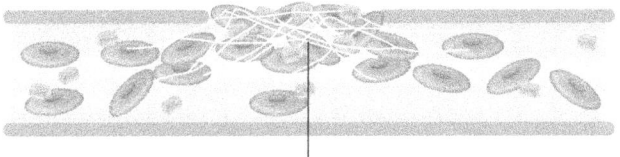

The threads (fibrin) that help build the clot

Fig. 1.49: Formation of blood clots.

- Secondary hemostasis defects typically present with bleeds into soft tissue (muscle) or joints (hemarthrosis).
- Direct defects in small blood vessels typically present with palpable purpura and ecchymosis. These may collect and become larger to develop a hematoma **(Fig. 1.49)**.

Also, laboratory testing involving PTT or PT/INR can be divided by the physiological mechanisms:
- Disorders exclusively effecting primary hemostasis do not affect the PT/INR or PTT, they only increase bleeding time
- Disorders that affect the extrinsic pathway of secondary hemostasis affect the PT/INR
- Disorders that affect the intrinsic pathway of secondary hemostasis affect the PTT.

STRUCTURE AND FUNCTIONS OF SENSORY ORGANS: EYE, EAR, NOSE, TONGUE SPECIAL SENSES (FIG. 1.50)

Aristotle (384-322 BC) is credited with the traditional classification of the five sense organs—*sight, smell, taste, touch, and hearing*. As far back as the 1760's, the famous philosopher Immanuel Kant proposed that our knowledge of the outside world depends on our modes of perception. In order to define what is 'extrasensory' we need to define what is 'sensory'. Each of the five senses consists of organs

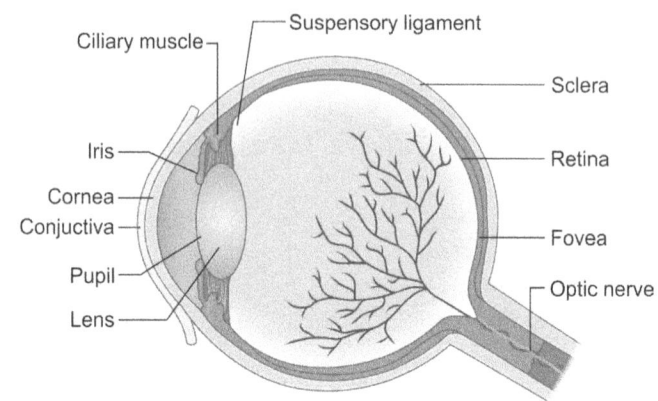

Fig. 1.50: Structure of an eye.

with specialized cellular structures that have receptors for specific stimuli. These cells have links to the nervous system and thus to the brain. Sensing is done at primitive levels in the cells and integrated into sensations in the nervous system. Sight is probably the most developed sense in humans, followed closely by hearing.

Sight

The eye is the organ of vision. It has a complex structure consisting of a transparent lens that focuses light on the retina. The retina is covered with two basic types of light-sensitive cells— *rods* and *cones*. The cone cells are sensitive to color and are located in the part of the retina called the fovea, where the light is focused by the lens. The rod cells are not sensitive to color, but have greater sensitivity to light than the cone cells. These cells are located around the fovea and are responsible for peripheral vision and night vision. The eye is connected to the brain through the *optic nerve*. The point of this connection is called the 'blind spot' because it is insensitive to light. Experiments have shown that the back of the brain maps the visual input from the eyes.

The brain combines the input of our two eyes into a single three-dimensional image. In addition, even though the image on the retina is upside-down because of the focusing action of the lens, the brain compensates and provides the right-side-up perception. Experiments have been done with subjects fitted with prisms that invert the images. The subjects go through an initial period of great confusion, but subsequently they perceive the images as right-side up.

The range of perception of the eye is phenomenal. In the dark, a substance produced by the rod cells increases the sensitivity of the eye so that it is possible to detect very dim light. In strong light, the iris contracts reducing the size of the aperture that admits light into the eye and a protective obscure substance reduces the exposure of the light-sensitive cells.

The spectrum of light to which the eye is sensitive varies from the red to the violet. Lower electromagnetic frequencies in the infrared are sensed as heat, but cannot be seen. Higher frequencies in the ultraviolet and beyond cannot be seen either, but can be sensed as tingling of the skin or eyes depending on the frequency. The human eye is not sensitive to the polarization of light, i.e., light that oscillates on a specific plane. Bees, on the other hand, are sensitive to polarized light, and have a visual range that extends into the ultraviolet. Some kinds of snakes have special infrared sensors that enable them to hunt in absolute darkness using only the heat emitted by their prey. Birds have a higher density of light-sensing cells than humans do in their retinas, and therefore, higher visual acuity.

Color blindness or '*Daltonism*' is a common abnormality in human vision that makes it impossible to differentiate colors accurately. One type of color blindness results in the inability to distinguish red from green. This can be a real handicap for certain types of occupations. To a color blind person, a person with normal color vision would appear to have extrasensory perception. However, we want to reserve the term '*extrasensory perception*' for perception that is beyond the range of the normal.

Hearing (Fig. 1.51)

The ear is the organ of hearing. The outer ear protrudes away from the head and is shaped like a cup to direct sounds toward the tympanic membrane, which transmits vibrations to the inner ear through a series of small bones in the middle ear called the *malleus*, *incus* and *stapes*. The inner ear, or cochlea, is a spiral-shaped chamber covered internally by nerve fibers that react to the vibrations and transmit impulses to the brain via the auditory nerve. The brain combines the input of our two ears to determine the direction and distance of sounds.

The inner ear has a vestibular system formed by three semicircular canals that are approximately at right angles to each other and which are responsible for the sense of balance and spatial orientation. The inner ear has chambers filled with a viscous fluid and small particles (otoliths) containing calcium carbonate. The movement of these particles over small hair cells in the inner ear sends signals to the brain that are interpreted as motion and acceleration.

The human ear can perceive frequencies from 16 cycles per second, which is a very deep bass, to 28,000 cycles per second, which is a very

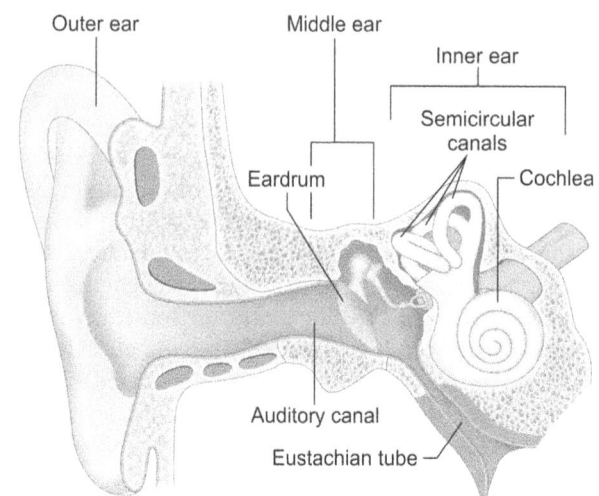

Fig. 1.51: Structure of ear (organ of hearing).

high pitch. Bats and dolphins can detect frequencies higher than 100,000 cycles per second. The human ear can detect pitch changes as small as 3 hundredths of 1% of the original frequency in some frequency ranges. Some people have '*perfect pitch*', which is the ability to map a tone precisely on the musical scale without reference to an external standard. It is estimated that less than one in ten thousand people have perfect pitch, but speakers of tonal languages, such as Vietnamese and Mandarin show remarkably precise absolute pitch in reading out lists of words because pitch is an essential feature in conveying the meaning of words in tone languages. The Eguchi Method teaches perfect pitch to children starting before they are 4 years old. After age 7, the ability to recognize notes does not improve much.

Taste

The receptors for taste, called *taste buds*, are situated chiefly in the tongue, but they are also located in the roof of the mouth and near the pharynx **(Fig. 1.52)**. They are able to detect four basic tastes—*salty, sweet, bitter, and sour*. The tongue also can detect a sensation called '*umami*' from taste receptors sensitive to amino acids. Generally, the taste buds close to the tip of the tongue are sensitive to sweet tastes, whereas those in the back of the tongue are sensitive to bitter tastes. The taste buds on top and on the side of the tongue are sensitive to salty and sour tastes. At the base of each taste bud, there is a nerve that sends the sensations to the brain. The sense of taste functions

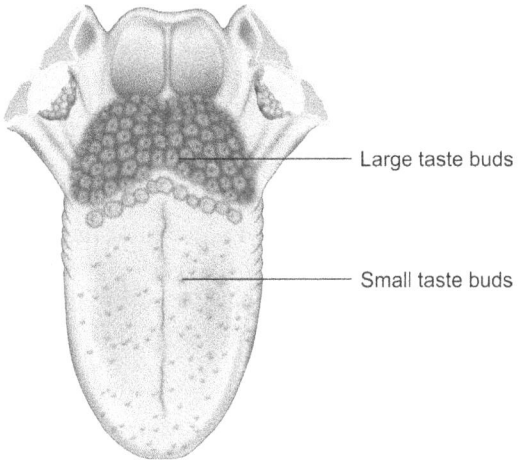

Fig. 1.52: Taste buds of tongue.

in coordination with the sense of smell. The number of taste buds varies substantially from individual to individual, but greater numbers increase sensitivity. Women, in general, have a greater number of taste buds than men. As in the case of color blindness, some people are insensitive to some tastes.

Smell

The nose is the organ responsible for the sense of smell **(Fig. 1.53)**. The cavity of the nose is lined with mucous membranes that have smell

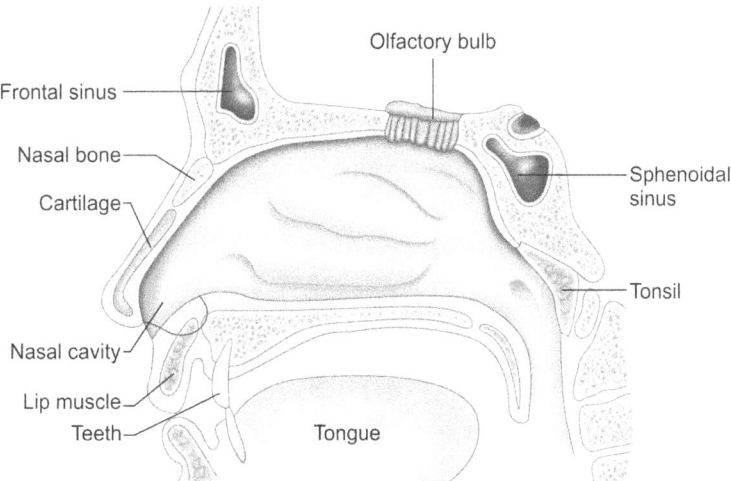

Fig. 1.53: Nasal cavity.

receptors connected to the olfactory nerve. The smells themselves consist of vapors of various substances. The smell receptors interact with the molecules of these vapors and transmit the sensations to the brain. The nose also has a structure called the vomeronasal organ (VNO) whose function has not been determined, but which is suspected of being sensitive to pheromones that influence the reproductive cycle. The smell receptors are sensitive to seven types of sensations that can be characterized as camphor, musk, flower, mint, ether, acrid, or putrid. The sense of smell is sometimes temporarily lost when a person has a cold. Dogs have a sense of smell that is many times more sensitive than man's.

Touch

The sense of touch is distributed throughout the body **(Fig. 1.54)**. Nerve endings in the skin and other parts of the body transmit sensations to the brain. Some parts of the body have a larger number of nerve endings and, therefore, are more sensitive. Four kinds of touch sensations can be identified—*cold, heat, contact, and pain*. Hairs on the skin magnify the sensitivity and act as an early warning system for the body. The fingertips and the sexual organs have the greatest concentration of nerve endings. The sexual organs have '*erogenous*

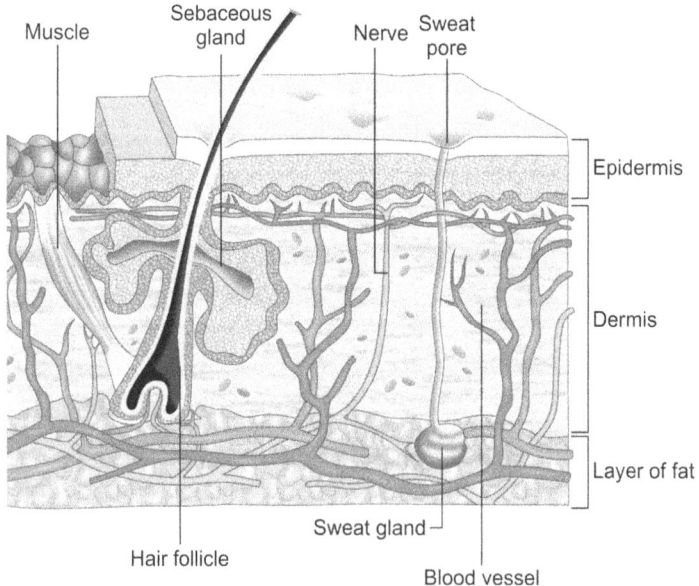

Fig. 1.54: The skin (sense of touch).

zones' that when stimulated start a series of endocrine reactions and motor responses resulting in orgasm.

Beyond the Five Sense Organs

In addition to sight, smell, taste, touch, and hearing, humans also have awareness of balance (equilibrioception), pressure, temperature (thermoception), pain (nociception), and motion all of which may involve the coordinated use of multiple sensory organs. The sense of balance is maintained by a complex interaction of visual inputs, the proprioceptive sensors (which are affected by gravity and stretch sensors found in muscles, skin, and joints), the inner ear vestibular system, and the CNS. Disturbances occurring in any part of the balance system, or even within the brain's integration of inputs, can cause the feeling of dizziness or unsteadiness.

Kinesthesia

It is the precise awareness of muscle and joint movement that allows us to coordinate our muscles when we walk, talk, and use our hands. It is the sense of kinesthesia that enables us to touch the tip of our nose with our eyes closed or to know which part of the body we should scratch when we itch.

Synesthesia

Some people experience a phenomenon called *synesthesia* in which one type of stimulation evokes the sensation of another. For example, the hearing of a sound may result in the sensation of the visualization of a color, or a shape may be sensed as a smell. Synesthesia is hereditary and it is estimated that it occurs in 1 out of 1000 individuals with variations of type and intensity. The most common forms of synesthesia are link numbers or letters with colors.

CARDIAC SYSTEM

Structure of Heart

The **heart** is a *muscular organ* in humans and other *animals*, which pumps *blood* through the *blood vessels* of the *circulatory system*. Blood provides body with the *oxygen* and *nutrients*, and also assists in the removal of *metabolic wastes*. The heart is located in the middle compartment of the *mediastinum* in the chest **(Fig. 1.55)**.

In humans, other mammals, and birds, the heart, is divided into four chambers—upper left and right *atria*; and lower left and right *ventricles*. Commonly, the right atrium and ventricle are referred

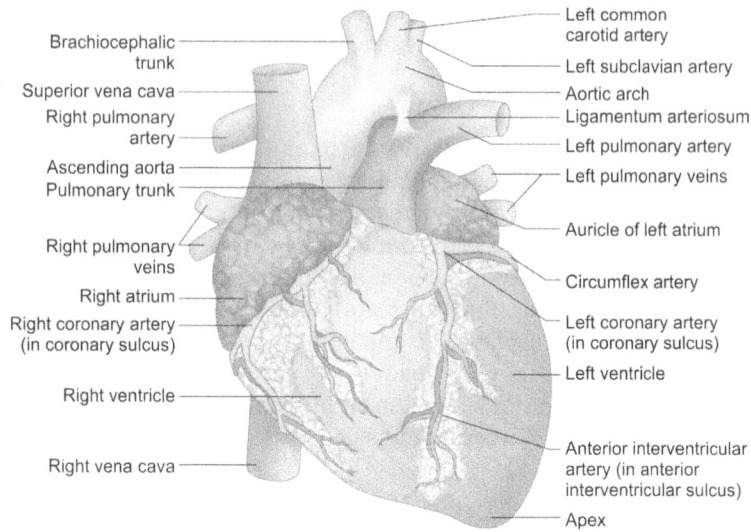

Fig. 1.55: Gross anatomy of the heart (anterior view).

together as the *right heart* and their left counterparts as the *left heart*. Fish in contrast have two chambers, an atrium and a ventricle, while reptiles have three chambers. In a healthy heart, blood flows one way through the heart due to *heart valves*, which prevent *backflow*. The heart is enclosed in a protective sac, the *pericardium*, which also contains a small amount of *fluid*. The wall of the heart is made up of three layers—*epicardium, myocardium,* and *endocardium*.

The heart pumps blood throughout the body. The heart receives blood low in oxygen from the *systemic circulation* enters the right atrium from the *superior* and *inferior venae cavae* and passes to the right ventricle. From here, it is pumped into the *pulmonary circulation*, through the *lungs* where it receives oxygen and gives off carbon dioxide. Oxygenated blood then returns to the left atrium, passes through the left ventricle and is pumped out through the *aorta* to the systemic circulation—where the oxygen is used and *metabolized* to *carbon dioxide*. In addition, the blood carries nutrients from the *digestive tract* to various organs of the body while transporting *waste* to the liver and *kidneys*. Normally with each *heartbeat* the right ventricle pumps the same amount of blood into the lungs as the left ventricle pumps to the body. *Veins* transport blood to the heart and carry deoxygenated blood except for the pulmonary and *portal veins*. *Arteries* transport blood away from the heart, and apart from the pulmonary artery hold oxygenated blood. Their increased distance from the heart cause veins to have lower *pressures* than arteries.

The heart contracts at a resting *rate* close to 72 beats per minute. *Exercise* temporarily increases the rate, but lowers *resting heart rate* in the long term, and is good for heart health.

The heart sits within a fluid-filled cavity called the *pericardial cavity*. The walls and lining of the pericardial cavity are a special membrane known as the pericardium. Pericardium is a type of serous membrane that produces serous fluid to lubricate the heart and prevent friction between the ever beating heart and its surrounding organs. Besides lubrication, the pericardium serves to hold the heart in position and maintain a hollow space for the heart to expand into when it is full. The pericardium has 2 layers—a visceral layer that covers the outside of the heart and a parietal layer that forms a sac around the outside of the pericardial cavity.

Structure of the Heart Wall

The heart wall is made of 3 layers—epicardium, myocardium and endocardium **(Fig. 1.56)**.

1. **Epicardium:** The epicardium is the outermost layer of the heart wall and is just another name for the visceral layer of the pericardium. Thus, it is a thin layer of serous membrane that helps to lubricate and protects the outside of the heart. Below the epicardium is the second, thicker layer of the heart wall: The myocardium.

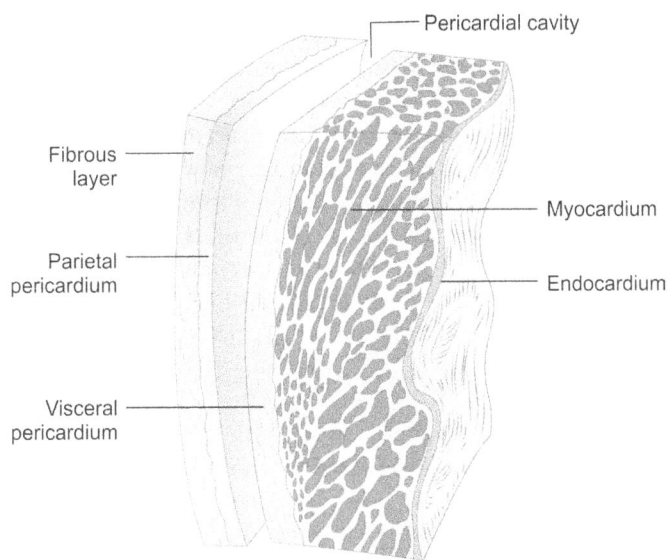

Fig. 1.56: Layers of heart.

2. **Myocardium:** The myocardium is the muscular middle layer of the heart wall that contains the cardiac muscle tissue. Myocardium makes up the majority of the thickness and mass of the heart wall and is the part of the heart which is responsible for pumping the blood. Below the myocardium is the thin endocardium layer.
3. **Endocardium:** It is the simple squamous endothelium layer that lines the inside of the heart. The endocardium is very smooth and is responsible for keeping blood from sticking to the inside of the heart and forming potentially deadly blood clots.

The thickness of the heart wall varies in different parts of the heart. The atria of the heart have a very thin myocardium because they do not need to pump blood very far—only to the nearby ventricles. The ventricles, on the other hand, have a very thick myocardium to pump blood to the lungs or throughout the entire body. The right side of the heart has less myocardium in its walls than the left side because left side has to pump blood throughout the entire body while the right side only has to pump to the lungs.

Chambers of the Heart

The heart contains 4 chambers—the right atrium, left atrium, right ventricle, and left ventricle. The atria are smaller than the ventricles and have thinner, less muscular walls. The atria act as receiving chambers for blood, so they are connected to the veins that carry blood to the heart. The ventricles are the larger, stronger pumping chambers that send blood out of the heart. The ventricles are connected to the arteries that carry blood away from the heart.

The chambers on the right side of the heart are smaller and have less myocardium in their heart wall when compared to the left side of the heart. This difference in size between the sides of the heart is related to their functions and the size of the two circulatory loops. The right side of the heart maintains pulmonary circulation to the nearby lungs while the left side of the heart pumps blood all the way to the extremities of the body in the systemic circulatory loop.

Valves of the Heart

The heart functions by pumping blood both to the lungs and to the systems of the body. To prevent blood from flowing backwards or 'regurgitating' back into the heart, a system of one-way valves are present in the heart. The heart valves can be broken down into two types—atrioventricular and semilunar valves.

Atrioventricular Valves

The atrioventricular (AV) valves are located in the middle of the heart between the atria and ventricles and only allow blood to flow from the atria into the ventricles. The AV valve on the right side of the heart is called the *tricuspid valve* because it is made of three cusps (flaps) that separate to allow the blood to pass through and connect to block regurgitation of blood. The AV valve on the left side of the heart is called the *mitral valve* or *the bicuspid valve* because it has two cusps. The AV valves are attached on the ventricular side to tough strings called *chordae tendineae*. The chordae tendineae pull on the AV valves to keep them from folding backwards and allowing blood to regurgitate past them. During the contraction of the ventricles, the AV valves look like domed parachutes with the chordae tendineae acting as the ropes holding the parachutes taut.

Semilunar Valves

The semilunar valves, so named for the crescent moon shape of their cusps, are located between the ventricles and the arteries that carry blood away from the heart. The semilunar valve on the right side of the heart is the pulmonary valve, so named because it prevents the backflow of blood from the pulmonary trunk into the right ventricle. The semilunar valve on the left side of the heart is the aortic valve, named for the fact that it prevents the aorta from regurgitating blood back into the left ventricle. The semilunar valves are smaller than the AV valves and do not have chordae tendineae to hold them in place. Instead, the cusps-of the semilunar valves are cup-shaped to catch regurgitating blood and use the blood's pressure to snap shut.

Conduction System of the Heart

The heart is able to both set its own rhythm and to conduct the signals necessary to maintain and coordinate this rhythm throughout its structures. About 1% of the cardiac muscle cells in the heart are responsible for forming the conduction system that sets the pace for the rest of the cardiac muscle cells.

The conduction system **(Fig. 1.57)** starts with the pacemaker of the heart—a small bundle of cells known as the *sinoatrial (SA) node*. The SA node is located in the wall of the right atrium inferior to the superior vena cava. The SA node is responsible for setting the pace of the heart as a whole and directly signals the atria to contract. The signal from the SA node is picked up by another mass of conductive tissue known as the atrioventricular (AV) node.

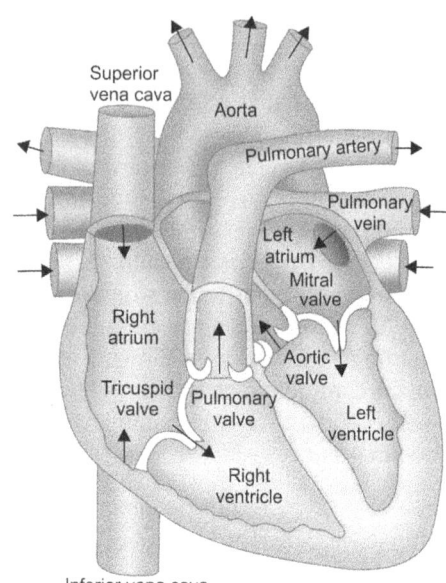

Fig. 1.57: Conduction system.

The AV node is located in the right atrium in the inferior portion of the interatrial septum. The AV node picks up the signal sent by the SA node and transmits it through the AV bundle. The AV bundle is a strand of conductive tissue that runs through the interatrial septum and into the interventricular septum. The AV bundle splits into left and right branches in the interventricular septum and continues running through the septum until they reach the apex of the heart. Branching off from the left and right bundle branches are many Purkinje fibers that carry the signal to the walls of the ventricles, stimulating the cardiac muscle cells to contract in a coordinated manner to efficiently pump blood out of the heart.

Coronary Systole and Diastole

At any given time, the chambers of the heart may found in one of two states:
1. **Systole:** During systole, cardiac muscle tissue is contracting to push blood out of the chamber.
2. **Diastole:** During diastole, the cardiac muscle cells relax to allow the chamber to fill with blood. Blood pressure increases in the major arteries during ventricular systole and decreases during ventricular diastole. This leads to the two numbers associated with blood pressure—systolic blood pressure is the higher number and

diastolic blood pressure is the lower number. For example, a blood pressure of 120/80, describes the systolic pressure (120) and the diastolic pressure (80).

The Cardiac Cycle

The cardiac cycle includes all of the events that take place during one heartbeat. There are three phases to the cardiac cycle—atrial systole, ventricular systole, and relaxation.

1. **Atrial systole:** During the atrial systole phase of the cardiac cycle, the atria contract and push blood into the ventricles. To facilitate this filling, the AV valves stay open and the semilunar valves stay closed to keep arterial blood from re-entering the heart. The atria are much smaller than the ventricles, so they only fill about 25% of the ventricles during this phase. The ventricles remain in diastole during this phase.
2. **Ventricular systole:** During ventricular systole, the ventricles contract to push blood into the aorta and pulmonary trunk. The pressure of the ventricles forces the semilunar valves to open and the AV valves to close. This arrangement of valves allows for blood flow from the ventricles into the arteries. The cardiac muscles of the atria repolarize and enter the state of diastole during this phase.
3. **Relaxation phase:** During the relaxation phase, all four chambers of the heart are in diastole as blood pours into the heart from the veins. The ventricles fill to about 75% capacity during this phase and will be completely filled only after the atria enter into systole. The cardiac muscle cells of the ventricles repolarize during this phase to prepare for the next round of depolarization and contraction. During this phase, the AV valves open to allow blood to flow freely into the ventricles while the semilunar valves close to prevent the regurgitation of blood from the great arteries into the ventricles.

Blood Flow through the Heart (Fig. 1.58)

Deoxygenated blood returning from the body first enters the heart from the superior and inferior vena cava. The blood enters the right atrium and is pumped through the tricuspid valve into the right ventricle. From the right ventricle, the blood is pumped through the pulmonary semilunar valve into the pulmonary trunk.

The pulmonary trunk carries blood to the lungs where it releases carbon dioxide and absorbs oxygen. The blood in the lungs returns to the heart through the pulmonary veins. From the pulmonary veins, blood enters the heart again in the left atrium.

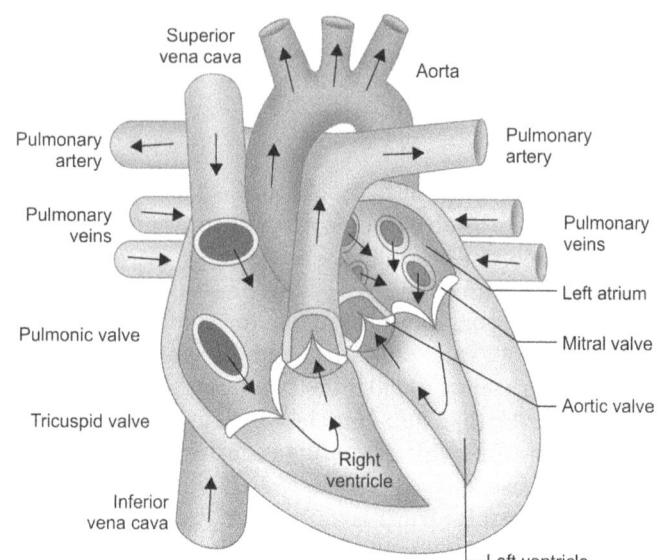

Fig. 1.58: Blood flow within heart.

The left atrium contracts to pump blood through the bicuspid (mitral) valve into the left ventricle. The left ventricle pumps blood through the aortic semilunar valve into the aorta. From the aorta, blood enters into systemic circulation throughout the body tissues until it returns to the heart via the vena cava and the cycle repeats.

Blood Vessels

Blood vessels are the body's highways that allow blood to flow quickly and efficiently from the heart to every region of the body and back again. The size of blood vessels corresponds with the amount of blood that passes through the vessel. All blood vessels contain a hollow area called the *lumen* through which blood is able to flow. Around the lumen is the wall of the vessel, which may be thin in the case of capillaries or very thick in the case of arteries.

All blood vessels are lined with a thin layer of simple squamous epithelium known as the *endothelium* that keeps blood cells inside of the blood vessels and prevents clots from forming. The endothelium lines the entire circulatory system, all the way to the interior of the heart, where it is called the *endocardium*.

There are three major types of blood vessels (Fig. 1.59): Arteries, capillaries and veins. Blood vessels are often named after either the region of the body through which they carry blood or for nearby structures.

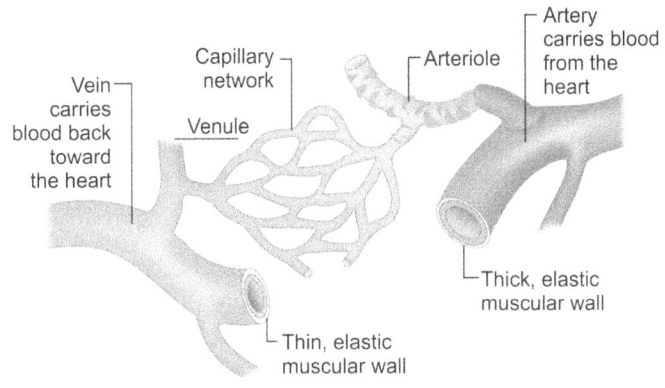

Fig. 1.59: Artery and vein.

For example, the brachiocephalic artery carries blood into the brachial (arm) and cephalic (head) regions. One of its branches, the subclavian artery, runs under the clavicle; hence, the name subclavian. The subclavian artery runs into the axillary region where it becomes known as the axillary artery.

Arteries and Arterioles

Arteries are blood vessels that carry blood away from the heart. Blood carried by arteries is usually highly oxygenated, having just left the lungs on its way to the body's tissues. The pulmonary trunk and arteries of the pulmonary circulation loop provide an exception to this rule—these arteries carry deoxygenated blood from the heart to the lungs to be oxygenated.

Arteries face high levels of blood pressure as they carry blood being pushed from the heart under the great force. To withstand this pressure, the walls of the arteries are thicker, more elastic, and more muscular than those of other vessels. The largest arteries of the body contain a high percentage of elastic tissue that allows them to stretch and accommodate the pressure of the heart.

Smaller arteries are more muscular in the structure of their walls. The smooth muscles of the arterial walls of these smaller arteries contract or expand to regulate the flow of blood through their lumen. In this way, the body controls how much blood flows to different parts of the body under varying circumstances. The regulation of blood flow also affects blood pressure, as smaller arteries give blood a less area to flow through and therefore increases the pressure of the blood on arterial walls.

Arterioles are narrower arteries that branch off from the ends of arteries and carry blood to capillaries. They face much lower blood pressures than arteries due to their greater number, decreased blood volume, and distance from the direct pressure of the heart. Thus, arteriole walls are much thinner than those of arteries. Arterioles, like arteries, are able to use smooth muscle to control their aperture and regulate blood a flow and blood pressure.

Capillaries

Capillaries are the smallest and thinnest of the blood vessels in the body and also the most common. They can be found running throughout almost every tissue of the body and border the edges of the body's avascular tissues. Capillaries connect to arterioles on one end and venules on the other.

Capillaries carry blood very close to the cells of the tissues of the body in order to exchange gases, nutrients, and waste products. The walls of capillaries consist of only a thin layer of endothelium so that there is the minimum amount of structure possible between the blood and the tissues. The endothelium acts as a filter to keep blood cells inside of the vessels while allowing liquids, dissolved gases, and other chemicals to diffuse along their concentration gradients into or out of tissues.

Precapillary sphincters are bands of smooth muscle found at the arteriole ends of capillaries. These sphincters regulate blood flow into the capillaries. Since, there is a limited supply of blood, and not all tissues have the same energy and oxygen requirements, the precapillary sphincters reduce blood flow to inactive tissues and allow free flow into active tissues.

Veins and Venules (Table 1.3)

Veins are the large return vessels of the body and act as the blood return counterparts of arteries. Because the arteries, arterioles, and capillaries absorb most of the force of the heart's contractions, veins and venules are subjected to very low blood pressures. This lack of pressure allows the walls of veins to be much thinner, less elastic, and less muscular than the walls of arteries.

Veins rely on gravity, inertia, and the force of skeletal muscle contractions to help push the blood back to the heart. To facilitate the movement of blood, some veins contain many one-way valves that prevent blood from flowing away from the heart. As skeletal muscles in the body contract, they squeeze nearby veins and push blood through valves closer to the heart.

Table 1.3: Comparison of arteries and veins.

	Arteries	Veins
Direction of blood flow	Conducts blood away from the heart	Conducts blood toward the heart
General appearance	Rounded	Irregular, often collapsed
Pressure	High	Low
Wall thickness	Thick	Thin
Relative oxygen concentration	• Higher in systemic arteries • Lower in pulmonary arteries	• Lower in systemic veins • Higher in pulmonary veins
Valves	Not present	Present most commonly in limbs and in veins inferior to the heart

When the muscle relaxes, the valve traps the blood until another contraction pushes the blood closer to the heart. *Venules* are similar to arterioles as they are small vessels that connect capillaries, but unlike arterioles, venules connect to veins instead of arteries. Venules pick up blood from many capillaries and deposit it into larger veins for transport back to the heart.

LYMPHATIC SYSTEM

Hodgkin lymphoma (HL) is a type of cancer that starts in the lymphatic system. The lymphatic system works with the circulatory system and the immune system. The complex group of cells and organs that defend the body against infection, disease and foreign substances. The body's natural defense against infection and disease. It is made up of spleen, thymus, tonsils, adenoids, bone marrow and a network of lymph nodes throughout the body that are connected by the lymph vessels **(Fig. 1.60)**. Lymphatic tissue (which stores infection-fighting cells) is also found in other parts of the body, including the stomach, intestines and skin.

❖ **Lymph:** It (lymph fluid) is a clear, yellowish fluid that carries white blood cells (WBCs). White blood cells—a type of blood cell that helps the body to fight with infection and diseases. (lymphocytes—a type of (WBCs) that fights with viruses, bacteria, foreign substances or abnormal cells (including cancer cells). Antibodies—a type of protein made by the immune system that disarms or destroys a specific foreign substance (antigen) when it appears in the body

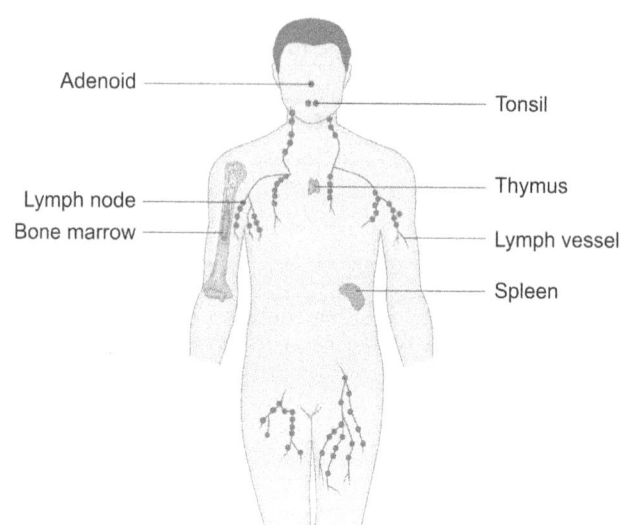

Fig. 1.60: Points showing presence of lymph.

and nutrients throughout the body. The lymph flows through the network of lymph nodes and vessels.

❖ **Lymphocytes:** Lymphocytes are a type of WBC that important to the immune system. There are two types:
1. B cells (B lymphocytes)—make antibodies to fight an infection
2. T cells (T lymphocytes)—regulate the immune system.

Lymphocytes start to develop in the bone marrow. The B and T cells mature in different places:
- B cells—bone marrow or lymphatic organs
- T cells—thymus.

❖ **Lymph vessels:** There are three main types of lymph vessels:
1. Lymphatic capillaries—microscopic, closed-ended tubes where fluid from body tissues enters the lymphatic system
2. Lymph vessels—tubes that move lymph to and from the lymph nodes
3. Collecting ducts—tubes that return lymph to the bloodstream

❖ **Lymph nodes:** Lymph nodes are small, bean-shaped organs that filter lymph. Lymph nodes vary in size but are usually less than 2.5 cm (1 inch) across. There are many lymph nodes throughout the body. The number of lymph nodes varies from one part of the body to another. Lymph nodes contain two types of WBCs that fight invading the microorganisms:
- Lymphocytes—attack viruses, bacteria and other microorganisms

- Macrophages—engulf and destroy foreign substances, damaged cells and bits of broken cells
- Lymph nodes are located in groups in the following major locations:
  - Neck—cervical nodes
  - Chest (thoracic) cavity—thoracic and mediastinal nodes
  - Armpit—axillary nodes
  - Abdominal cavity—para-aortic (peri-aortic) and mesenteric nodes
  - Groin—inguinal nodes
- The main functions of the lymph nodes are to:
  - Filter harmful particles, such as bacteria, viruses and foreign substances, from the lymph before returning it to the bloodstream
  - Activate the immune system.

If a large number of particles are filtered through a lymph node or group of nodes, they may swell and become tender to the touch. For example, a sore throat may cause the lymph nodes under the jaw and in the neck to swell.

❖ **Spleen:** The spleen is the largest lymphatic organ. It is located in the upper-left abdomen. The spleen:
- Makes, stores and removes lymphocytes
- Filters the blood
- Stores red blood cells (RBCs)
- Destroys old RBCs

❖ **Thymus:** The thymus is located in the chest behind the breastbone (sternum). It is where the T lymphocytes mature and multiply.

❖ **Tonsils:** The tonsils are two small masses of lymphatic tissue in the throat that contain lymphocytes.

❖ **Adenoids:** The adenoids are actually a single, small mass of lymphatic tissue in the back of the nose [nasopharynx— the upper part of the pharynx (throat) behind the nose and above the soft palate (the back, soft part of the roof of the mouth)] that contains lymphocytes. Although there is only one adenoid, it is often referred to as adenoids. The adenoid is also sometimes called the pharyngeal tonsil. The adenoids are present in infants and children, and start to shrink just before puberty. They are usually absent in adults.

❖ **Bone marrow:** It is soft, spongy tissue in the center of certain bones. It contains immature blood cells called stem cells. Stem cells develop into:
- Red blood cells—a type of blood cell that carries oxygen to and carbon dioxide from tissues in the body. RBCs contain

hemoglobin (a protein that carries oxygen and gives blood its red color) and are made in the bone marrow.
- Deliver oxygen to the body
- White blood cells (including lymphocytes)
- Protect the body from infection
- Platelets—a type of blood cell that helps blood to clot. Platelets are made in the bone marrow.
- Helps blood to clot.

Function

The main functions of the lymphatic system are to:
- Move excess fluid from tissues and return it to the bloodstream
- Help in defend the body against disease
- Provide an alternate route for transporting hormones, nutrients and waste products.

CHAPTER 2

Pathology, Pharmacology and Microbiology

Chapter Outline

- Acute and Chronic Inflammation and Healing of Wound
- Apoptosis and Necrosis
- Shock
- Disorders of Blood Coagulation System
- Disorders of Immune System of Body
- Disease Transmission and Prevention of Infection
- Sterilization and its methods
- Bacteria, Virus and Fungi
- Routes of Drug Administration
- Adverse Effects and Side Effects of Drugs
- Analgesics: Opioid and NSAIDs
- Drugs used in Cough and Expectorations
- Drugs used in Bronchial Asthma and COPD
- Drugs used in Gastrointestinal Tract
- Basic Idea of Antimicrobials
- Basic Idea of Antihistamine and Corticosteroids
- Drugs used in Treatment of Anemia
- Anesthetic Agents (LA and GA)
- Muscle Relaxant.

INFLAMMATION

- Inflammation is a defensive host response to foreign invaders and necrotic tissue.
- Can be acute or chronic.

Acute Inflammation

- Immediate and early response to tissue injury (physical, chemical, microbiologic, etc.).
- Acute inflammation has two major components:
  1. Vascular changes
  2. Cellular events

Vascular Change

The main vascular reactions of acute inflammation are increased blood flow followed by vasodilation and increased vascular permeability:
- Warmth and redness
- Opens microvascular beds and protein-rich fluid moves into extravascular tissues
- Migration of leukocytes (principally neutrophils)

Increased Vascular Permeability

- This will leads to the movement of protein-rich fluid and blood cells into the extravascular tissue. The resulting protein-rich accumulation is called an exudate.
- Increases interstitial osmotic pressure contributing to edema.

Vascular Leakage

Several mechanisms may contribute to increased vascular permeability:
- Endothelial cell contraction that leading to intracellular gaps of venules. This occur after binding of histamines and bradykinins, and many other mediators and is usually short-lived (15–30 min).
- Cytokine mediators (TNF, IL-1) induce endothelial cell junction retraction through cytoskeleton reorganization.
- This reaction may take 4–6 hours to develop, and lasting for 24 hours or more.
- Endothelial injuries result in vascular leakage by causing direct endothelial cell necrosis, detachment making them leaky until they are repaired or may cause delayed damage as in thermal, certain bacterial toxins or ultraviolet injury.
- Certain mediators such as vascular endothelial growth factor (VEGF) may cause increased transcytosis via. intracellular vesicles which travel from the luminal to basement membrane surface of the endothelial cell.
- All or any combination of these events may occur in response to a given stimulus.

Leukocyte Cellular Events

Leukocytes leave the vascular lumen to the extravascular space through the following sequence of events:
- Margination and rolling along the vessel wall
- Firm adhesion and transmigration between endothelial cells
- Chemotaxis and activation

Margination and Rolling

- With increased vascular permeability, fluid leaves the vessel causing leukocytes to settle-out of the central flow column and "marginate" along the endothelial surface.
- Endothelial cells and leukocytes have complementary surface adhesion molecules which briefly stick and release causing the leukocyte to roll along the endothelium until it eventually comes to a stop as mutual adhesion reaches a peak.
- Early rolling adhesion mediated by selectin family of adhesion molecules:
  - E-selectin (on endothelium cell)
  - P-selectin (present on platelets, endothelium)
  - L-selectin (on the surface of most leukocytes)

Adhesion

- The rolling leukocytes are able to sense change on the endothelium that initiate the next step in the reaction of leukocytes, which is firm adhesion to endothelial surface.
- Occur as leukocytes adhere to the endothelial surface and is mediated by the interaction of integrins on leukocytes binding to IG-family adhesion proteins on the endothelium.

Transmigration (Diapedesis)

- Is the movement of leukocyte across the endothelial surface.
- Occurs after firm adhesion and mediated by platelet endothelial cell adhesion molecules-1 (PECAM-1) on both leukocyte and endothelium).

Chemotaxis

- Leukocytes follow chemical gradient to site of injury this process called (chemotaxis).
- Chemotactic factors for neutrophils, produced at the site of injury, include:
  - Bacterial products
  - Components of complement system especially (C5a)
  - Cytokines

Phagocytosis

- Phagocytosis is the ingestion of particulate material by phagocytic cell.
- Neutrophils and monocytes-macrophages are the most important phagocytic cells

- Phagocytosis consists of three steps:
  1. Recognition and attachment of the particle
  2. Engulfment (form phagocytic vacuole)
  3. Killing and degradation of the ingested materials.

Defects of Leukocyte Function

Defects of leukocyte adhesion:
- **Leukocyte adhesion deficiency type I:** Is associated with recurrent bacterial infections.
- **Leukocyte adhesion deficiency type 2:** Is associated with recurrent bacterial infections and result from mutations in the gene that required for the synthesis of Sialyl Lewis X on neutrophils.
- **Defects of chemotaxis/phagocytosis:** Microtubule assembly defect leads to impaired locomotion and lysosomal degranulation (Chediak-Higashi Syndrome).

Possible Outcomes of Acute Inflammation
- **Complete resolution of tissue structure and function:**
  - When the injury is limited or short-lived.
  - There has been no or little tissue damage
  - When the injured tissue is capable of regeneration
- **Scarring (fibrosis):**
  - When inflammation occur in tissues that do not regenerate
  - The injured tissue is filled with connective tissue
- Abscess formation occurs with some bacterial or fungal infections.
- Progression to chronic inflammation.

Chronic Inflammation

- Is inflammation of prolonged duration (week to years) in which continuing inflammation, tissue injury, and healing, often by fibrosis, proceed simultaneously.
- Is characterized by a different set of reactions:
  - Lymphocyte, macrophage, plasma cell (mononuclear cell) infiltration
  - Tissue destruction by inflammatory cells
  - Repair with fibrosis and angiogenesis (new vessel formation)
- Chronic inflammation may arise in the following setting:
  - Persistent injury or infection (ulcer, TB)
  - Prolonged toxic agent exposure (silica)
  - Autoimmune disease states (RA, SLE)

Chronic Inflammatory Cells and Mediators
Macrophages
- The dominant cells.
- Scattered all over (Kupffer cells, sinus histiocytes, alveolar macrophages, etc.)
- Derived from circulating blood monocytes and reach site of injury within 24-48 hours and transform to macrophages. Two major pathways of macrophage activation:
  1. *Classical macrophage activation:* Induced by T cell-derived cytokines, endotoxins, and other products of inflammation.
  2. *Alternative macrophage activation:* Induced by cytokines produced by T lymphocytes and other cell including mast cell and eosinophils.
- Macrophages have several roles in host defense and inflammatory reaction:
  - Ingest and eliminate microbes and dead tissue.
  - Initiate the process of tissue repair.
  - Secrete mediators of inflammation such as cytokines.

Lymphocytes (T-B)
Antigen-activated (via. macrophages and dendritic cells)
Lymphocytes and macrophages interact in a bidirectional way and these interaction play an important role in propagating chronic inflammation. Lymphocyte release macrophage-activating cytokines (in turn, macrophages release lymphocyte-activating cytokines until inflammatory stimulus is removed).

Eosinophils
- Found especially at sites of parasitic infections, and as part of immune reaction mediated by IgE
- Typically associated with allergies.

Granulomatous Inflammation
- Is a distinctive pattern of chronic inflammation characterized by aggregates of activated macrophages and scattered lymphocytes.
- Granulomatous inflammation can form under three setting:
  1. Persistence T-cell response to certain microbes (such as TB)
  2. In some immune-mediated inflammatory diseases (Crohn disease)
  3. In sarcoidosis disease in response to relatively inert foreign bodies (suture or splinter)

Systemic Effects

- **Fever:** The most prominent manifestation of acute-phase response.
- Fever is produced in response to pyrogens which stimulate prostaglandin synthesis.
- PGE stimulate the production of neurotransmitters to reset the temperature at a higher level.
- Leukocytosis is a common feature of inflammatory reaction, especially those induced by bacterial infection. Elevated white blood cell count.
- Other manifestations include:
  - Increased heart rate and blood pressure.
  - Decreased sweating.
  - Sepsis in severe bacterial infection.

HEALING

Healing is the process of the restoration of health to an unbalanced, diseased or damaged organism. With physical damage or disease suffered by an organism, healing involves the repair of living tissue, marks and the biological system as a whole and resumption of normal functioning. It is the process by which the cells in the body regenerate and repair to reduce the size of a damaged or necrotic area and replace it with new living tissue. The replacement can happen in two ways: (1) By regeneration in which the necrotic cells are replaced by new cells that form similar tissue as was originally there; or (2) by repair in which injured tissue is replaced with scar tissue. Most organs will heal using a mixture of both mechanisms.

Wound Healing

In response to an incision or wound, a wound healing cascade is unleashed. This cascade takes place in four phases: Clot formation, inflammation, proliferation, and maturation.

Clotting Phase

Healing of a wound begins with clot formation to stop bleeding and to reduce infection by bacteria, viruses and fungi. Clotting is followed by neutrophil invasion 3-24 hours after the wound has been incurred, with mitoses beginning in epithelial cells after 24-48 hours.

Inflammation Phase

In the inflammatory phase, macrophages and other phagocytic cells kill bacteria, debride damaged tissue and release chemical factors such as growth hormones that encourage fibroblasts, epithelial cells and endothelial cells which make new capillaries to migrate to the area and divide.

Proliferative Phase

In the proliferative phase, immature granulation tissue containing plump active fibroblasts forms. Fibroblasts quickly produce abundant type III collagen, which fills the defect left by an open wound. Granulation tissue moves, as a wave, from the border of the injury towards the center.

As granulation tissue matures, the fibroblasts produce less collagen and become more spindly in appearance. They begin to produce the much stronger type I collagen. Some of the fibroblasts mature into myofibroblasts which contain the same type of action found in smooth muscle, which enables them to contract and reduce the size of the wound.

Maturation Phase

During the maturation phase of wound healing, unnecessary vessels formed in granulation tissue are removed by apoptosis, and type III collagen is largely replaced by type I. Collagen which was originally disorganized is cross-linked and aligned along tension lines. This phase can last a year or longer. Ultimately a scar made of collagen, containing a small number of fibroblasts is left **(Fig. 2.1)**.

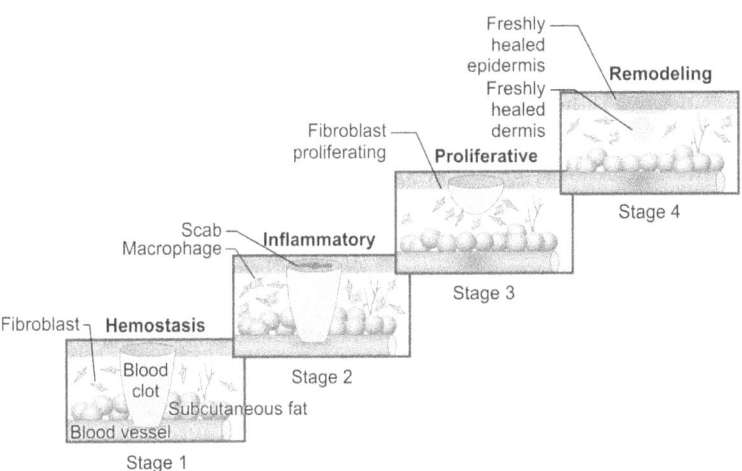

Fig. 2.1: Wound healing process.

Healing of Tissue Damaged by Inflammation

After inflammation has damaged tissue (when combating bacterial infection for example) and proinflammatory eicosanoids have completed their function, healing proceeds in four phases.

1. **Recall phase:** In the recall phase the adrenal glands increase production of cortisol which shuts down eicosanoid production and inflammation.
2. **Resolution phase:** In the resolution phase, pathogens and damaged tissue are removed by macrophages (white blood cells). Red blood cells are also removed from the damaged tissue by macrophages. Failure to remove all of the damaged cells and pathogens may retrigger inflammation. The two subsets of macrophage M1 and M2 plays a crucial role in this phase, M1 macrophage being a proinflammatory while as M2 is a regenerative and the plasticity between the two subsets determines the tissue inflammation or repair.
3. **Regeneration phase:** In the regeneration phase, blood vessels are repaired and new cells form in the damaged site similar to the cells that were damaged and removed. Some cells such as neurons and muscle cells (especially in the heart) are slow to recover.
4. **Repair phase:** In the repair phase, new tissue is generated which requires a balance of anti-inflammatory and proinflammatory eicosanoids. Anti-inflammatory eicosanoids include lipoxins, epilipoxins, and resolvins, which cause release of growth hormones.

Steps of the Wound Healing Process

1. **Rapid hemostasis:** This refers to the mechanism that stops the actual bleeding. Most of the time, your body will accomplish this through a process called vasoconstriction, in which your blood vessels are closed tight. It similar to how you might turn a level as to stop a leaky faucet **(Fig. 2.2)**.
2. **Inflammation:** Inflammation is your body's way of alerting you of an injury. Beyond that, it helps dictate where the next barrage of healthy cells should be headed. As such, inflammation is vital in the wound care process, but if it goes on for too long, it can actually prevent regeneration.
3. **Proliferation and migration:** When inflammation occurs, the body releases several kinds of cells, including those that are responsible for migration and proliferation. The former function actually refers to the movement of the cells, a carefully coordinated process that involves cells moving in a specific order. Meanwhile, proliferation is similar to hemostasis, as cells work to further constrict your blood vessels.

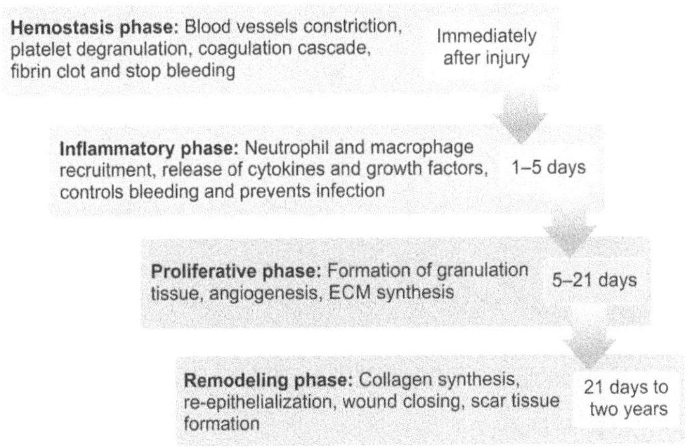

| Hemostasis phase: Blood vessels constriction, platelet degranulation, coagulation cascade, fibrin clot and stop bleeding | Immediately after injury |

| Inflammatory phase: Neutrophil and macrophage recruitment, release of cytokines and growth factors, controls bleeding and prevents infection | 1–5 days |

| Proliferative phase: Formation of granulation tissue, angiogenesis, ECM synthesis | 5–21 days |

| Remodeling phase: Collagen synthesis, re-epithelialization, wound closing, scar tissue formation | 21 days to two years |

Fig. 2.2: Stages of healing process.

4. **Angiogenesis:** Once the bleeding is under control, the body then begins the process of rebuilding tissue. Angiogenesis, as it is called, involves the formation of new blood vessels. This process occurs when your body's cells begin to replace the veins and arteries that were damaged, either creating new sections or adding onto existing portions. It is a decidedly complex endeavor, with many chemicals activating to facilitate these all-new veins.
5. **Re-epithelialization:** Once your body has begun to regrow veins, its time to begin regrowing damaged skin. Your epidermis is comprised of cells called keratinocytes, and during the re-epithelialization process, your body has to begin forging these chemical components. The process involves the creation of several layers, each working in tandem to offer protection and prevent fluid loss.
6. **Synthesis:** Though it is seen as the last step, synthesis often happens almost simultaneously. In this process, certain proteins form blood clots, which helps further prevent bleeding as new skin and veins are formed. There are a number of proteins at play, and certain people lack those necessary proteins to form blood clots.

APOPTOSIS (FIG. 2.3)

Apoptosis is the process of programmed cell death. It is used during early development to eliminate unwanted cells; for example, those between the fingers of a developing hand. In adults, apoptosis is used to rid the body of cells that have been damaged beyond repair. Apoptosis also plays a role in preventing cancer. If apoptosis is for

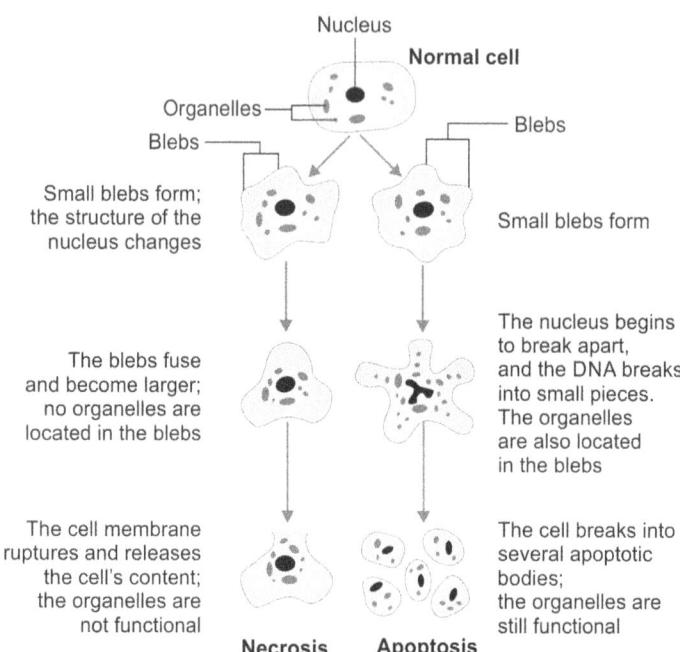

Fig. 2.3: Necrosis and apoptosis.

some reason prevented, it can lead to uncontrolled cell division and the subsequent development of a tumor.

NECROSIS

Necrosis is the death of body tissue. It occurs when too little blood flows to the tissue. This can be from injury, radiation, or chemicals. Necrosis cannot be reversed.

When large areas of tissue die due to a lack of blood supply, the condition is called gangrene.

Patterns of Necrosis

When body's cells die of necrosis, they form different patterns and appearances. The dead cells appear in one of six ways. These patterns include:

Coagulative Necrosis

With coagulative necrosis, the dead cells remain firm and look normal for days after death. Lack of blood flow or oxygen to any part of your body except your brain can cause coagulative necrosis.

Liquefactive Necrosis

With liquefactive necrosis, the dead cells partially or completely dissolve within hours of death. Then they transform into a thick, sticky liquid. The cells sometimes appear creamy yellow because pus is forming. Infections and lack of oxygen to your brain can cause liquefactive necrosis.

Fat Necrosis

With fat necrosis, damaged cells release enzymes, causing them to turn to liquid. The liquid cells combine with calcium, creating chalky, white deposits on the cells. Acute pancreatitis is the most common cause of fat necrosis. It can also occur in breast tissue.

Caseous Necrosis

With caseous necrosis, the dead cells look white and soft. They've been described as looking like cheese—the word caseous means "cheese-like." Caseous necrosis is uniquely seen in the infectious lung disease tuberculosis.

Fibrinoid Necrosis

With fibrinoid necrosis, the dead cells appear pink and lack structure. This is because plasma proteins (fibrins) are leaking out of your blood vessel walls. Fibrinoid necrosis occurs when an autoimmune disease or infection damage your blood vessels.

Gangrenous Necrosis

With gangrenous necrosis, your skin appears black and is beginning to rot. Lack of blood flow to your legs can cause gangrenous necrosis. It can sometimes affect your arms and fingers too.

Types of Necrosis

Necrosis can affect many different areas of your body, including your bones, skin and organs. The different types of necrosis include:

Avascular Necrosis (Osteonecrosis)

Avascular necrosis goes by many names. Osteonecrosis, aseptic necrosis and bone necrosis are all other terms for avascular necrosis. Avascular necrosis occurs when blood flow to your bone tissue is blocked. Lack of blood flow to your bones causes them to break down and eventually die. Hip necrosis is the most common form of avascular necrosis.

Osteonecrosis of the Jaw

Osteonecrosis of the jaw (ONJ) is a type of avascular necrosis. ONJ is a mouth (oral) disorder that occurs when cells in your jaw bone die. Osteonecrosis of the jaw can cause severe mouth and jaw pain. In addition, pus may ooze from your mouth and jaw.

Pancreatic Necrosis

Pancreatic necrosis is a serious complication that can develop due to acute pancreatitis. When the blood supply to your pancreas is cut off, it can cause your pancreatic tissue to die. When this happens, your pancreas can become infected. The infection can spread into your blood (sepsis) and cause organ failure.

Fat Necrosis of the Breast

Fat necrosis of the breast is a noncancerous (benign) condition that can occur when fatty breast tissue is damaged. Your body usually replaces damaged breast tissue with scar tissue. With fat necrosis, some fat cells die instead of forming scar tissue. This forms a pocket of greasy fluid called an oil cyst.

Acute Tubular Necrosis

Acute tubular necrosis (ATN) or tubular necrosis is a kidney disorder. When the tubule cells of your kidneys are damaged, it can lead to acute kidney failure. The tubules are the tiny ducts in your kidneys that help filter your blood when it passes through your kidneys.

Radiation Necrosis

Radiation necrosis is a rare side effect of high-dose radiation to your brain, head or neck. It can result in the permanent death of brain tissue.

Renal Papillary Necrosis

Renal papillary necrosis is a kidney disorder that occurs when the renal papillae of your kidneys die. The renal papillae are the openings of the tubes (ducts) that enter your kidneys and pass pee (urine) into your bladder.

Skin Necrosis

Skin necrosis (gangrene) occurs when blood flow to your body tissues or internal organs is blocked. It can also occur due to a bacterial infection. It most commonly affects your fingers, toes, hands and feet but can affect any part of your body.

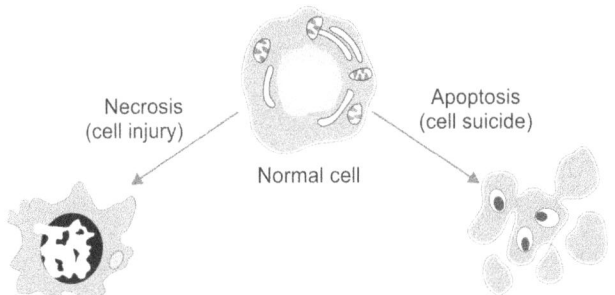

Fig. 2.4: Difference between necrosis and apoptosis.

Spider Bite Necrosis

Spider bite necrosis can occur when a recluse spider bites you. The venom from a recluse spider bite can cause a skin-decaying wound. However, necrosis from a spider bite is rare.

Pulp Necrosis

Pulp necrosis happens when the soft flesh (pulp) inside your tooth dies. Inside each of your teeth is a chamber that holds small pieces of flesh. Inside each chamber are blood vessels and nerves. If a tooth is injured or decayed, the flesh can get infected and die.

Difference Between Apoptosis and Necrosis

Apoptosis and necrosis are both ways cells die. Apoptosis is the normal, healthy way cells die. They die naturally to maintain cellular balance in your body. Apoptosis is needed for your body to function normally. Apoptosis very rarely needs treatment **(Fig. 2.4)**.

Cells die through necrosis accidentally due to internal or external factors. These factors may include diseases, infections, injuries or other conditions. These conditions lead to damage in your cell walls, which makes them unable to function normally. Necrosis generally needs treatment.

SHOCK

Definition

Shock is defined as inadequate tissue perfusion, perfusion can be caused by various disorder that result in decreased oxygenation at the cellular level.

Cause

Shock is commonly discussed under three major categories:
1. Hypovolemic shock
2. Distributive shock
3. Cardiogenic shock

Hypovolemic Shock

It is a shock that occurs due to fluid loss from body.

Causes

- **Hemorrhage:** Which lead to the loss of blood if 500-1500 mL of circulatory blood gets lost, it leads shock.
- **Burns:** Hypovolemic shock due to burns occurs most of clients with large partial thickness of full thickness burns.
- **Dehydration:** If there is excessive fluid loss occurs through sweating, vomiting or less intake of oral fluids.

Signs and Symptoms

- Decreased tissue perfusion.
- Cold clammy skin.
- Cyanosis may be there.
- Pallor.

First aid

- Lie down the patient on the floor.
- Give psychological support to the patient and family.
- Check the skin turgor of the patient by pinching and see whether the skin goes back to its original position within 1 second or not.
- Loosen the clothes of the patient.
- If there is excessive sweating to the patient than ventilate the room and switch on the fans.
- If patient is conscious and if he can tolerate then give oral fluid to the patient.
- Down the head of the patient and raise his legs end side so that to increase circulation towards heart.
- If there is any bleeding through the wound area then press it, wrap any pressure bandage or any cloths, to stop bleeding.
- Shift the patient to the hospital as soon as possible.
- Arrange the blood for the patent if needed.
- In hospital start in fluid to regenerate fluid volume.

Distributive Shock

It is also called vasogenic shock result from inadequate vascular toro. With this shock, blood volume remains same. The size of vessels increases due to disproportion of the blood availability and size of capillary space.

Causes

- **Anaphylactic shock:** Distributive shock induced by vasoactive substances released during an allergic reactions is called anaphylactic shock. It is due to:
  - Pollen
  - Particular food
  - Wasp sting
  - Bee sting
- **Septic shock:** Shock resulting from massive septic and the release of toxic or vasoactive substance leads to septic or toxic shock.
- **Neurogenic shock:** Shock occurs as the result of loss of innervations to the vessels as from spinal card injury or spinal anesthesia.

Signs and Symptoms

- Headache
- Anxiety
- Dizziness
- Disorientation
- Loss of consciousness
- Lump in the throat
- Laryngeal edema
- Hoarseness
- Dyspnea
- Itching of body
- Subnormal temperature
- Vomiting
- Rapid pulse
- Swelling of face and neck
- Diarrhea

First Aid

- Place person in a head down or recumbent position.
- Reassure the patient and family.
- Clean the mouth of patient with clean cloth.
- Check the respiration of the patient.

- If it is not normal or if needed then do mouth to mouth respiration.
- Maintain the temperature of the patient by regulating the temperature of the room.
- Keep the patient to reduce the wastage of energy caused by shivering and by sweating.
- Shift the patient to the hospital as soon as possible so that the shock can be prevented and patient can be improved.

Cardiogenic Shock

Client with hypovolemic shock may develop the cardiogenic shock. This happen because the rapid pulse initiated to compensate for decrease volume and to increase the cardiac output does not allow time for the coronary at arteries to fill with blood because these arteries supply blood to the myocardium, myocardial oxygen supply impaired also the increased heart rate, increase the myocardium need for oxygen. Decreased coronary artery perfusion and inadequate oxygenation of the myocardium finally shock **(Fig. 2.5)**.

Causes

The causes of cardiogenic shock are:
- Myocardial infarction.
- Valvular insufficiency and cardiac dysrhythmias.
- Obstructive conditions, e.g., pulmonary embolism.

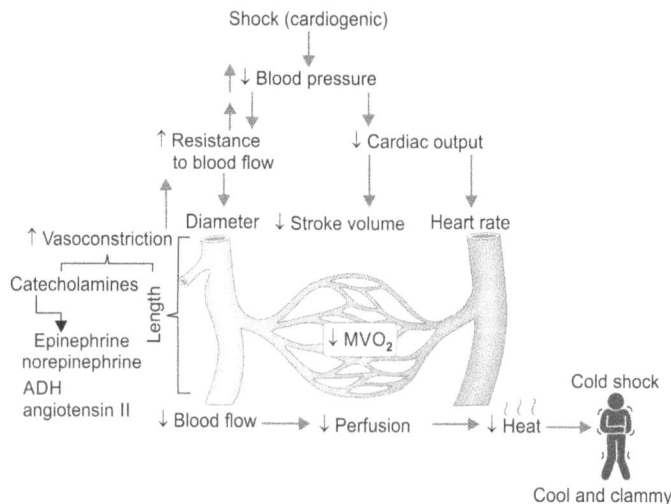

Fig. 2.5: Cardiogenic shock.

Signs and Symptoms

- Low blood pressure
- Dilated pupils
- Thirsty, dry mucus membrane
- Cyanosis may be present
- Thready pulse, slow capillary refills
- Restless, anxiety
- Cold clonary skin
- Decrease level of consciousness
- Anuria
- Pallor skin
- Irritability
- Flat neck veins
- Weakness

First Aid

- Observe the patient closely for signs and symptoms of shock.
- Give position to the patient, including elevating the legs, leaving the trunk flat and elevating the head and shoulders slightly.
- Check the respiration of the patient. Ventilate the room by opening door and windows.
- Clean the mouth of the patient, if there is any secretion in the mouth.
- Tilt the head towards outside so that the patient does not aspirate the secretions.
- To maintain the normal respiratory rate 24/min if needed. To mouth to mouth respiration in emergency.
- If there is any bleeding, i.e., cardiac shock due to bleeding then press the bleeding area so that to resolve the blood volume.
- Do cardiopulmonary resuscitation (CPR) to the patient so that the patient gains his cardiac function.
- Shift the patient to the hospital as soon as possible.

DISORDERS OF BLOOD COAGULATION SYSTEM

Introduction

The coagulation system is made up of blood cells and proteins and is responsible for creating blood clots, which are an important part of the body's healing process. When this system does not work properly, it can cause blood clots to form at inappropriate times, blocking the flow of blood to vital parts of the body **(Fig. 2.6)**.

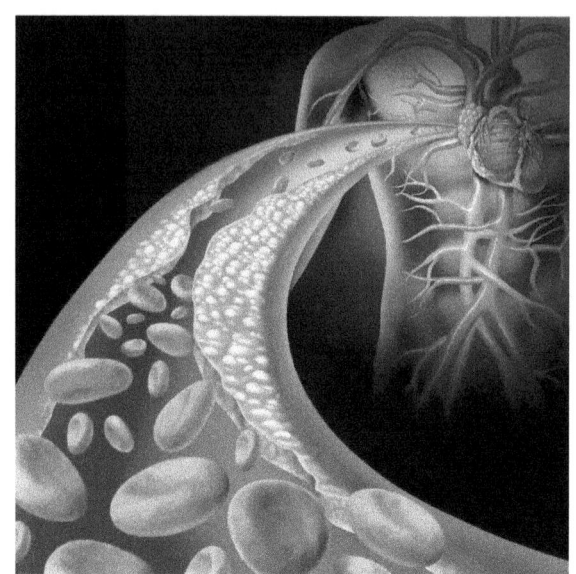
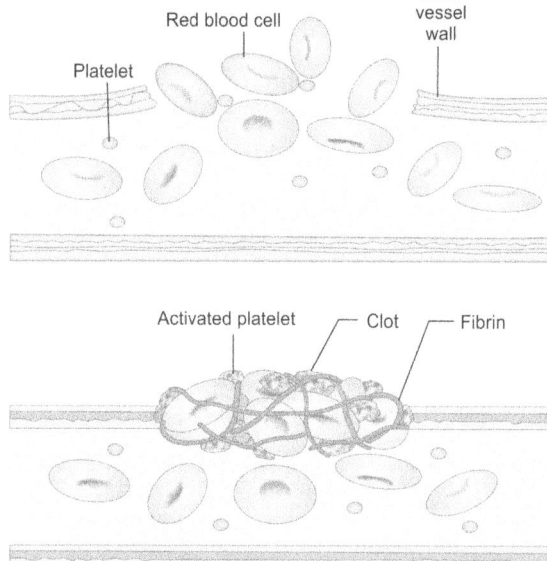

Fig. 2.6: Coagulation of blood.

Coagulation disorders refer to conditions that affect how the body controls blood clotting. If a person's blood does not clot, or coagulate, normally, they may experience complications from bleeding too much after injury or surgery or having blockages that prevent blood flow.

Coagulation disorders cause the body to form too many or too few blood clots. They are usually due to a genetic mutation and are often treatable with medications. Coagulation disorders can cause excessive bleeding if the body is unable to form blood clots properly. In other cases, they may cause the body to produce blood clots too readily and increase the risk of blocked blood vessels.

Definition

Coagulation disorders are when the body has issues controlling blood clots. Coagulation refers to the process of forming blood clots—our bodies rely on this vital process to help prevent excessive bleeding from an injured blood vessel.

Common Coagulation Disorders

Hemophilia

A genetic disorder that passes through families. It causes excessive bleeding, swelling, and bruising. The most common types are hemophilia A and B, where the body lacks certain proteins in the blood for clotting.

Von Willebrand's Disease

Another genetic disorder that prevents clotting due to insufficient von Willebrand factor, a blood-clotting protein. Females are more likely to notice the condition than males due to heavy or bleeding that characterizes the condition during menstrual periods or birth.

Liver Disease-associated Bleeding

People with liver disease can experience scarring that increases the risk of bleeding disorders or thrombosis.

Vitamin K Deficiency Bleeding

The body requires vitamin K to form blood clots. Babies born with low vitamin K levels who do receive supplements may develop vitamin K deficiencies, which can lead to excessive internal or external bleeding.

Causes and Risk Factors

Some risk factors for coagulation disorders can include—age, such as newborns for vitamin K deficiency or older adults in hemophilia A:
- A family history of the condition
- Being male
- Other medical conditions, such as cancer, autoimmune diseases, or liver disease
- Blood transfusions
- Obesity
- Infections
- Medications, such as antibiotics, blood thinners, or interferon alfa
- Surgery
- Hormone-based medications, such as birth control pills
- Pregnancy and giving birth
- Physical inactivity and sitting for long periods
- Medical devices that increase blood flow.

Symptoms

People with bleeding disorders can experience symptoms that include:
- Excessive bleeding that does not stop with pressure
- Easy bruising
- Blood in urine or stool
- Heavy bleeding during menstruation or after childbirth
- Bleeding under the skin
- Redness and swelling around the body
- Umbilical stump bleeding in newborns

Diagnosis

- A D-dimer test, which tests for venous thromboembolism
- A partial thromboplastin or prothrombin time test, which measure how long it takes for a blood clot to form
- Clotting factor tests to identify any missing clotting factors
- A complete blood count (CBC), which measures the amount of red and white blood cells in your body
- A platelet aggregation test, which checks how well your platelets clump together
- A bleeding time test, which determines how quickly your blood clots to prevent bleeding
- Von Willebrand factor tests
- Genetic testing to identify genes that can cause coagulation disorders

- Medical scans, such as ultrasounds or CT scans, to check for blood clots

Treatment

The best treatment approach will depend on the type of coagulation disorder, its severity, and the person's overall health. Treatments typically aim to manage symptoms and reduce the risk of complications. Doctors might recommend one or more medications, including:
- Antifibrinolytic drugs to treat bleeding after childbirth or surgeries
- Birth control pills to reduce menstrual bleeding
- Desmopressin
- Immunosuppressive medicines
- Vitamin K supplements
- Blood thinners to reduce the risk trusted source of clotting in people with hypercoagulable states
- Thrombin inhibitors or thrombolytics
- Doctors may also recommend other treatments, such as factor replacement therapy. This involves replacing missing clotting factors using blood donations or replacements from a laboratory.
- Treatment options vary depending on the type of bleeding disorder and its severity. Though treatments can't cure bleeding disorders, they can help relieve the symptoms associated with certain disorders.

Iron Supplementation

Doctor may prescribe iron supplements to replenish the amount of iron in your body if you have significant blood loss. A low iron level can result in iron deficiency anemia. This condition can make you feel weak, tired, and dizzy. You may need a blood transfusion if symptoms do not improve with iron supplementation.

Blood Transfusion

A blood transfusion replaces any lost blood with blood taken from a donor. The donor blood has to match your blood type to prevent complications. This procedure can only be done in the hospital.

Other Treatments

Some bleeding disorders may be treated with topical products or nasal sprays. Other disorders, including hemophilia, can be treated with factor replacement therapy. This involves injecting clotting factor concentrates into your bloodstream. These injections can prevent or control excessive bleeding.

■ DISORDERS OF IMMUNE SYSTEM OF BODY

Introduction

Immune system is a complex network of cells, tissues, and organs. Together they help the body fight infections and other diseases.

When germs such as bacteria or viruses invade your body, they attack and multiply. This is called an infection. The infection causes the disease that makes you sick. Your immune system protects you from the disease by fighting off the germs.

Types of Immunity

There are three different types of immunity **(Fig. 2.7)**:
1. **Innate immunity**, is the protection that you are born with. It is your body's first line of defense. It includes barriers such as the skin and mucous membranes. They keep harmful substances from entering the body. It also includes some cells and chemicals which can attack foreign substances.
2. **Active immunity**, also called adaptive immunity, develops when you are infected with or vaccinated against a foreign substance. Active immunity is usually long-lasting. For many diseases, it can last your entire life.

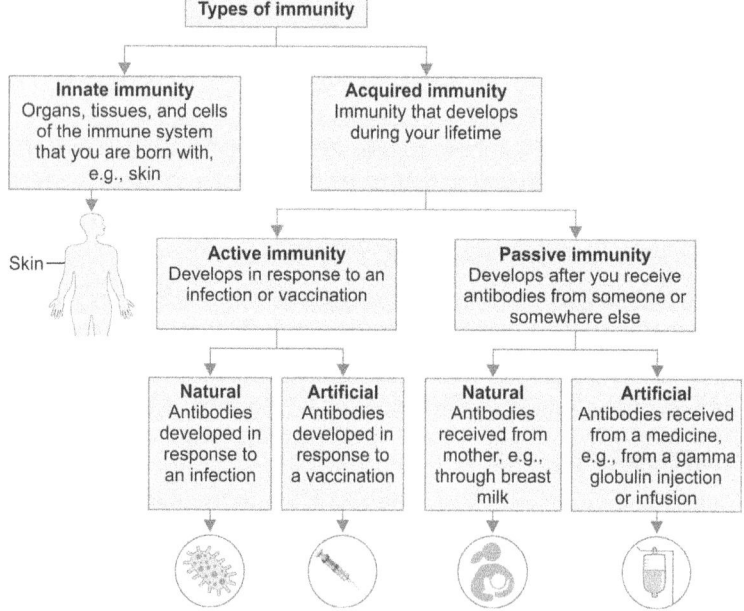

Fig. 2.7: Types of immunity.

3. **Passive immunity,** happens when you receive antibodies to a disease instead of making them through your own immune system. For example, newborn babies have antibodies from their mothers. People can also get passive immunity through blood products that contain antibodies. This kind of immunity gives you protection right away. But it only lasts a few weeks or months.

Parts of the Immune System (Fig. 2.8)

The main parts of the immune system are:
- White blood cells
- Antibodies
- Complement system
- Lymphatic system
- Spleen
- Bone marrow
- Thymus

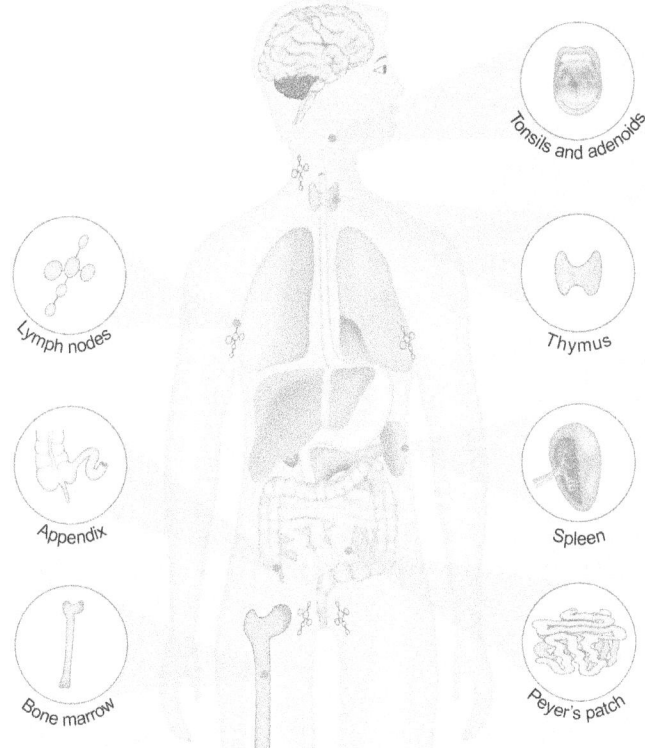

Fig. 2.8: Parts of immune system.

White Blood Cells

White blood cells are the key players in your immune system. They are made in your bone marrow and are part of the lymphatic system.

White blood cells move through blood and tissue throughout your body, looking for foreign invaders (microbes) such as bacteria, viruses, parasites and fungi. When they find them, they launch an immune attack.

White blood cells include lymphocytes (such as B-cells, T-cells and natural killer cells), and many other types of immune cells.

Antibodies

Antibodies help the body to fight microbes or the toxins (poisons) they produce. They do this by recognizing substances called antigens on the surface of the microbe, or in the chemicals they produce, which mark the microbe or toxin as being foreign. The antibodies then mark these antigens for destruction. There are many cells, proteins and chemicals involved in this attack.

Complement System

The complement system is made up of proteins whose actions complement the work done by antibodies.

Lymphatic System (Fig. 2.9)

The lymphatic system is a network of delicate tubes throughout the body. The main roles of the lymphatic system are to:
- Manage the fluid levels in the body
- React to bacteria
- Deal with cancer cells
- Deal with cell products that otherwise would result in disease or disorders
- Absorb some of the fats in our diet from the intestine.

The lymphatic system is made up of:
- **Lymph nodes (also called lymph glands)**—which trap microbes
- **Lymph vessels**—tubes that carry lymph, the colorless fluid that bathes your body's tissues and contains infection-fighting white blood cells.
- **White blood cells** (lymphocytes).

Spleen

The spleen is a blood-filtering organ that removes microbes and destroys old or damaged red blood cells. It also makes disease-

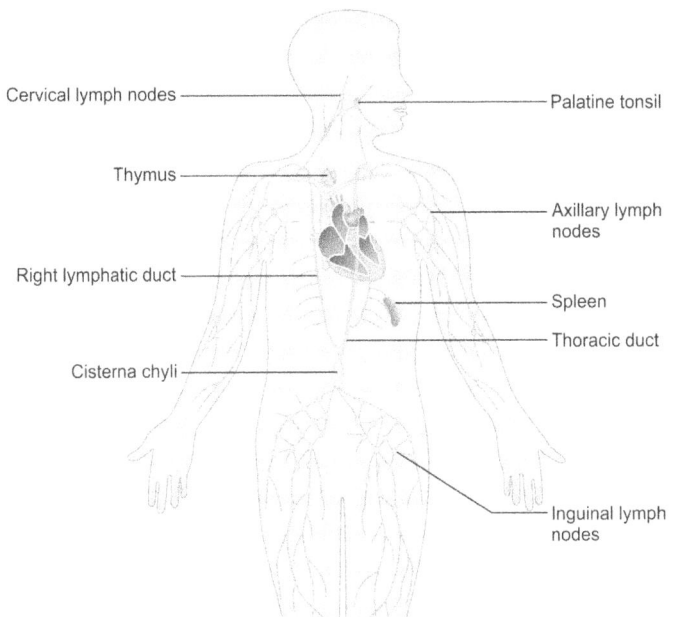

Fig. 2.9: Lymphatic system.

fighting components of the immune system (including antibodies and lymphocytes).

Bone Marrow

Bone marrow is the spongy tissue found inside your bones. It produces the red blood cells our bodies need to carry oxygen, the white blood cells we use to fight infection, and the platelets we need to help our blood clot.

Thymus

The thymus filters and monitors your blood content. It produces the white blood cells called T-lymphocytes.

The body's other defenses against microbes:

As well as the immune system, the body has several other ways to defend itself against microbes, including:

- **Skin**—a waterproof barrier that secretes oil with bacteria-killing properties.
- **Lungs**—mucous in the lungs (phlegm) traps foreign particles, and small hairs (cilia) wave the mucous upwards so it can be coughed out.

- **Digestive tract**—the mucous lining contains antibodies, and the acid in the stomach can kill most microbes.
- **Other defenses**—body fluids like skin oil, saliva and tears contain antibacterial enzymes that help reduce the risk of infection. The constant flushing of the urinary tract and the bowel also helps.

Fever is an immune system response: A rise in body temperature, or fever, can happen with some infections. This is actually an immune system response. A rise in temperature can kill some microbes. Fever also triggers the body's repair process.

IMMUNE DISORDERS

Definition

A condition that affects the immune system. The immune system is made up of cells, tissues, and organs that help the body fight infections and other diseases. There are many different types of immune system disorders, including immunodeficiency disease, autoimmune disorders, and allergic disorders.

Common Disorders of the Immune System

It is common for people to have an over- or underactive immune system. Overactivity of the immune system can take many forms, including:

- **Allergic diseases**—where the immune system makes an overly strong response to allergens. Allergic diseases are very common. They include allergies to foods, medications or stinging insects, anaphylaxis (life-threatening allergy), hay fever (allergic rhinitis), sinus disease, asthma, hives (urticaria), dermatitis and eczema.
- **Autoimmune diseases**—where the immune system mounts a response against normal components of the body. Autoimmune diseases range from common to rare. They include multiple sclerosis, autoimmune thyroid disease, type 1 diabetes, systemic lupus erythematosus, rheumatoid arthritis and systemic vasculitis.

Underactivity of the immune system, also called immunodeficiency, can:

- Be inherited—examples of these conditions include primary immunodeficiency diseases such as common variable immunodeficiency (CVID), X-linked severe combined immunodeficiency (SCID) and complement deficiencies.
- Arise as a result of medical treatment—this can occur due to medications such as corticosteroids or chemotherapy.
- Be caused by another disease, such as HIV/AIDS or certain types of cancer.

- Severe combined immunodeficiency: This is an example of an immune deficiency that is present at birth. Children are in constant danger of infections from bacteria, viruses, and fungi. This disorder is sometimes called "bubble boy disease." In the 1970s, a boy had to live in a sterile environment inside a plastic bubble. Children with SCID are missing important white blood cells.

Temporary acquired immune deficiencies. Your immune system can be weakened by certain medicines, for example. This can happen to people on chemotherapy or other drugs used to treat cancer. It can also happen to people following organ transplants who take medicine to prevent organ rejection. Also, infections like the flu virus, mono (mononucleosis), and measles can weaken the immune system for a brief time. Your immune system can also be weakened by smoking, alcohol, and poor nutrition.

AIDS

HIV, which causes AIDS, is an acquired viral infection that destroys important white blood cells and weakens the immune system. People with HIV/AIDS become seriously ill with infections that most people can fight off. These infections are called "opportunistic infections" because they take advantage of weak immune systems.

Some conditions caused by an overactive immune system are:
- **Asthma:** The response in your lungs can cause coughing, wheezing, and trouble breathing. Asthma can be triggered by common allergens like dust or pollen or by an irritant like tobacco smoke.
- **Eczema:** An allergen causes an itchy rash known as atopic dermatitis.
- **Allergic rhinitis:** Sneezing, a runny nose, sniffling, and swelling of your nasal passages from indoor allergens like dust and pets or outdoor allergens like pollens or molds.

Types of Autoimmune Disorders

Autoimmune disorders can affect nearly every organ and system of the body. Some autoimmune disorders include:
- **Diabetes (Type I)**—affects the pancreas. Symptoms include thirst, frequent urination, weight loss and an increased susceptibility to infection.
- **Graves' disease**—affects the thyroid gland. Symptoms include weight loss, elevated heart rate, anxiety and diarrhea.
- **Inflammatory bowel disease**—includes ulcerative colitis and possibly, Crohn's disease. Symptoms include diarrhea and abdominal pain.

- **Multiple sclerosis**—affects the nervous system. Depending on which part of the nervous system is affected, symptoms can include numbness, paralysis and vision impairment.
- **Psoriasis**—affects the skin. Features include the development of thick, reddened skin scales.
- **Rheumatoid arthritis**—affects the joints. Symptoms include swollen and deformed joints. The eyes, lungs and heart may also be targeted.
- **Scleroderma**—affects the skin and other structures, causing the formation of scar tissue. Features include thickening of the skin, skin ulcers and stiff joints.
- **Systemic lupus erythematosus**—affects connective tissue and can strike any organ system of the body. Symptoms include joint inflammation, fever, weight loss and a characteristic facial rash.

Risk Factors for Autoimmune Disorders

The exact causes of autoimmune disorders are not known. The risk factors seem to include:

- **Genetics**—a predisposition to autoimmune disorders seems to run in families. However, family members can be affected by different disorders; for example, one person may have diabetes, while another has rheumatoid arthritis. It seems that genetic susceptibility alone is not enough to trigger an autoimmune reaction, and other factors must contribute.
- **Environmental factors**—a family's susceptibility to autoimmune disorders may be linked to common environmental factors, perhaps working in conjunction with genetic factors.
- **Gender**—around three quarters of people with autoimmune disorders are women.
- **Sex hormones**—autoimmune disorders tend to strike during the childbearing years. Some disorders seem to be affected, for better or worse, by major hormonal changes such as pregnancy, childbirth and menopause.
- **Infection**—some disorders seem to be triggered or worsened by particular infections.

Diagnosis of Autoimmune Disorders

It can be hard to diagnose an autoimmune disorder, especially in its earlier stages and if multiple organs or systems are involved. Depending on the disorder, diagnosis methods may include:
- Physical examination
- Medical history
- Blood tests, including those to detect autoantibodies

- Biopsy
- X-rays

Treatment for Autoimmune Disorders

Autoimmune disorders in general cannot be cured, but the condition can be controlled in many cases. Historically, treatments include:
- **Anti-inflammatory drugs**—to reduce inflammation and pain
- **Corticosteroids**—to reduce inflammation. They are sometimes used to treat an acute flare of symptoms
- **Pain-killing medication**—such as paracetamol and codeine
- **Immunosuppressant drugs**—to inhibit the activity of the immune system
- **Physical therapy**—to encourage mobility
- **Treatment for the deficiency**—for example, insulin injections in the case of diabetes
- **Surgery**—for example, to treat bowel blockage in the case of Crohn's disease
- **High dose immunosuppression**—the use of immune system suppressing drugs (in the doses needed to treat cancer or to prevent the rejection of transplanted organs) have been tried recently, with promising results. Particularly when intervention is early, the chance of a cure with some of these conditions seems possible.

An underactive immune system does not function correctly and makes people vulnerable to infections. It can be life-threatening in severe cases.

People who have had an organ transplant need immunosuppression treatment to prevent the body from attacking the transplanted organ.

Immunoglobulin Therapy

Immunoglobulins (commonly known as antibodies) are used to treat people who are unable to make enough of their own, or whose antibodies do not work properly. This treatment is known as immunoglobulin therapy.

Until recently, immunoglobulin therapy in Australia mostly involved delivery of immunoglobulins through a drip into the vein—known as intravenous immunoglobulin (IVIg) therapy. Now, subcutaneous immunoglobulin (SCIg) can be delivered into the fatty tissue under the skin, which may offer benefits for some patients. This is known as subcutaneous infusion or SCIg therapy.

Subcutaneous immunoglobulin is similar to intravenous immunoglobulin. It is made from plasma—the liquid part of blood containing important proteins like antibodies.

Immunization

Immunization works by copying the body's natural immune response. A vaccine (a small amount of a specially treated virus, bacterium or toxin) is injected into the body. The body then makes antibodies to it. If a vaccinated person is exposed to the actual virus, bacterium or toxin, they won't get sick because their body will recognize it and know how to attack it successfully.

DISEASE TRANSMISSION AND PREVENTION OF INFECTION

Modes of Transmission of Infection

Pathogenic organisms can spread from one host to another by a variety of mechanisms. These include:

- **Contact:** Infection may be acquired by contact, which may be direct or indirect.
  - *Direct contact* such as sexually transmitted diseases
  - *Indirect contact* may be through the agency of fomites, which are inanimate objects such as clothing, pencils or toys which may be contaminated by a pathogen from one person and act as a vehicle for its transmission to another.
- **Inhalation:** Respiratory infection such as common cold, influenza, measles, mumps, tuberculosis and whooping cough are acquired by inhalation.
- **Ingestion:** Intestinal infections are generally acquired by the ingestion of food or drink contaminated by pathogens. Infection transmitted by ingestion may be waterborne (cholera), foodborne (food poisoning) or handborne (dysentery).
- **Inoculation:** The disease agent may be inoculated directly into the skin or mucosa, e.g., rabies virus deposited subcutaneously by dog bite, tetanus spores implanted in deep wounds, and arboviruses injected by insect vectors. Infection by inoculation may be iatrogenic when unsterile syringes and surgical equipment are employed, e.g., hepatitis B and the human immunodeficiency virus (HIV).
- **Inserts (*See* under sources of infection):** Vector is defined as an arthropod or any living carrier (e.g., snail) that transports an infectious agent to a susceptible individual.
- **Congenital (Vertical transmission):** Some pathogens are able to cross the placental barriers and reach the feces in utero. This is known as vertical transmission. For example, so called to RCH agent (*Toxoplasma gondii rubella virus, Cytomegalovirus,* and Herpes

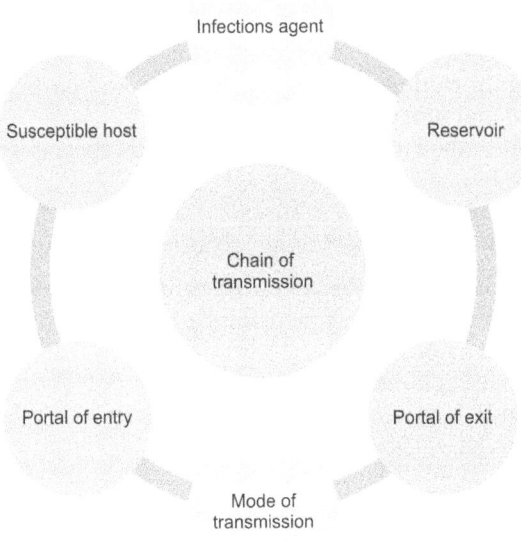

Fig. 2.10: Chain of transmission.

virus, varicella virus, syphilis, hepatitis B, coxsackie *B* and AIDS) **(Fig. 2.10)**.

❖ **Iatrogenic and laboratory infections:** If meticulous care in asepsis in not taken, infections like AIDS and hepatitis B may sometime be transmitted during administration of injections, lumbar and catheterization.

Prevention of Infection

According to the World Health Organization (WHO), infection prevention and control (IPC) is a scientific approach and practical solution designed to prevent harm caused by infection to patients and health workers. It is a subset of epidemiology, but also serves an essential function in infectious diseases, social sciences and global health.

Infection control and prevention is a global issue and there are many protocols and guidelines that can be followed to minimize the spread of infection between people, within a population and globally. Identifying at-risk groups such as children, older people and those with chronic conditions can also help guide relevant strategies to protect these vulnerable groups. The first step when looking at infection control can start at the community level by changing behavior, including:

- Regular hand washing
- Appropriate use of face-masks (protect from and prevent spread of respiratory infections)
- Using insect repellents
- Ensuring up-to-date routine vaccinations and participating in immunization programs
- Taking prescribed medications, such as antibiotics, as directed by health professionals
- Social distancing—avoiding contact with others
- Using condoms when having sex, especially with a new partner

Other steps that can be taken to control the spread within communities include environmental measures such as:
- Modifying environments
- Surveillance of diseases
- Food safety
- Air quality

Medical Interventions

As well as simple steps to prevent and control infections, there are biochemical interventions that can be implemented to speed up the recovery process and in some cases prevent viral infections completely. The development of antibiotics, antivirals and vaccinations have been shown to speed up recovery, slow down the progression and in some cases eradicate infectious diseases from entire populations.

Antibiotics

Antibiotics are prescribed for bacterial infections and support the body's natural defense system to eliminate the disease-causing bacterial agent. They are designed to either kill bacteria or stop them from reproducing. However, poor use of antibiotics, over-prescribing and the mutation of bacteria has led the development of resistant bacteria. In these cases, either stronger doses are required or the combination of one or more antibiotics.

Vaccinations

Vaccinations are designed to improve immunity to a particular disease. Vaccines work by introducing small amounts of the disease-causing virus or bacteria into the host, allowing them to build up natural immunity. The introduction of regular vaccines have slowed down and in some cases eradicated certain diseases such as polio, measles, mumps, whooping cough and rubeola (measles). There are also vaccinations for chickenpox, but this is not given routinely and is reserved for those at risk of spreading the disease to those with a weakened immune system

This is due to the fact that it is prevalent in children under 10 years of age and symptoms are usually mild; this method allows them to build up natural immunity and contributes to improving the immunization of a community. This type of protection is known as **herd immunity**.

Antivirals

Antibiotics provide no defense for infectious diseases that are caused by viral agents such as influenza, HIV, herpes, and hepatitis B. In these cases, antiviral medications are the most effective at slowing down the progression of the disease and boosting the immune system. Unfortunately, as with antibiotics, viruses can mutate over time and become resistant to these antiviral drugs.

Infection Control in Healthcare Facilities

Another important factor in controlling and preventing infection is by improving practices in healthcare facilities. It is the duty of healthcare professionals worldwide to ensure they develop strategies and implement policies that protect those who may be immunocompromised in order to keep susceptible patients safe from healthcare-associated infections (HAIs). Globally, up to 7% of patients in developed and 10% in developing countries will acquire at least one HAI.

HAIs are one of the most common detrimental effects in care delivery and both the endemic burden and the occurrence of epidemics are a major public health concern. HAIs have a significant impact on morbidity, mortality and quality of life and present an economic burden at the societal level. However, a large proportion of HAI are preventable and there is a growing body of evidence to help raise awareness of the global burden of harm caused by these infections, including strategies to reduce their spread.

Standard Precautions for all Nursing Care

- Perform hand hygiene
- Use personal protective equipment (PPE) to prevent exposure to infection
- Follow respiratory hygiene/cough etiquette principles
- Ensure appropriate patient placement and isolation precaution
- Properly handle, clean, and disinfect patient care equipment and medical instruments
- Handle and sterilize textiles and laundry carefully
- Follow safe injection practices and proper handling of sharps/needles
- Ensure healthcare worker safety via IPC and postexposure prophylaxis

- Prevention of intervention-related infections (catheter-associated urinary tract infections, intravascular catheter-related infections, surgical site infections)
- The implementation of the specific isolation precaution when diagnosing some syndromes.
- Improving the communication between healthcare workers especially when referring potentially contagious patients
- In pediatric departments or ambulatory settings, there should be efforts to decrease infection from contaminated toys. Families can be encouraged to bring their own toys.

STERILIZATION

Heat is the reliable and short period process of sterilization. Proteins of bacteria coagulate at high temperature resulting in death of bacteria. Majority of bacteria die in moist heat at 50–70°C in 2-3 minutes. *Streptococcus faecalis* is destroyed on high temperature. Vegetative forms are killed at low temperature but spores required high temperature. High temperature required less period.

Two types of heat are used:
1. Dry heat
2. Moist heat

Dry Heat

Is used to sterilize metal made instruments such as needles, syringes, test tube, etc. Scalpel, forceps, needle, glass slide, cover slip are placed directly on flame and sterilized without becoming red. Bunsen burner is used in this method. Platinum loop and vaccinating instruments are also sterilized by this procedure. Test tube, pipette, petri dish are kept in hot air oven wrapped in paper. These instruments operated by electricity and controlled by heat regulator.

Moist Heat

Three manners are adopted for sterilization by moist heat.
- **Heating:** Heating liquid on 100°C
- **Boiling:** Instruments are kept in water contained by sterilizer which is boiled on 100°C. Syringes, needles, knives or other surgical instruments are sterilized by the procedure.
- **Vapor sterilization:**
  - Sterilization by vapor at 100°C is an effective method. It is done with the help of steamer. Broth or agar is retained in vapor for one and half hours.

- Vapor is used several times on short intervals in intermittent vapor sterilization. Vapor at 100°C is used for 3 days continuously at an interval of 20-20 minutes. Sugar and gelatin are sterilized by this method. Twice sterilization kills vegetative bacteria and spores completely.
- Sterilization is done at above 100°C in pressure cooker or autoclave. Water boils at 121°C temperature in presence of 15 lbs (pounds) vapor pressure.

Chemical Sterilization (Tables 2.1 to 2.3)

- ❖ **Glutaraldehyde:** Endoscope is sterilized by 2% liquid.
- ❖ **Formaldehyde gas:** Sterilizes endoscope.
- ❖ **Ethylene gas:** It sterilizes heart lung machine, respirator, and dental instruments. These are retained in gas for 2-4 hours. It is also used in fumigating atmosphere.
- ❖ **Beta propiolactone:** Its 0.2% gas is also used for sterilization.

Ultraviolet Radiation

- ❖ Low pressure mercury vapor lamp is used to destroy Gram-negative and Gram-positive bacteria.
- ❖ Sunray has capacity to kill bacteria due to presence of ultraviolet ray. TB causing bacteria are killed on exposure to sunlight (by sitting in sunlight).
- ❖ Besides these, disposable medical materials are sterilized by X-ray, β-rays and γ-rays. Filtration is also a process for sterilizing

Table 2.1: Classification of chemical sterilizing agents.

Chemical disinfectant	Examples
Interfere with membrane functions	
• Surface acting agents	Quaternary ammonium compounds Tween 80 Soaps and fatty acids
• Phenols	Phenol, cresol, hexylresorcinol
• Organic solvent	Chloroform, alcohol
• Acids and alkalis	Organic acids Hydrochloric acids, sulfuric acids
Destroy functional groups of properties	
• Heavy metals	Copper, silver, mercury
• Oxidizing agents	Iodine, chlorine, hydrogen peroxide
• Dyes	Acridine orange, acriflavine
• Alkylating agents	Formaldehyde, ethylene oxide

Table 2.2: Applications and in-use dilution of chemical disinfectants.

Agent	Common use	Use dilution (%)
Alcohols	Skin antiseptic Surface disinfectant	70
Mercurials	Skin antiseptics Surface disinfectant	0.1
Silver nitrate	Antiseptics (eyes and burns)	1
Phenolic compounds	Antiseptics skin washes	5
Iodine	Disinfect inanimate object Skin antiseptic	2
Chlorine compounds	Water treatment Disinfect inanimate object	5
Quaternary ammonium compounds	Skin antiseptic Disinfects inanimate object	<1
Glutaraldehyde	Heat sensitive instruments	1–2

Table 2.3: Applications and in-use dilution of chemical disinfectants.

Autoclaving	Hot air oven	Ethylene oxide	Autoclaving	Ethylene oxide
• Animal cages • Sugar tubes • Lab coats • Cotton • Filters • Instruments • Culture media • Rubber • Gloves • Stopper • Tubing • Oils • Slides • Syringe and Wax needles	• Glassware • Beakers • Flasks • Petri dish • Pipette • Slides • Syringes • Test tubes • Glycerine • Needles • Scissors • Paper • Matrix band • Saliva ejector	• Fabric • Bedding • Blanket • Clothing • Mattresses • Pillows • Disposable Instruments • Blades • Knives • Scalpels • Scissors • Talcum power • Books • Cups, plates	• Test tubes • Enamel metal trays • Wire baskets • Wood • Tongue depressor • Applicator • Endodontic Instruments • Catheters • Orthodontic kits • Saliva ejector • Hand pieces • Cavitron heads • Steel burs • Steel tumbler • Hand instruments	• Plastics • Flasks • Petri dish • Tubes • Tubing • Rubber • Drains • Special items • Broncho-scope • Gloves • Heart lung machine

liquid materials. An apparatus, namely, Seitz filter is used for sterilization of medium components, preparation of vaccine and separation of bacteria from toxic liquid.

Preferred methods of sterilization for the sterilization of a small and closed common use articles are given in **Table 2.3**.

BACTERIA: VIRUS AND FUNGI

Bacteria

Bacteria are unicellular, prokaryotic and multiply their number by binary fission.

Classification
- **On the basis of shape:**
    - *Coccus*: Spherical or oval, e.g., staphylococci in groups, streptococci in chain, pneumococci, etc.
    - *Bacillus*: Rod-shaped, e.g., *E.coli*, diphtheria.
    - *Coccobacilli*: Same in length and width, e.g., *Brucella*.
    - *Vibrio:* Comma (,) shaped, e.g., Cholerae.
    - *Spirilla:* Spiral, e.g., *Spirilum minus*.
    - *Spirochaete*: Nonrigid, spiral form, e.g., *Treponema, Leptospira, Borrelia*.
    - *Mycoplasma pneumoniae*: Indefinite in shape.
    - *Actinomycetes*: Branched and filamentous.
- **On the basis of staining:** Gram staining
    - *Gram positive*: Retains violet color, e.g., staphylococci, streptococci.
    - *Gram negative*: Do not retain violet color, e.g., *N. gonorrhoeae*.
    - *Acid fast stain*: Appears red colored on staining with Ziehl-Neelsen technique, e.g., *Mycobacterium tuberculosis*.
    - *Gram positive bacilli*: Spore forming, e.g., *Clostridium*.
    - *Gram negative bacilli*: Non-spore forming, e.g., *Corynebacterium*.
- **On the basis of arrangement:**
    - *Diplococci*: Cocci in pair, e.g., pneumococcal (Gram-positive). *Neisseria* (Gram-negative).
    - *Staphylococci*: In the form of bunches.
    - *Sarcina*: In group of 8 cocci.
    - *Streptobacilli*: Bacilli in the form of chain.

Fungi

Fungal infections are collectively called mycosis. These are classified on the basis of affected part of body.
- **Superficial mycosis:** Commonly called ring worm or tinea infection such as:
    - *Tinea capitis*: Scalp
    - *Tinea corporis*: Nonhairy skin of body

- *Tinea cruris*: Groin and perineum
- *Tinea barbae*: Bearded areas of face and neck
- *Tinea pedis*: Toe clefts (athlete's foot).

❖ **Cutaneous mycosis:**
- *Trichophytons:* Infect skin, hair and nails.
- *Microsporum:* Infects hair and skin but not nails.
- Epidermophytosis: Infect skin and nails but not hair.

❖ **Subcutaneous mycosis:** Cause tissue destruction and sinus formation.
- *Madurella mycetomatis:* Caused by some actinomycetes and filamentary fungi.
- Sporotrichum.

❖ **Systematic mycosis**: Infect internal organs, acquired by inhalation.
- *Candida albicans*: Oral thrush, vaginitis.
- *Cryptococcus neoformans.*
- *Coccidioides.*
- *Aspergillus fumigatus.*

❖ **Opportunistic fungi**: Become active in case of low immunity.
- *Candida albicans*
- *Geotrichum*
- *Mucor*
- *Aspergillus*
- *Penicillium.*

Viruses

❖ **Ribonucleic acid (RNA) viruses:**
- Poliovirus
- Rhinovirus
- Hepatitis virus
- Influenza virus
- Mumps virus
- Rabies virus
- HIV virus
- Rotavirus.

❖ **DNA viruses:**
- Poxvirus
- *Herpes virus*
- Adenovirus
- Papillomavirus.

Table 2.4: Similarities and differences between bacteria and virus.

Bacterium	Virus	
Living attributes	Living	Opinions differ on whether a virus is a form of life or organic structure that interacts with living organisms
Cell number	Unicellular (one cell)	No cells; not living
Structures	DNA, RNA, cell wall, cell membrane	DNA or RNA enclosed inside a coat of protein
Ribosomes	Present	Absent
Enzymes	Yes	Yes—in some
Nucleus	No	No
May cause disease	Yes	Yes
Treatment	Antibiotics	Vaccines—prevent the spread and antiviral medicines help to slow reproduction but cannot stop it completely
Beneficial	Some beneficial—certain bacteria produce vitamins in gut; used to make yogurt, cheese	Specific viruses may be able to destroy tumors and may be useful in genetic engineering
Reproduction	Fission—form of asexual reproduction	Invades host cell and takes over the cell causing it to make copies of the viral DNA or RNA. Destroys the host cell releasing new viruses
Size	Larger (1,000 nm)	Smaller (20–400 nm)

ROUTES OF DRUG ADMINISTRATION

Modes of Drug Administration

Drug may be administered by various routes. The choice of the route in a given patients depends on the properties of the drug and the patient's requirements. The routes can be broadly divided into:
- Enteral
- Parenteral
- Local

Enteral Route (Oral Ingestion)

This is the common oldest and safest route of drug administration. The large surface area of the gastrointestinal tract. The mixing of its constants and the differences in pH at different parts of the gut which help in defective absorption of drugs given orally.

Advantages
- Safest route.
- Most convenient.
- Most economical.
- Can be self-administrated.
- Non-invasive route.

Disadvantages
- Onset of action is slower as absorption needs time.
- Irritant of unpalatable drugs can be administered.
- There may be irregularities in absorption.
- Irritation to the gastrointestinal track may leads to vomiting.
- Some drug may be destroyed by gastric juices as insulin.
- Cannot be given to unconscious and uncooperative patients.

Parenteral Route

Route of administration other than the enteral route are known as parenteral routes. These drugs are directly delivered into tissue fluids or blood.

Advantages
- Action is more rapid than oral administration.
- These routes can be employed in an unconscious or uncooperative patient.
- Gastric irritant can be given parenterally of these for irritation to the gastrointernal tract can be avoided.

Disadvantages
- Asepsis must be maintained.
- Injection may be painful.
- More expensive, less safe and inconvenient.
- Injury ensues other tissue may occur.

Injections
The drug is injected into the large skin by:
- Raising a bleb, e.g., BCG vaccine test frugally
- By multiple punctures of the epidermis through a drop of the drug, e.g., smallpox vaccine only a small quantity can be administrated this route, and it may be painful.

Subcutaneous Injection

There the drug is deposited in the SC tissue, e.g., insulin heparin. As the tissue is less vascular absorption is slow of largely uniform and this makes the drug long active.

Advantage
It is reliable and routes can be trained for self-administration.

Disadvantages
- As SC tissue is richly supplied by nerves irritant drugs cannot be injected.
- In shock absorption is not dependable because of nasal constriction.

Drug can also be administrated subcutaneously as:
- **Dermojet:** In this method a high velocity jet of drug solution is projected from a five office using a gun needle is not required in this method so its painless.
- **Pellet implantation:** Small pellets packed with drug are implanted subcutaneously. The drug is slowly released for weeks or month to provide constant blood levels, e.g., testosterone.
- **Silastic implant:** The drug is packed in silastic tubes and implanted subcutaneously the drug gets absorbed over maths to provide constant blood levels, e.g., hormone of contraceptives.

Intramuscular (IM)

The drug is injected directly into the muscles used sites for intramuscular injection are:
- Deltoid
- Gluteus maximus

Intravenous (IV)

Here the drug is injected into one of the superficial veins so that, it immediately available for action.

Advantages
- Intravenous route is the most useful route in emergencies because the drug is immediately available for action.
- Provided predictable blood concentration with 100% bioavailability.
- Large volume solution can be given.

Disadvantages
- Once injected the drug can be withdraw.
- Irritation of veins may cause thrombosis phlebitis.
- The solution should be sterile of strict aseptic measure should be taken.

Inhalation

Volatile liquids and gases are given by inhalation, e.g., general anesthetics

In addition, drug can be administered as solid particles, i.e., as solution of drug particles, and the fine droplets are inhaled as aerosols, e.g., salbutamol.

Advantages
- Almost instantaneous absorption of the drug is achieved because of the large surface area of the lungs.
- Duration of action is prolonged
- Provides constant plasma drug levels
- Patient compliance is good

Disadvantages
- Irritant gases may enhance pulmonary secretions and should be avoided by this route
- Transdermal route
- Highly lipid soluble drug can be applied over the skin for slow of prolonged absorption, e.g., nitroglycerin ointment in even angina pectoris.

Transmucosal

Drug are absorbed across the mucous membrane, transmucosal administration includes sublingual, nasal of rectal route.

Topical

Drug may be applied on the skin for local action as ointment, cream, gel, powder, paste, etc.

Linctuses

Are sweet viscous liquids they contain syrup and may also have glycerin as a vehicle which has demulcent effect on mucous membrane and throat, e.g., linctus codeine.

Drops: These are liquid preparations which may be usually orally or for local effect like eye drops, nasal drops and ear drops, e.g., paracetamol drop cephalexin (sporidex) drops.

ADVERSE EFFECTS AND SIDE EFFECTS OF DRUGS

Adverse effect is an undesired harmful effect resulting from a medication or other intervention, such as surgery.

An adverse effect may be termed as a "side effect".

Common Causes of Adverse Drug Reaction/Effect

- Failing to take the correct dosages at the correct time.
- Overdosing
- Allergies to chemical component of the medicine.
- Combining the medicine with alcohol.
- Taking other drugs or preparation that interact with the medicine.

Factors Affecting Adverse Drug Reaction

Patient-related Factors

- Age
- Sex
- Genetic influences
- Concurrent diseases (renal, liver, cardiac)
- Compliance with dosing regimen
- Total no. of medication
- Diet, smoking, environmental exposure

Age

- **Children:** Are more often at risk because their capacity to metabolize drugs is usually not fully developed.
- **Elderly:** Reasons for ADRs in the elderly:
  - Regular uses of several medication
  - Decreased drug ADME activity due to age.
- **Pregnancy:**
  - Sulfonamides—jaundice and brain damage in the fetus.
  - Warfarin—birth defect
  - Lithium—defect of the heart, lethargy, etc.

Drug-related Factors

- Dose
- Duration
- Inherent toxicity of the agent
- Pharmacodynamics properties
- Pharmacokinetics properties

Types of Adverse Effect of Drug

- **Type A:** Augmented
- **Type B:** Bizarre
- **Type C:** Continuous

- **Type D:** Delayed
- **Type E:** Ending of use
- **Type F:** Failure of efficacy

Type Based on Onset

Onset of event:
- **Acute:** Within 60 minute
- **Subacute:** 1–24 hours
- **Latent:** 2 days

Type (A) Reaction (or) Augmented

- **Extension effect:**
  - Predictable
  - Dose-related responses
  - *Prevention:* Adjustment of dosage regimen
- **Example:**
  - *Benzodiazepines:* Sedation
  - *Furosemide:* Water and electrolyte imbalance
  - *Heparin, warfarin:* Spontaneous bleeding
  - *Insulin:* Hypoglycemia

Type (B) Reaction (or) Bizarre

Example:
1. Hypersensitivity reaction
2. Hemolytic anemia
3. Stevens-Johnson syndrome

Type (C) Reaction (or) Continuous

Long-term effect are usually related to the dose and duration of treatment.

Example:
- **Ethambutol:** Retinopathy
- **NSAIDs:** Nephrotoxicity

Type (D) Reaction (or) Delayed

- Carcinogenesis
- Teratogenesis

Example: Thalidomide

Type (E) Reaction (or) Ending of Use

Withdrawal syndrome

Example:
- ❖ **Benzodiazepines:** Rebound insomnia
- ❖ **Clonidine:** Rebound hypertension
- ❖ **Corticosteroids:** Acute adrenal insufficiency

Type (F) Reaction (or) Failure of Efficacy

Example:
- ❖ Counterfeit medicines
- ❖ Under dosing of medication
- ❖ Drug interaction

SIDE EFFECTS OF DRUGS

Many side effects of medications may not be reported. Always consult your doctor or healthcare specialist for medical advice. A side effect is usually regarded as an undesirable secondary effect which occurs in addition to the desired therapeutic effect of a drug or medication. Side effects may vary for each individual depending on the person's disease state, age, weight, gender, ethnicity and general health.

Side effects can occur when commencing, decreasing/increasing dosages, or ending a drug or medication regimen. Side effects may also lead to noncompliance with prescribed treatment. When side effects of a drug or medication are severe, the dosage may be adjusted or a second medication may be prescribed. Lifestyle or dietary changes may also help to minimize side effects.

Prescription Medicines can Cause Side Effects

All medicines can cause unwanted side effects. For example, some antibiotics can cause allergic reactions in around 5% of the population. Skin rashes are a common reaction. But, it is not always easy to tell if the reaction is caused by the medicine or the illness.

Interactions between other medicines the person may be taking is a further complication. Interactions can happen between prescription, over-the-counter and complementary medicines.

Complementary Medicines also Cause Side Effects

About 60% of Australians use complementary medicines at least once a year. Many people believe that they are safer because they come from natural sources. This is not always true.

Some herbal remedies act on the body as powerfully as any conventional medicine, and unwanted side effects can occur.

Some examples of complementary medicines that can cause side effects include:
- **Echinacea**—more than 20 different types of reactions have been reported. Some include asthma attacks, hives, swelling, aching muscles and gastrointestinal upsets.
- **Feverfew**—pregnant women should not use this herb, as it can trigger uterine contractions. In animal experiments, feverfew triggered spontaneous abortions (miscarriages).

Complementary Medicines can Interact with Prescription Medicines

About 1 in 5 Australians take both complementary and prescription medicines. Active ingredients in these medicines can interact, increasing the risk of side effects.

Some medicines have similar active ingredients, which may act in the same way. Other complementary medicines may make the prescription medicine more or less effective.

Some combinations that can put people's health at risk include:
- Echinacea may interact with medications broken down by the liver.
- Many complementary medicines (including feverfew, ginkgo and chamomile) may increase the risk of bleeding in people taking anticoagulant medicines (such as warfarin) and anti-inflammatory medicines (such as aspirin).
- St John's wort increases serotonin. If taken with other medicines that increase serotonin (such as antidepressants) it can cause serotonin toxicity. Serotonin toxicity can range from mild to life-threatening. Symptoms include tremors, high temperature and low blood pressure.

For advice about complementary medicines, speak with your doctor or other health professional.

Alcohol Used with Medicines can Cause Side Effects

Drinking alcohol with some medicines can also cause unwanted (and sometimes dangerous) side effects. For example:
- Alcohol can cause drowsiness or dizziness when taken with (some) antihistamines, antidepressants, sleeping tablets or medicines for anxiety.
- Alcohol can affect medicines for high blood pressure and travel sickness.
- When alcohol is mixed with strong prescription medicines like opioid pain medicines, the combination can increase the chances

of overdose. Alcohol with opioids can slow down a person's breathing rate and lead to drowsiness and loss of consciousness.
- ❖ Some antibiotics interact negatively with alcohol and some can cause a severe reaction. Symptoms can include upset stomach, skin flushing, headache, a fast or irregular heartbeat, drowsiness or dizziness.

Remember that alcohol can stay in system for several hours after your last drink, so it is important to be aware that interactions can occur long after you stop drinking.

Talk to your doctor or other health professional for advice about your medication and drinking alcohol.

If the person experience side effects when taking medication:
- ❖ In an emergency, always call triple zero (000).
- ❖ Note the side effects and consult your doctor or pharmacist if you have any concerns. They may need to adjust the dose or type of medicine you use.
- ❖ Call the NPS Medicines Line Tel. 1300 633 424 or the Adverse Medicines Events Line Tel. 1300 134 237 for advice. These phoneline services allow consumers to report or receive advice on side effects. They are not emergency services.

Reduce the Risk of Side Effects

To reduce your risk of experiencing side effects:
- ❖ Take all medicines as prescribed by your doctor.
- ❖ Do not take anyone else's medicines.
- ❖ Learn about your medication. All prescription medicines have an information leaflet called consumer medicine information (CMI). This gives detailed information on the medicine in plain English, including how to use it, side effects and precautions. Your pharmacist can also give you the CMI for your medicine.
- ❖ Speak to your pharmacist if you buy over-the-counter or complementary medicines. They can advise you about side effects and interactions with other medicines you are taking. Be aware that medicines you buy in the supermarket can also cause side effects.
- ❖ Tell your doctor about all the medicines you take, including prescription, over-the-counter and complementary medicines.
- ❖ Have an annual review of all the medicines you take. This is important for older people as they are more likely to experience side effects. A review can take place in a pharmacy or at home. Ask your doctor for more information about medication reviews.

Other things you can do to reduce your risk of side effects from medicines include:
- Ask your doctor if improving your lifestyle could reduce your need for medication. Some conditions can be better managed with changes to your diet and regular exercise.
- Return unwanted and out-of-date medicines to your pharmacy for safe disposal. This is a free service.
- Talk to your pharmacist about dosage aids that can help you organize your pill taking. You may be at risk of making mistakes if you take many different medicines at different times.
- Ask your doctor or pharmacist questions so you understand the benefits and risks of your medicines.

ANALGESICS

Opioids Drug

Fentanyl
- Very commonly used opioid in anesthesia.
- 100 times more patient than morphine.

Advantages
- Rapid onset and rapid recovery.
- Opioid of choice for hepatic and renal diseases.
- With bupivacaine used epidural for painless labor.

Disadvantages
- Respiration depression.
- Chest wall rigidity.
- Used for induction of anesthesia.

Pentazocine (Fortwin)
- Against at copper and delta receptors and antiaging at mu receptor.
- Manly act on receptor at spinal level.
- 1/3 as patient as morphine.

Commonly Used as
- Analgesic in moderate to seven pain.
- Preanesthetic medication.
- Pre and postoperative medication.

Doses
- 30–60 mg IM.
- 30 mg IV.

Maximum dose is 360 mg/day.
* Not recommended in children below year
* Contraindicated in head injury/brain damage.

Side Effects
* Sedation.
* Nausea.
* Constipation.
* Vomiting.
* Dizziness.

NSAIDs

These drugs are common pain and fever relievers. NSAID is used to relieve headache, body aches, swelling, stiffness and fever.

Most Common NSAIDs

* Aspirin (available as a single ingredient known by various brand names such as Bayer® or St. Joseph® or combined with other ingredients known by brand names such as Anacin®, Ascriptin®, Bufferin®, or Excedrin®).
* Ibuprofen (known by brand names such as Motrin® and Advil®).
* Naproxen sodium (known by the brand name Aleve®).

Common Side Effects of NSAIDs

It may cause side effects if taken large doses of NSAIDs, or if taken them for a long time. Some side effects are mild and go away, while others are more serious and need medical attention. Unless doctor tells to do so, do not take an over-the-counter NSAID with a prescription NSAID, multiple over-the-counter NSAIDs or more than the recommended dose of an NSAID. Doing so could increase risk of side effects.

The side effects listed below are the most common, but there may be others. Ask doctor if you have questions about your specific medication.

The most frequently reported side effects of NSAIDs are gastrointestinal (stomach and gut) symptoms, such as:
* Gas.
* Feeling bloated.
* Heartburn.
* Stomach pain.
* Nausea.
* Vomiting.
* Diarrhea and/or constipation.

These gastrointestinal symptoms can generally be prevented by taking the drug with food, milk or antacids (such as Maalox® or Mylanta®).

Call doctor if these symptoms continue for more than a few days even if you're taking the NSAID with food, milk or antacid. The NSAID may need to be stopped and changed.

Other side effects of NSAIDs include:
- Dizziness.
- Feeling lightheaded.
- Problems with balance.
- Difficulty concentrating.
- Mild headaches.

If these symptoms go on for more than a few days, stop taking the NSAID and call your doctor.

NSAIDs for High Blood Pressure

NSAIDs can cause high blood pressure (hypertension) in some people. You may have to stop taking NSAIDs if you notice your blood pressure increases even if you're taking your blood pressure medications and following your diet. Ask your doctor about this before you start taking NSAIDs.

NSAIDs cause Allergic Reactions

Rarely, an NSAID can cause a generalized allergic reaction known as anaphylactic shock. If this happens, it usually occurs soon after the person starts taking the NSAID. The symptoms of this reaction include:
- Swollen eyes, lips or tongue.
- Difficulty swallowing.
- Shortness of breath.
- Rapid heart rate.
- Chest pain or tightness.

If any of these symptoms occur, call 9-1-1 or have someone drive you to the nearest emergency room immediately.

Remember, before any medication is prescribed, tell doctor:
- If you are allergic to any medications, foods or other substances.
- If you currently take any other medications (including over-the-counter medications) and/or herbal or dietary supplements.
- If you are pregnant, planning to become pregnant, or are breast-feeding.
- If you have problems taking any medications.
- If you have anemia, kidney or liver disease, stomach or peptic ulcers, heart disease, high blood pressure, bleeding or clotting problems, asthma or growth in the nose (nasal polyps).

DRUGS USED IN COUGH AND EXPECTORATION

Cough is protective reflex that remove the irritant matter and secretion from the respiratory tract. It could be due to infection allergy pleural diseases and malignancy. Because it is a protective mechanism, unnecessary suppression of cough can cause more harm than any benefit. Only in some condition as in dry cough it may not be useful in such situations and antitussives or cough suppressants may be used.

DRUGS FOR COUGH

Central Cough Suppressant (Antitussives Agent)

Tussive cough means, antitussive are the drug that acts in the CNS to raise the threshold of cough center or act peripherally in the respiratory tract to reduce tussal impulses. Used only if cough is hazardous.

- **Codeine:** An opioid is a good antitussive with less addiction liability nausea constipation and drowsiness is common. Dose 10-15 mg every 6 hours.
- **Noscapine:** It is a potent antitussive; no other CNS effect is prominent in therapeutic doses. Nausea is the only occasional side effect. Dose 15-30 mg every 6 hours.
- **Dextromethorphan and pholcodine:** These are synthetic opioid derivatives with antitussive actions like codeine but with fewer side effects.

Classification of Antitussive

- Opioid antitussive, e.g., codeine, pholcodine, morphine, ethyl morphine, hydrocodone, oxycodone.
- Nonopioid antitussive, e.g., noscapine, dextromethorphan, oxepin, propoxyphene.
- **Antihistamine:** These are used in cough due to allergy except that due to bronchial asthma, e.g., chlorpheniramine, diphenhydramine, promethazine, etc.
- **Benzonatate:** It is chemically related to the local anesthetic proiaine. Doses 100 mg thrice daily.
- **Peripherally acting antitussive:**
  - *Mucosal anesthetics:* Benzonatate, chlophedianol
  - *Hydrating agents:* Steam, aerosols
  - *Pharyngeal demulcent:* These drugs increases the flow of saliva which produces a soothing effect on the pharyngeal mucosa and reduce afferent impulses arising from irritated mucosa, e.g., glycerine, liquorice

- **Expectorant or mucokinetics:** These are the drug which increases bronchial secretion or reduce its viscosity, facilitating its removal by coughing.
- **Mucolytics:** It depolymerizes the mucopolysaccharides, thus breaks down this mucus plug and removed out by coughing.
- **Bronchodilators:** Bronchospasm induce or aggravate cough bronchodialators reduce the spasm, dilates the bronchiole and bronchus, this should be used only if bronchoconstriction is present.
- **Steam inhalation:** Offers and effective and alternative to drug
- **Mucoactive agent:** Hypertonic 7% saline, dry powder mannitol.

DRUGS USED IN BRONCHIAL ASTHMA AND COPD

Antiasthmatic Drugs

Antiasthmatic are the drugs which can be used to terminate acute attack of asthma or prevent the occurrence of an attack. Bronchial asthma is characterized by dyspnea and wheezing due to increase resistance to the flow of air through the bronchi. Bronchospasm, mucosal congestion and edema result in increase resistance the tracheobronchial smooth muscle is hyper-responsive to various stimuli such as dust, allergens, cold air, infection and drug.

Classification

1. **Bronchodilators:** These are helpful in individuals with cough and bronchoconstriction due to bronchial hyperactivity. They have by improving the effectiveness of cough in clearing secretions.
    - *Sympathomimetics (adrenergics):*
        - Selective beta 2 stimulant (beta 2 agonist):
            - Salbutamol
            - Bambuterol
            - Formoterol
            - Terbutaline
        - Nonselective beta stimulant (beta agonist):
            - Adrenaline
            - Ephedriner
            - Isoprenaline
    - *Methylxanthines (phosphodiesterase inhibitors):*
        - Theophyllinate
        - Choline theophillinate
        - Hydroxyethyl theophyllinate

- ♦ Aminophylline
- ♦ Theophylline ethanoate of piperazine
- ■ *Anticholinergic:*
  - ♦ Atropine methonitrate
  - ♦ Ipratropium bromide
  - ♦ Tiotropium bromide
2. **Anti-inflammatory drugs:** Anti-inflammatory is the property of a substance or treatment that reduces inflammation or swelling.
   - ■ *Leukotriene antagonist:* Leukotriene are one of the important mediators of inflammations. They bring about bronchospasm, mucosal edema, increase the influx of inflammatory cells and respiratory mucous production by their action on leukotrienes receptors, e.g.:
     - ♦ Montelukast
     - ♦ Zafirlukast
   - ■ *Mast cell stabilizers:* Cromolyn inhibits the release of medicators of inflammations. It thus prevents bronchospasm and inflammation following exposure to allergens. It is therefore used for prophylaxis, e.g.:
     - ♦ Sodium cromoglycate
     - ♦ Ketotifen
   - ■ *Corticosteroids:* Corticosteroids do not relax airway smooth muscles directly but reduce bronchial reactivity, increase airway caliber, suppress inflammatory response to antigen antibody reacton or triggers stimuli and reduce the frequency of asthma excerbation.

     Systemic steroids: Systemic steroids are used in both severe chronic asthma and in acute emergency of asthma, e.g.:
     - ♦ Hydrocortisone
     - ♦ Prednisolone

     Inhalational steroid: Inhalational steroid, beclomethasone is a halogenated corticosteroid ester used in aerosol form. It suppress asthma by a topical anti-inflammatoiry action without causing any systemic side effects, e.g.:
     - ♦ Budesonide
     - ♦ Beclomethasone dipropionate
     - ♦ Fluticasone propionate
     - ♦ Flunisolide
   - ■ *Anti IgE antibodies:* Omalizumab is monoclonal antibody against IgE. Omalizumab binds to IgE to form a complex and such bound IgE antibodies cannot find to IgE receptors on mast cells and basophiles, so allergic process inhibited.
     - ♦ Omalizumab

- *Other:* Roflumilast is phosphodiesterase 4 inhibitors effective orally. It has anti-inflammatory properties and may be used in COPD.

DRUGS USED IN GASTROINTESTINAL TRACT

Antiemetic

Vomiting center is located in lateral reticular formation in the brain. Chemoreceptor trigger zone on stimulation induces vomiting. Distension of viscera can also lead to afferent pathway stimulation which can lead to emesis.

Vomiting is a protective mechanism to eliminate the unwanted harmful material from the stomach.

Vomiting as a symptom is associated with many diseases. The removal of primary cause is the best way to treat vomiting.

But in some situations, vomiting may not serve any useful purpose and may only be troublesome. In such circumstances, vomiting needs to be suppressed. Repeated vomiting can lead to imbalance of electrolyte, dehydration, exhaustion, aspiration of vomitus into lungs and gastric hemorrhage. However, for symptomatic relief antiemetics are given.

Antiemetics are the drugs used to prevent motion sickness and severe nausea and vomiting induced by chemotherapy, radiation therapy, and vital illnesses.

Action

These drugs are potent dopamine antagonist with antiemetic properties. These act by inhibiting vomiting center stimulation by suppressing hyperstimulated labyrinth.

These drugs suppress end organ receptors or inhibit central cholinergic pathway.

Dose

Dimenhydrinate:
- ❖ **Adult:** 50–100 mg TDS
- ❖ **Child:** 5 mg/kg BD or TDS
- ❖ **Metoclopramide:** 10 mg TDS
- ❖ **Chlorpromazine:** 25 mg TDS
- ❖ **Domperidone:** Adult—20–40 mg TDS, child—0.3 mg/kg TDS before meal at bed time
- ❖ **Ondansetron:** 8 mg as slow IV before chemotherapy or radiations therapy or 8 mg orally 1–2 hours before. This is followed by 8 mg orally every 12 hours.

Route
Orally: IV, IM

Indications
- Nausea and vomiting associated with electroshock therapy
- Anesthesia and surgery.
- Motion sickness.
- Vertigo.
- Gastric motility disorders such as reflux esophagitis and duodenogastric dyspeptic symptoms.
- Nausea and vomiting of pregnancy.
- Vomiting and nausea associated with cytotoxic radiotherapy and chemotherapy.
- Radiation sickness and postpenetration syndrome.
- Prophylaxis and treatment of postoperative vomiting and nausea.
- Sea sickness.
- Meniere's syndrome.
- Migraine.
- Labyrinthitis.
- Schizophrenia and other psychotic disorder
- Anticancer drugs.
- Uremia.
- Anxiety/tension.
- Alcohol withdrawal syndrome.
- Gastritis, hiccups.

Contraindications
- Hypersensitivity.
- Domperidone contraindicated in pregnancy
- Granisetron and ondansetron are contraindicated in children below 2 years.
- Prochlorperazine contraindicated in lactation and pregnancy.
- Promethazine theoclate is contraindicated in narrow angle glaucoma; epilepsy, concomitant therapy with MAO inhibitors. lactation.
- Parkinson's disease.
- Acute asthma attack.
- Drowsiness.
- Coma.
- Extrapyramidal reactions.
- Hepatic/renal disease.

- Severe depression due to alcohol.
- Pheochromocytoma.
- Asthmatics.

Dosage

Granisetron—Adult

10 mcg/kg IV within 30 minutes before initiation of chemotherapy. This should be given only on the day of chemotherapy.

Children

2-16 years of age—10 mcg/kg.

Oral—Adult

2 mg once daily (up to 1 hour before chemotherapy) or 1 mg twice daily (first 1 mg to be given up to one hour before chemotherapy and the second tablet to be given 12 hours after the first dose). The drug should be administered on the days of chemotherapy.

Prochlorperazine

5-10 mg BD or TDS.

In migraine—20 mg stat followed by 10 mg 2 hours Later. In schizophrenia and other psychotic disorders 75-100 mg daily

In divided doses. In children—0.25 mg/kg body weight. BD or TDS. IM route not recommended for children.

Promethazine Theoclate

25 mg thrice daily. In motion sickness 25 mg 1-2 hours before journey.

Drug interactions:

- Antihistamines and phenothiazines interact with anticholinergic type drugs.
- Reduces absorption of oral digoxin.
- Increase absorption of aspirin, PCM and oral diazepam.
- Enhances CNS depression by phenothiazine
- Increased risk of cardiac arrhythmias with terfenadine and astemizole
- Additive anticholinergic effects with antihistamines, tricyclic antidepressants and drug used in Parkinsonism.
- Potentiates other CNS depressants (sedative, hypnotics, antihistamines opiates and alcohol).
- Antacids decreases trifluoperazine bioavailability.

Side Effects
- Impaired alertness
- Sedation
- Dizziness
- Dry mouth
- Serum prolactin level may rise resulting in galactorrhea in females and less frequently gynecomastia in males.
- Headache
- Constipation
- Rarely allergic reactions
- Anxiety
- Fever
- Headache
- Elevation of liver enzymes (AST and ALT).
- Nasal stuffiness
- GI upset
- Restlessness
- Agitation
- Blood disorders
- Insomnia
- Drowsiness
- Asthenia
- Somnolence
- Dizziness
- Tachycardia
- Epigastric distress
- Hypotension
- Anorexia
- Dystonia
- Akathisia

Adverse effects:
- Phenothiazine causes extrapyramidal side effects
- Paradoxical CNS stimulation
- Jaundice
- Seizures
- Blurred vision
- Blood dyscrasias
- Ventricular tachyarrhythmias
- Urinary retention

Toxicity: Masked ototoxicity produced by aminoglycosides antibiotics.

Role of nurse:
- Antihistamine, antiemetics should be used cautiously with other CNS depressants. Administer with food or milk.
- Monitor BP assess for orthostatic hypotension.
- In a conscious patient, the cause of vomiting should be elicited through history.
- In medicolegal cases vomitus must be preserved.
- In unconscious state, the patient should be tilted to one side so as prevent aspiration of the vomitus.
- Patient is advised to take frequent small meals and excess of fluids.
- Reassurance helps.
- In pregnancy, dry biscuits in the morning prevent vomiting.
- If vomiting is severe, patient should be administered drugs which do not have teratogenic effect, e.g., pyridoxine is given and is found to be effective.

Emetics

Emetics are the drugs that induce vomiting by irritating the stomach and stimulating the vomiting center in the brain. When a toxic substance is ingested, vomiting has to be induced.

Action mechanism: Vomiting is a complex series of actions involving the stomach, esophagus and pharynx with the voluntary muscles of the chest and abdomen and results in the ejection of the stomach contents. A vomiting center in the medulla of the brain coordinates these actions.

This center can be stimulated:
- Directly from the labyrinth of the ear in conditions such as sea sickness or vertigo.
- By gastric irritation or distension.
- By mental activity (e.g., being sick with fright, imaging something extremely unpleasant).
- Via the chemoreceptor trigger zone (CTZ) which lies close to the vomiting center in the brainstem and which is stimulated by a number of circulating substances, including certain drugs.
- By stimulation of the 5-hydroxytryptamine (5-HT) receptors of the CTZ. Circulating cytotoxic drugs release 5-HT from nerve endings, and this activates the CTZ receptors. From the CTZ, Impulses travel to the vomiting center and activate it by acting on muscarinic acetylcholine (ACH) receptors.

Before the act of vomiting occurs, stimulation of the vomiting center produces a sensation known as nausea, which is often associated with increased secretions by the salivary and bronchial glands.

Emetics are rarely used in medication practice except in cases of poisoning. They may be divided into two types:
1. Reflex emetics, e.g., ipecacuanha.
2. Central emetics, e.g., apomorphine.

Reflex Emetics

This group of drugs produce vomiting by irritating the stomach. The only one in common use is ipecacuanha, a plant extract, which is dispensed as ipecacuanha emetic mixture and vomiting should occur in 15–30 min. It may be used as first-aid treatment for overdose provided that:
1. The patient is fully conscious.
2. Overdose is not corrosive substances or petroleum products when inhalation of vomit could be fatal.

Ipecacuanha can be used up to 1 hour after ingestion of poison and longer for some substances, such as tricyclic antidepressants and salicylates, when gastric emptying is delayed. It is not as effective as a stomach washout, but is particularly useful in children, when the upset caused by the process of lavage should be avoided if possible, and in removing such objects as berries, which cannot be washed out of the stomach. In general, the use of emetics in poisoning is decreasing because there is little evidence, even if used soon after ingestion of poison, that they usefully reduce absorption.

Central Emetics (Those Acting on the Brain)

Apomorphine stimulates dopamine receptors in the CTZ. It is closely related to morphine but has none of its analgesic effects. It has, however, a very powerful emetic action and also produces some cerebral depression. It was formerly used as an emetic but because of its depressing action it should not be used in treating patients who have taken an overdose. At present its use is confined to patients with resistant Parkinson's disease.

Dosage:
Ipecacuanha: 15–20 mL followed by 200–300 mL water.

Apomorphine: 6 mg in adults: 0.05 mg/kg IM is given in children.

Route: Ipecac—Orally as syrup. Apomorphine—IM.

Indications: Accidental overdoses of drugs, poisoning with noncaustic substances by stimulating vomiting center in medulla.

Contraindications:
- Unconscious
- Semiconscious
- Corrosive poisoning
- Poisoning by CNS stimulants as convulsions may be precipitated.
- Poisoning due to petroleum products as these can cause pneumonitis.

Drug interactions: Interacts with activated charcoal, alcohol and CNS depressants

Adverse reactions:
- Prolonged vomiting.
- Dysrhythmias
- Dehydration.

Side effects:
- Convulsions.
- Lethargy.
- Diarrhea.
- Respiratory distress.
- Shock
- Delirium.
- Circulatory disorders.

Toxicity: No systemic toxicity.

Role of nurse:
- Never administer ipecac syrup to treat poisoning of caustic substances.
- Never administer pure ipecac, it can cause death.
- If emesis does not occur with ipecac syrup within 30 mins, a further dose can be administered.
- Know how to administer ipecac syrup.
- For children under age of one year, administer 10 mL syrup followed by a glass of water.
- For children over the age of one year, administer 15 mL syrup followed by glass of water.
- For adults, administer 15-30 mL syrup followed by several glasses of water.

Purgative (Purges)

Purges may be defined as drugs that loosen the bowel. They are also called cathartics or laxatives.

These drugs cause evacuation of the bowel and facilitate smooth bowel elimination in those having defecation problem

With continued use of purgatives the muscle of the bow become flabby and dependency of purgatives develop. It is more dangerous to use purges for all types of abdominal pain.

Bowel evacuation may be achieved using orally administered purges or by the use of enemas and suppositories.

An ideal purgative should be:
❖ Dependable.
❖ Devoid of systemic effects.
❖ Not produce any griping pain.
❖ Not be habit forming
❖ Not cause after constipation.

Composition:
❖ **Bulk purges** that are high residue foods, e.g., bran: ispaghula (Isogel).
❖ **Stool softners**, e.g., docusate sodium.
❖ **Osmotic purges**, e.g., magnesium sulfate, lactulose.
❖ **Stimulant purges**, e.g., anthracenes, bisacodyl.

Action mechanism:
❖ Bulk purges increases the contents of the bowel and the stimulate peristalsis.
❖ The emollient (stool softening) purges and the passage of fecal material by their lubricating action.
❖ The stimulant purges increase peristalsis and thus the intestinal contents pass more rapidly through the bowel and remain more fluid.
❖ The osmotic purges promote peristalsis by drawing water into the intestine and distending the bowel.

Dosage

❖ **Bulk forming**: 1-2 tsp in water, swallowed immediately. 1-2 times daily with meals or milk.
❖ **Stool softners**: Docusate sodium: 50-500 mg daily in divided doses.
 Liquid paraffin: 15-30 mL/day.
❖ **Stimulant purgatives:** Bisacodyl-5-15 mg at bedtime.
 Phenolphthalein: 60-130 mg at bedtime.
❖ **Osmotic purgatives:** 4-10 mg or (30-50 mL) thrice daily

Route: Orally as these are available in forms of tablets, syrup and powder. Enema or suppositories through anal route.

Indications:

❖ For purgation in pregnant woman at term. This induces labor.
❖ Constipation.
❖ Irritable colon syndrome.

- ❖ Habitual geriatric.
- ❖ Obstetric and pediatric constipation.
- ❖ Recent MI.
- ❖ Severe hypertension.
- ❖ Abdominal hernia.
- ❖ Piles, fissures.
- ❖ Bed ridden patients.
- ❖ Hemorrhoidal complaints.
- ❖ Portal systemic encephalopathy.
- ❖ Chronic or habitual constipation.
- ❖ Postoperative cases.
- ❖ Hypertension.

Contraindications:
- ❖ Organic intestinal obstruction.
- ❖ Not to be used under 3 years.
- ❖ Acute surgical abdomen.
- ❖ Spastic constipation.
- ❖ Electrolyte imbalance.
- ❖ Lactation.
- ❖ Galactosemia.
- ❖ Patients on low galactose diets.
- ❖ Disaccharides deficiency.
- ❖ Hypersensitivity.
- ❖ Severe hepatic impairment.
- ❖ Abdominal adhesions.

Drug interactions: Dioctyl sodium sulfosuccinate enhances absorption of laxatives. Clinically no significant drug-interactions have been observed.

Side effects
- ❖ Cramps and abdominal pain.
- ❖ Nausea.
- ❖ Perianal irritation.
- ❖ Flatulence.
- ❖ Vomiting
- ❖ Skin rashes.
- ❖ Abdominal discomfort because of impaction and obstruction.
- ❖ Soreness in the anal region due to leakage of the suppository base
- ❖ Regular use (4-12 months) causes colonic atony and mucosal pigmentation (melanosis).
- ❖ Dizziness
- ❖ Migraine.
- ❖ Back pain.

- ❖ Headache.
- ❖ Weakness.
- ❖ Bitter taste.
- ❖ Fixed drug eruption.

Adverse effects:
- ❖ Hypovolemia.
- ❖ Increased blood sugar.
- ❖ Dehydration.
- ❖ Electrolyte imbalance.
- ❖ Atonic colon.
- ❖ Proctitis.
- ❖ Weight loss.
- ❖ Tachycardia.
- ❖ Ileus.

Toxicity: Hepatotoxicity is feared on prolonged use.

Nursing care:
- ❖ Assess bowel elimination habits.
- ❖ Teach the patient the benefits of proper diet containing roughage and exercise are important strategies in addition to purgatives.
- ❖ Never give purges to patients with undiagnosed abdominal pain.
- ❖ Bulk purges that swell in water must be mixed with water before oral use.
- ❖ Powerful stimulant purges should be avoided in pregnancy.
- ❖ Saline purges such as magnesium sulfate should be taken on an empty stomach.
- ❖ Liquid paraffin should be stopped once a regular pattern of evacuation is achieved.
- ❖ Mineral oil enemas are the best for those who are elderly, had recent heart attack and those with increased intracranial pressure.
- ❖ Monitor fluid intake and output and electrolyte levels.
- ❖ Monitor the frequency of laxative use in those patients with anorexia and bulimia.

Antacids

Antacids are basic substances. Given orally, they neutralize the gastric acid and raise the pH of gastric contents. Peptic activity is also reduced. Therefore, relieve heartburn and stomach pain associated with gastric disorders.

Antacids were once widely used in the treatment of peptic ulcers and other forms of dyspepsia. They are very effective at temporarily relieving the pain from an ulcer, but unless used. intensively, don't accelerate healing. They are also used in various minor gastric upsets.

Composition:
- Magaldrate.
- Aluminum hydroxide.
- Magnesium hydroxide/carbonate/trisilicate.
- Calcium carbohydrate.
- Sodium bicarbonate

Action: Antacids have acid neutralizing effect which raises the pH of gastric contents and decreases pepsin activity in the stomach.

Dosage:
- **Sodium bicarbonate:** 1-4 g. Patient should be advised to keep this drug as a stand by for emergency treatment of acute pain but should not use this routinely.
- **Magaldrate:** 480 mg
- **Magnesium hydroxide:** 150-250 mg.
- **Aluminum hydroxide:** 300 mg.

Route: Orally

Indications:
- Heartburn.
- Peptic ulcer.
- Abdominal surgeries
- Hyperacidity.
- Reflux esophagitis.
- Hyperphosphatemia in chronic renal failure.
- Indigestion.
- Stress ulcers.

Contraindications:
- Sodium preparations are contraindicated in cardiac diseases and hypertension.
- Calcium carbonate prepare continued in patient with peptic ulcer.
- Rarely in case of diabetes.

Drug interactions: Antacids may interfere with the absorption of digoxin, tetracycline, iron salts, indometacin. Antibiotics and isoniazide given orally at same time. As a rule these drugs should be given two hours apart from antacids.

Side effects:
- Rebound hyperacidity.
- Electrolyte disturbances such as hypermagnesemia. Hypophosphatemia (caused by aluminum containing antacids).
- Hyponatremia.

Adverse reaction:
- Magnesium preparations cause diarrhea.
- Aluminum preparations cause constipation.
- Magnesium based antacids cannot be excreted from body in case of dysfunctional kidneys.

Toxicity: The risk of toxicity is more with warfarin, antidepressants, theophylline, phenytoin, propranolol and lidocaine, etc.

Nursing care:
- Antacids should be given on schedule.
- Antacids impair the absorption of other drugs, enteric-coated drugs should be administered separately by 1 hour.
- Shake well the syrup/gel bottle before administration.
- Give 6 to 8 oz of water after administering antacid. Advise the patient to take sips of water.
- If chewable, advise the patient to chew well, follow with water.
- Avoid giving calcium carbohydrate for long term, as it will cause gastric hypersecretion and acid rebound.

Antidiarrheals

Diarrhea is the frequent passage of liquid stools. It can be due to a variety of causes like:
- Infection.
- Toxins.
- Anxiety.
- Drugs.
- Irritant food.
- Malabsorption.

Acute diarrhea is one of the major causes of death in infants. Death in diarrhea is mostly due to dehydration. A nurse can prevent such death by proper hydration of the child and educating the parents regarding the dangers of dehydration.

In diarrhea, there is an increase in motility and secretions in the gut with absorption of water and electrolyte. Hence the steps in the treatment of diarrhea include:
1. Replacement of fluid and electrolytes.
2. Treatment of cause.
3. Antidiarrheal agents.

Replacement of fluid and electrolyte:
- Correction of fluid and electrolyte disturbances can be life-saving in most cases especially infants.
- Oral rehydration with sodium chloride, glucose and water is useful.

- In the ileum, glucose and sodium citrate enhance sodium absorption and water follows.
- Oral rehydration salts are available to be mixed with water for mild to moderate cases.
- ORS with sodium bicarbonate and with sodium citrate are available.
- Trisodium citrate is used in place of bicarbonate because use of citrate makes ORS more stable, absorption of glucose and stool control is better.
- If ORS powder is not available, a mixture of 5 g table salt with 20 g sugar dissolved in 1 L of boiled and cooled water may be used till regular ORS is available.
- In severe degrees of dehydration, prompt intravenous rehydration is required.
- The correct type of IV solution should be selected depending on the patient's requirements.

Treatment of the cause:
- Acute diarrhea could often be due to viral, bacterial or protozoal infection.
- The pathogen should be identified whenever possible and treated accordingly.
- Gastroenteritis is often due to virus and does not require antibiotics.
- Mild bacterial gastroenteritis also subsides by itself but some infections like typhoid, cholera and amebic dysentery need antibiotics.

Antidiarrheal agents: These agents are the group of drugs used to relieve symptoms of diarrhea and the effects of it but do not cure the problem.

Composition: Nalidixic acid with metronidazole.

Action:
- **Opium preparations**: Inhibits peristalsis by acting on the brain. Decreases expulsive contractions and increases anal sphincter and ileocecal valve tone.
- **Synthetic opiates**: Decreases GI motility by depressing intestine muscle action.
- **Absorbents:** Binds with toxins to sooth intestinal mucosa.

Dosage: 1 tablet of 500 mg twice daily for 5–10 days.

Route: IV orally.

Indications/uses:
- Treatment of dysentery and diarrhea.
- Amebic infections.
- Appendicitis and cholecystitis like other GI infections.

- Postoperative infections.
- Bronchiectasis.
- Lung abscess.
- Empyema.
- Cystic fibrosis.
- Acute and chronic bone and joint infections.
- Diabetic infections, especially of the foot.
- Infections in immunocompromised patients.
- Patients taking steroids.
- Anticancer drugs or antimetabolites.
- Chronic diarrhea in HIV patients.
- Irritable bowel syndrome.
- Ulcerative colitis.
- Ileocolitis.
- Symptomatic relief of diarrhea.

Contraindications:
- Hypersensitivity
- Children below 2 years
- Porphyria.
- Intestinal and urinal obstruction.
- Atropine intolerance.
- Jaundice.
- Acute infective diarrhea.
- Ulcerative colitis.
- Electrolyte imbalance.
- Pregnancy and lactation.

Drug interactions:
- Disulfiram like reaction when used with alcohol.
- Probenecid reduces urinary excretion of antidiarrheal drug.
- Effects of oral anticoagulant are increased.
- Theophylline level increases.
- Nitrofurantoin antagonizes the effect of drug.

Side effects:
- Nausea.
- Headache.
- Dizziness.
- Fatigue.
- Abdominal pain.
- Discomfort.
- Dyspepsia.
- Insomnia.
- Heart burn.

- Metallic taste.
- Anorexia.
- Drowsiness.
- Lethargy.

Adverse effects:
- Fecal impaction.
- Constipation.
- Dysphoria.
- Abdominal distension.
- Skin rashes or allergy.
- Dry mouth.

Toxicity: No systemic toxicity.

Role of nurse:
- Assess fluid and electrolyte loss.
- Notify physician if diarrhea persists for more than 48 hours.
- If food poisoning is suspected avoid the use of antidiarrheals. Since toxic substances need to exit GI tract.
- Allow patient to use lot of fluids and electrolytes.

Histamine

"Histos tissue" is an amine formed in many tissues.
- Histamine is present in animal as well as plants.
- Venom of bees and wasps contains histamine.
- Mast cells release large quantities of this agent.
- Tissue injury causes release of histamine.
  It is said to be responsible for symptoms of allergy and anaphylactic shock. There are three types of receptors, on which histamine acts: H1R, H2R, H3R and H4R.
- Histamine is released:
  - By drugs such as morphine, d-tubocurarine and chlortetracycline.
  - By especially cold and chemical injury.
  - Allergic conditions: Antigen antibody reactions.
  - By proteolytic enzymes.

Action:
- Histamine dilates the smaller blood vessels.
- It constricts larger blood vessels.
- Produces fall in blood pressure of short duration.
- When injected into skin it produces itching, pain and various other changes collectively called triple response.
  - Vasodilation producing flush or reddening of the area.
  - Flare-spread of redness and edema formation.

- Smooth muscles of the bronchi and gut are contracted by these agents.
- Due to stimulation of H, receptors
  - It produces cardiac irregularities-ventricular tachycardia
  - Secretions of gastric juice are increased.
  - Secretions of all exocrine glands, pancreatic, bronchial salivary and lachrimal are increased.

Dose: 0.5 mg/kg.

Route: IV. orally

Indications:
- For diagnose of achlorhydria and pernicious anemia.
- In diagnosis of leprosy.
- Rarely, it is employed for diagnosis of pheochromocytoma.
- Meniere's syndrome.

Contraindications:
- Peptic ulcer.
- Bronchial asthma.

Side effects:
- Bronchial asthma.
- Headache.
- Visual disturbances.

Adverse reactions: Effect on gastric secretions is more marked than other effects. Therefore, the adverse reactions are limited.

Histamine H_2 Antagonists

These drugs block histamine effects on acid producing cells of stomach to decrease acid production in the stomach. Histamines are well absorbed after oral and IM administration. These are metabolized in liver and eliminated by the kidneys.

Action: Inhibits the action of histamine at the H, receptor site located primarily in gastric parietal cells, resulting in inhibition of gastric acid secretion.

In addition, ranitidine bismuth citrate has some antibacterial action against *H. pylori*.

Indications:
- Short-term treatment of active duodenal ulcers and benign gastric ulcers.
- Prophylaxis of duodenal ulcer
- Management of GERD

- Treatment and prevention of heart burn, acid indigestion, sour stomach.
- Management of gastric hypersecretory states.
- Prevention and treatment of stress-induced upper GI bleeding in critically ill patients.
- Management of GI symptoms associated with the use of NSAIDs side effects.
- Prevention of stress ulceration.
- Aspiration pneumonitis.
- Prevention of acid inactivation of supplemental pancreatic enzymes in patients with pancreas insufficiency.
- Management of urticaria.
- Severe esophagitis.

Contraindications:
- Hypersensitivity
- Cross-sensitivity may occur
- Porphyria
- Renal impairment
- Geriatric patients
- Pregnancy or lactation

Adverse reactions and side effects:
- Confusion
- Dizziness
- Drowsiness
- Hallucinations
- Headache
- Arrhythmias
- Altered taste
- Black tongue
- Constipation
- Dark stools
- Diarrhea
- Drug-induced hepatitis
- Nausea
- Decreased sperm count
- Impotence
- Gynecomastia
- Agranulocytosis
- Aplastic anemia
- Neutropenia
- Thrombocytopenia

- ❖ Hypersensitivity
- ❖ Vasculitis
- ❖ Pain at IM site.

Indications:
- ❖ Clarithromycin increases ranitidine levels.
- ❖ Cimetidine inhibits drug metabolizing enzymes.
- ❖ All agents decrease absorption of ketoconazole.
- ❖ Antacids and sucralfate decrease absorption of all age.

Dosage:
1. **Cimetidine:** 300–600 mg BD: q4hr, q6hr.
2. **Famotidine**: 20–40 mg OD, BD, q6hr.
3. **Nizatidine**: 150–300 mg BD.
4. **Ranitidine**: 150–300 mg OD, BD.

Route: IV, IM, oral.

Toxicity: These drugs may increase the levels and toxicity with the following: Benzodiazepines, beta-blockers, calcium channel blockers, carbamazepine, chloroquine, quinidine, metformin and phenytoin.

Nursing care:
- ❖ If antacids or sucralfate are used concurrently for relief of pain, avoid administration of antacids, within 30 min–1 hour of the histamine H, antagonist and take sucralfate 2 hours after histamine H_2 antagonist; may decrease the absorption of histamine H, antagonists.
- ❖ Administer with meals or immediately afterward and at bedtime to prolong effect.
- ❖ Doses administered once daily should be administered at bedtime to prolong effect.
- ❖ Cimetidine tablets have a characteristic odor.
- ❖ Shake oral suspension before administration. Discard unused suspension after 30 days.
- ❖ Remove foil from ranitidine tablets, dissolve in 6–8 OZ water before drinking.
- ❖ Instruct patient to take medication as directed for the full course of therapy, even if feeling better. Take missed doses as soon as remembered but not if almost time for next dose. Do not double doses.
- ❖ Advise patients taking OTC preparations not to take the maximum dose continuously for more than 2 weeks without consulting healthcare professional.

- Encourage patient to quit smoking or at least not to smoke after last dose of the day.
- Caution patient to avoid driving or other activities requiring alertness response to the drug in known.
- Advise patient to avoid alcohol, products containing aspirin or NSAIDs and foods that may cause an increase in GI irritation.
- Inform patient that increased fluid and fiber intake and exercise may minimize constipation.
- Advise patient to report onset of black, tarry stools, fever, sore throat, diarrhea, dizziness, rash, confusion or hallucinations to healthcare professional promptly.

BASIC IDEA OF ANTIMICROBIALS

Antimicrobials

Antimicrobials—including antibiotics, antivirals, antifungals and antiparasitics—are medicines used to prevent and treat infections in humans, animals and plants.

An **antimicrobial** is an agent that kills microorganisms or stops their growth. Antimicrobial medicines can be grouped according to the microorganisms they act primarily against. For example, antibiotics are used against bacteria, and antifungals are used against fungi. They can also be classified according to their function. Agents that kill microbes are **microbicides**, while those that merely inhibit their growth are called bacteriostatic agents. The use of antimicrobial medicines to treat infection is known as antimicrobial chemotherapy, while the use of antimicrobial medicines to prevent infection is known as antimicrobial prophylaxis.

The main classes of antimicrobial agents are disinfectants (non-selective agents, such as bleach), which kill a wide range of microbes on nonliving surfaces to prevent the spread of illness, antiseptics (which are applied to living tissue and help reduce infection during surgery), and antibiotics (which destroy microorganisms within the body). The term "antibiotic" originally described only those formulations derived from living microorganisms but is now also applied to synthetic agents, such as sulfonamides or fluoroquinolones. Though the term used to be restricted to antibacterials (and is often used as a synonym for them by medical professionals and in medical literature), its context has broadened to include all antimicrobials. Antibacterial agents can be further subdivided into bactericidal agents, which kill bacteria, and bacteriostatic agents, which slow down or stall bacterial growth. In response, further advancements in antimicrobial technologies have resulted in solutions that can go beyond simply inhibiting microbial growth. Instead, certain types of porous media have been developed to kill microbes on contact.

Treating Infections: Selective Toxicity

The aim of antimicrobial therapy is to kill or inhibit the infecting organism without damaging the host; this is known as selective toxicity. This is commonly accomplished through the use of antimicrobial drugs. The terminology surrounding the drugs used to treat infections is complex; a strict definition of the term antibiotic, for example, is that it is a substance produced by one living organism that kills or inhibits the growth of another. This definition excludes completely synthetic products which are antimicrobials, a broader term referring to any substance that has this effect.

Many of the antimicrobials in common use are true antibiotics, being isolated from bacteria and fungi, but some are not. For example, penicillin is made by a number of fungi in the genus *Penicillium* and vancomycin by a bacterium known as *Amycolatopsis orientalis*, and both are therefore true antibiotics, while ciprofloxacin and linezolid are synthetic products and so are technically antimicrobials. Some drugs, such as the newer penicillins, are semisynthetic, which means that they have a natural base that has been altered synthetically. In practice this makes very little difference, but it does have implications for the development of resistance, as it means that some resistance genes are found in the producing organism or the environment; for example, a bacterium producing an antibacterial substance must itself be resistant to the substance it is producing if it is not to kill itself. From a resistance perspective, this becomes problematic if these resistance genes spread into medically significant bacteria.

The aim of selective toxicity means that pharmaceutical companies developing antimicrobials have to identify structures or metabolic processes in the microorganism that is different to or absent from the host. In the case of bacteria, our evolutionary relationship is distant meaning we have had a lot of time to evolve to be different and there are many selective targets; however, this is not the case with fungi to which we are relatively similar on a cellular basis. Viruses present a more difficult problem again, as they do not have their own metabolic or growth capabilities; instead, they use those of the host cell; technically, they are known as obligate intracellular organisms. Therefore, damaging viruses or preventing their growth usually means damaging the infected host cells, and while the immune system is able to differentiate infected from non-infected cells, it is more difficult to find drugs that are able to do this. This explains why drug formularies contain many antibacterial drugs and far fewer antifungal and antiviral drugs and why some of the latter are associated with the toxicities and adverse effects resulting from poor selective toxicity; that is they damage the microorganism but also the host. Protozoa are even more problematic because they often have a complex life cycle, are relatively similar to human cells in many respects, and are often found in developing countries with limited healthcare budgets.

Bacteria

Many serious infections are caused by bacteria, and the first task in their treatment is their identification. There are many ways of identifying bacteria, for example, by shape; by their ability to take up and retain certain stains, (e.g., Gram's stain); by their susceptibility to antimicrobials (antibiogram); or, increasingly, by molecular methods. The first three of these are known as phenotypic traits, that is, they are observable characteristics; the latter are genotypic, being based on bacterial genetics. Although most tests used in everyday practice identify phenotypic characteristics, molecular and genetic methods such as the polymerase chain reaction (PCR) are becoming increasingly important.

Bacteria are prokaryotes, that is, they do not have a nucleus and, consequently, are relatively simple organisms. Because they are only distantly related to humans, there are a lot of selective targets, some of the more important of which are given in **Table 2.5**. The bacterial cell wall is an important target because it is a structure that is lacking from human cells and is made of a substance known as peptidoglycan, which again human cells do not have; thus, it is a very good selective target. Bacterial ribosomes are a target not because these are lacking in humans, but because they are of different sizes, so most drugs that bind to bacterial ribosomes do not bind to the human equivalents. Similarly, some of the enzymes involved in the reproduction of bacterial nucleic acid are different to their equivalents in humans. Folic acid synthesis is an example of a metabolic process that differs between bacteria and humans; while bacteria synthesise their own folic acid, humans gain theirs from the diet. Hence, blocking the synthesis of folic acid production is selective against bacteria.

The evolutionarily distant relationship of bacteria to humans means that there are lots of differences between human and bacterial cells and so lots of selective targets. However, the clinician still needs to identify the infecting organism, establish the best treatment and

Table 2.5: Common targets in bacteria (Tenover, 2006).

Target and mode of action	Examples of drug groups	Examples of drugs
Damage cell wall	β-lactams	Penicillins, cephalosporins
	Glycopeptides	Vancomycin
	β-lactam with β-lactamase inhibitor	Amoxicillin/clavulanic acid (co-amoxiclav)
Prevent protein synthesis by binding to ribosome	Macrolides	Erythromycin
	Chloramphenicol	Chloramphenicol
	Lincosamides	Clindamycin
	Streptogramins	Quinupristin-dalfopristin
	Oxazolidanones	Linezolid
	Aminoglycosides	Gentamicin
	Tetracyclines	Tetracycline
Prevent nucleic acid synthesis	Flouroquinolones	Ciprofloxacin
	Rifampicin	Rifampicin
Inhibit metabolic pathway	Sulfonamides	Sulfamethoxazole
	Folic acid analogues	Trimethoprim
Disrupt membrane structure	Polymyxins	Colistin
	Lipopeptides	Daptomycin

deliver that treatment in a way that can resolve the infection. Although the details differ, many of these principles are common to most infections and are considered later in the chapter.

Fungi

Because fungi are relatively closely related to humans, compared to bacteria, they have had less time to evolve differences, and so fewer selective targets exist **(Table 2.6)**. This means that there are far fewer drugs to treat fungal infections than there are to treat bacterial

Table 2.6: Main antifungal targets.

Target	Drugs
Cell wall—glucan inhibitors	Echinocandins (caspofungin, micafungin)
Cell membrane—ergosterol binders	Polyenes (amphotericin B, nystatin)
Cell membrane—ergosterol inhibitors	Azoles (ketoconazole, itraconazole, fluconazole, voriconazole, posaconazole, ravuconazole)

infections, and many of those which do exist, particularly older antifungal drugs, have toxicities associated with them. A further complication is that many people who have severe systemic fungal diseases also have comorbidities, in particular, immunodeficiencies, further compromising the ability to treat the infection. Fungi can take two main forms: a yeast-like form that usually grows on surfaces and a hyphal form where it grows as finger-like projections that can force their way between cells and so become invasive; this is sometimes referred to as being a 'mould' (one may see these growing on bread). *Candida* species are examples of the former, and *Aspergillus* the latter; in addition, some fungi can take both forms known as dimorphic fungi.

Most antifungal agents work by inhibiting the cell wall or membrane which is the main difference between fungal and human cells. Human cells do not have a cell wall, and the fungal cell wall, which contains glucan and chitin, is the target for a range of drugs. The other main target is ergosterol which is a component of the fungal cell membrane, a structure that humans do have, but in fungi the membrane sterol is ergosterol, in humans the equivalent is cholesterol. Although there is a difference between these two sterols, the difference is not great, reducing the selective toxicity and explaining some of the toxicities associated with the main drugs that bind to this, the polyene drugs amphotericin B and nystatin. Amphotericin, which has historically been the most important drug for treatment of severe fungal disease, has a range of toxicities including nausea, vomiting, rigors, fever and hypotension or hypertension. However, of most concern is its effect upon the renal system, where it can cause nephrotoxicity, particularly in those individuals with existing renal problems, on high doses, who are dehydrated or on other nephrotoxic drugs.

These adverse effects are reduced in those drugs that inhibit its production rather than bind to it and in liposomal preparations where the amphotericin molecules are enclosed in a lipid membrane. Additionally, polyenes are not absorbed through the gastrointestinal tract, making nystatin a safe drug for the topical treatment of superficial fungal infections. Less commonly used drugs include flucytosine which inhibits fungal nucleic acid synthesis, griseofulvin which has the same effect upon microtubules and the polyoxins and nikkomycin which inhibit chitin in the fungal cell wall.

Viruses

Viruses are simple organisms that have no metabolism of their own. Consequently, they have to use the metabolism of host cells to replicate, making them obligate intracellular pathogens.

This is problematic for treating viral infections because it means there are few selective targets, and while the immune system is able to differentiate infected from noninfected cells, it is hard to produce drugs that can damage or inhibit infected cells while leaving uninfected cells alone; and targeting all cells would lead to severe toxicity or even death. Consequently, most therapies in this area have tended to maximize immunity through immunization rather than treat established infections.

Viruses that can most successfully be treated are usually those which have something in their structure or replication cycle which is different to or not found in human cells. The first viruses to be successfully treated were the herpes viruses, in particular, cytomegalovirus (CMV), varicella-zoster virus (VZV) and herpes simplex virus type 1 (HSV1) and type 2 (HSV2). These can be treated using drugs such as acyclovir that inhibit viral DNA polymerase, which is the enzyme that copies viral DNA during replication. Its selective toxicity stems from its specificity for the viral polymerase rather than the human equivalent, and because the drugs are inactive in the form given needing to be activated by phosphorylation which is preferentially done by a viral enzyme known as thymidine kinase. Although humans also have this enzyme, the drug is specific for the viral version, hence its selective toxicity.

The treatment of influenza has undergone major changes in recent years. Earlier treatments, such as amantadine and rimantadine which are Matrix-2 (M2) inhibitors, are acted by binding to a viral protein; however, these are not recommended for general use today. Newer drugs in use today inhibit the activity of neuraminidase, which is needed by the virus to leave the infected cell and so complete its replication cycle, the two main drugs being oseltamivir and zanamivir.

Most research in the treatment of viral infections has been undertaken on HIV. HIV is a retrovirus, meaning that it uses a viral-specific enzyme known as reverse transcriptase to turn the viruses RNA genome into DNA which can be integrated into the genome of the infected cell. Although human cells make DNA copies of DNA when cells replicate and RNA copies of DNA for protein production, they never convert RNA to DNA in the way that retroviruses such as HIV do, and because of this reverse transcriptase is a highly selective and important target for anti-HIV drugs. There are two groups of drugs that target this enzyme, the nucleoside reverse transcriptase inhibitors (NRTI) and the non-nucleoside reverse transcriptase inhibitors (NNRTI). Another viral enzyme, protease, is the third major target as it is required for viral assembly and maturation and is again different to human enzymes. Drugs that target this enzyme are known as protease inhibitors (PIs).

Newer drugs target the process of viral binding and entry into the cell and the viral integrase enzyme that inserts viral DNA into the cellular genome. The former group is particularly important, as these drugs have the potential to prevent cells becoming infected in the first place, not merely preventing or reducing viral replication after infection. In order to maximize the effectiveness of these drugs and to reduce the risk of resistance developing, they are given in combinations of at least three drugs from two of the groups; these combinations are known as (highly active antiretroviral therapy or ART/HAART).

Different approaches to treating viruses are shown in the treatment of hepatitis B and C viruses. Because hepatitis B has both RNA and DNA polymerases, some of the reverse transcriptase inhibitors used for the treatment of HIV also have activity against it. Other approaches to the treatment of this virus and hepatitis C virus include therapies aimed at improving the immune response, known as immunomodulators; these include drugs such as interferons, which are antiviral substances produced by the body in response to viral infections.

Protozoa and Helminths

Protozoa, like fungi are relatively closely related to humans, and because of this and probably also the fact that most severe protozoal disease is suffered by those in developing countries, there are relatively few treatments for many protozoal diseases. Although it is rare to see severe protozoal disease in most developed countries, on a global scale they are responsible for significant morbidity and mortality. Helminths are worms, which rarely reproduce in humans but are transmitted through the environment and are often asymptomatic in the human host.

The most common protozoal disease is malaria, which in humans is caused by either *Plasmodium falciparum*, *Plasmodium vivax*, *Plasmodium ovale*, *Plasmodium malariae* or *Plasmodium knowlesi*. Because plasmodia are carried and transmitted by a mosquito which is not endemic to most of Europe, primary transmission does not occur here, malaria almost always being an imported disease. Most severe infection is associated with *Plasmodium falciparum*. Because the treatments are complex, and resistance patterns vary widely, it is necessary to consult the current guidelines whenever a case of malaria is encountered.

The most important intervention for the control of malaria is not treatment with drugs but efforts to reduce the incidence of the mosquito that carries the *Plasmodium* protozoa, such as the removal of still water pools, or to separate them from humans, particularly at times when they are most likely to bite, for example, by using bed nets. Visitors to malaria-endemic countries are advised to take antimalarial prophylaxis, but this is not always an option for the indigenous residents.

Delivering the Drug

Choosing the best drug to treat a particular infection is only part of the answer. The next part is to deliver the drug to the site of the infection in sufficient quantities or concentrations to achieve the desired outcome. The science of how drugs move from the site of administration to site of activity and their subsequent elimination is known as pharmacokinetics, while the concentration of the drug as it relates to its clinical effect is known as pharmacodynamics.

As most drugs are taken orally or given intravenously, getting a drug into the bloodstream is relatively straightforward. However, most infections occur in the tissues, and so the drug needs to be able to leave the bloodstream and get to the site of the infection. In some cases, where the blood supply is poor or absent, this can be particularly problematic. For example, the cornea has a limited blood supply, which is why many eye medications are given as eye drops. More problematic can be infections of implantable devices, such as orthopedic implants, necrotic tissue or abscesses, all of which have limited or no blood supply. Therefore, the serum concentration of a drug is unlikely to be representative of the actual concentration at the site of infection, unless this is the bloodstream. One way of remembering this is that whatever the blood results are saying about serum concentrations of antimicrobials, 'it is the tissue that is the issue'.

Another problematic type of infection is that which occurs on hard surfaces, such as orthopedic implants. Layers of bacteria and other microorganisms can form, known as biofilms. While those on the top of the film can be treated, those in the deeper layers of the biofilm are more difficult to treat, partly because of the physical protection of those above, but also because they are often metabolically less active. Biofilms that form on implantable devices, such as orthopedic implants, also benefit from the lack of blood supply making it difficult to deliver sufficient concentrations of the drug to the site of the infection, making them even more difficult to treat successfully.

Biofilms can be extremely complicated, and in some cases a number of different organisms can form a stable and difficult to treat community of organisms.

Antimicrobial Dosing

Most antimicrobial drugs express their effect either through being static, (e.g., bacteriostatic) or cidal (bactericidal). Static drugs stop the organism from growing but do not necessarily kill it; cidal drugs generally kill the microorganism at concentrations that can be achieved clinically.

Antimicrobials may also be concentration or time-dependent. Concentration dependent drugs usually have a longer action, and many are taken up by the target organism. In these cases, the important issue with regard to dosing is not how many doses a patient has, but what concentration of the drug can be achieved, so these are generally given in fewer but larger doses. With time-dependent drugs on the other hand, the important parameter is not the maximum dose, but the length of time that the drug persists above the MIC at the site of infection. These drugs tend to be given in smaller but more frequent doses. Gentamicin is an example of a concentration-dependent drug; hence, it is usually given in one large dose, while penicillin which is time-dependent is normally given a multiple daily doses to maximize its time over the MIC.

In general, the best approach to treatment is to give a single highly targeted antimicrobial. However, there are many exceptions to this rule, for example, in those who are immunosuppressed and for whom waiting for test results is not an option or who might be at an increased risk of polymicrobial infection with more than one organism. In these cases, the treatment approach might be to give combination empirical therapy (empirical meaning treatment based not on test results, but on knowledge and experience of what they are most likely to have). As there is limited information available, such therapies are often less targeted and broad spectrum antimicrobial medications are prescribed (the spectrum referring to the range of organisms targeted by the drug). In addition to broadening the spectrum of the therapy, combinations might also show synergy, that is, the drugs work better together than on their own. However, by increasing the spectrum of the therapy the risk of drug interactions and adverse reactions is increased, as is the cost of the treatment, and more damage is likely to be done to the normal flora of the body, increasing the risk of opportunistic infections such as *C. difficile*.

Resistance

Antimicrobial resistance has become a matter of increasing concern in recent years. It is important to be clear about the difference between intrinsic and acquired resistance. Intrinsic resistance occurs where some feature of an organism means that it is inherently undamaged by an antimicrobial. For example, Gram-negative bacteria have an outer membrane that prevents glycopeptides such as vancomycin from accessing the cell wall where the drug is active, making the bacteria intrinsically resistant to these drugs. This being a feature of this group of bacteria, there is nothing that can be done to prevent this. A more serious problem is that of acquired resistance, where a previously susceptible organism develops a new resistance to one or more groups of antibiotics. The latter is known as multiple resistance and is often seen in MRSA. One particularly concerning development is the acquisition of vancomycin resistance by MRSA, which may already be resistant to a range of antimicrobials including all β-lactams apart from perhaps the new 5th generation cephalosporins which are active against MRSA, macrolides, aminoglycosides, fluoroquinolones and tetracyclines; and for which vancomycin would normally be the treatment of choice.

Bacteria can become resistant in two main ways: the first is that they undergo a genetic mutation that changes an antimicrobial target in some way and the second is that they acquire resistance genes from another bacterium or the environment. While the first of these are chance events, the sheer number of bacteria means that such mutations probably occur quite frequently. Most of these will not cause resistance, and may actually be damaging to the bacterium, but a small number may confer resistance allowing that bacterium to survive or grow in the presence of the antimicrobial.

Probably more problematic than this is the acquisition of resistance genes, either from other bacteria or the environment. This most commonly occurs in one of three ways:
1. Acquisition of resistance genes from the environment, a process known as transformation (remember that many antimicrobials are produced by organisms which therefore need resistance genes to survive their own antibiotic).
2. Transfer of resistance genes from one bacterium to another by viruses, a process known as transduction.
3. The direct physical transfer of resistance genes from one bacterium to another, through a process known as conjugation.

Conjugation usually involves larger genetic elements that may contain a number of different resistance genes, or possible genes for toxins or other traits that aid bacterial survival. There are a number of different types of such genetic elements, the most complex being plasmids which may contain many different genes, and acquisition of such a plasmid by a bacterium might confer multiple resistances upon that bacterium. Plasmids may also contain genes encoding for toxins, in which case the bacterium may be capable of causing severe disease.

The development of resistance is almost inevitable when antimicrobials are used. This is because populations of microorganisms are heterogenous, that is to say all are a little different; for example, some will be very susceptible to an antimicrobial, while others may be a less susceptible. This is sometimes referred to as heteroresistance. Often a resistance mechanism reduces growth rates of organisms that have it, meaning that they are less likely to predominate than their susceptible equivalents. For example, a thickened cell-wall might reduce susceptibility but it might also take longer to grow. However, the use of that antimicrobial, particularly if the dose is not sufficient or it is not given for sufficient time may result in it killing the susceptible organisms but not the less susceptible ones, turning the disadvantage of resistance into an advantage and allowing them to 'take over'. Over time this leads to selection of resistant organism, the use of the antimicrobial resulting in 'selection pressure' for resistance. Although this may seem complicated, it is a simple Darwinian selection occurring as a result of antimicrobial use. This is the reason why antimicrobials are fundamentally different to all other medicines; they have both an individual effect (curing the infection) and a population effect (selection for resistance), and sometimes these conflict. The main mechanisms of resistance are given in **Table 2.7**.

The World Health Organization adopted a global action plan on antimicrobial resistance in 2015 (World Health Organization 2015), which contained five objectives:

1. To improve awareness and understanding of antimicrobial resistance
2. To strengthen the knowledge and evidence base through surveillance and research
3. To reduce the incidence of infection through effective sanitation, hygiene and infection prevention measures
4. To optimize the use of antimicrobial medicines in human and animal health
5. To increase investment in new medicines, diagnostic tools, vaccines and other interventions

Table 2.7: Mechanisms of resistance in bacteria (Giedraitienė et al. 2011; Kapoor et al. 2017).

Category of resistance	Example of resistance	Examples of organisms
Altered target prevents the drug from binding	Altered penicillin binding proteins in cell wall	Methicillin resistant *S. aureus*
	Change in cell wall structure	Glycopeptide resistant *S. aureus*
Decreased permeability or uptake prevents the drug from entering the cell	Change in outer membrane permeability	Multiple resistances in *Pseudomonas aeruginosa*
Efflux mechanisms pump the drug out of the cell	Acquired and chromosomally encoded efflux pumps	*Acinetobacter baumannii* multiple resistance
Enzymatic degradation breaks the drug down or changes its structure	β-lactamase enzymes that degrade β-lactam drugs	*Klebsiella pneumoniae* that produce extended spectrum β-lactamases
Target overproduction overwhelms the drug	Overproduction of cell wall components targeted by glycopeptides	Vancomycin intermediately resistant *S. aureus*

The last point, although perhaps the most obvious, is not without its difficulties, in particular the long development period required for human medicines and the relatively poor financial return that drug companies receive from antimicrobials compared to other drug groups.

Antimicrobial Policies

All healthcare organizations should have an antimicrobial policy, which aims to guide clinicians as to the best and most rational use of these drugs. Such policies have a number of aims, specifically to:
- Ensure that a sufficient range of antimicrobials remain available
- Guide prescribing
- Avoid their unnecessary use
- Reduce the emergence and spread of resistance
- Promote good practice
- Contain costs

Although the exact content will differ between institutions as the type of patient treated and local resistance patterns might vary, they should include guidance as to the treatment of common infections, including dosages and special considerations or cautions, details of who to contact for advice in the treatment of infection and details of restricted drugs, for example, new or expensive drugs, or those which for other reasons such as resistance are restricted. Some of this information is available on a national basis from the British National Formulary or other national formularies, although this needs to be read and interpreted in light of local conditions.

BASIC IDEA OF ANTIHISTAMINE AND CORTICOSTEROIDS

Antihistamine

Antihistamine is histamine antagonist. They can be H_1 receptor blocker and H_2 receptor block. Drugs that completely block H_1 histamine receptors are conventionally called the antihistamine. H_2 blockers are used in the treatment of peptic ulcer.

Indication of Antihistamines
- Allergic reactions
- Common cold
- Motion sickness
- Antiemetic
- Preanesthetic medication
- Hypnotic
- Parkinsonism
- Cough
- Purities

Classification of H_1 Blockers
- **First generations (sedative):**
    - Diphenhydramine
    - Dimenhydrinate
    - Promethazine
    - Pheniramine
    - Chlorpheniramine
    - Cyclizine
    - Meclizine
    - Buclizine
    - Mepyramine
    - Tripelennamine
- **Second generation (non-sedative):**
    - Fexofenadine
    - Loratadine

- Desloratadine
- Cetirizine
- Levocetirizine
- Acrivastine
- Azelastine
- Mizoplastine
- Levocabastine
- Mequitazine

Corticosteroids

Corticosteroids do not relax airway smooth muscles directly but reduce bronchial reactivity, increase airway caliber, suppress inflammatory response to antigen antibody reaction or triggers stimuli and reduce the frequency of asthma exacerbation.

Systemic Steroids

Systemic steroids are used in both severe chronic asthma and in acute emergency of asthma, e.g.:
- Hydrocortisone
- Prednisolone

Inhalational Steroid

Inhalational steroid beclomethasone is a halogenated corticosteroid ester used in aerosol form. It suppresses asthma by a topical anti-inflammatory action without causing any systemic side effects, e.g.:
- Budesonide
- Beclomethasone dipropionate
- Fluticasone propionate

▮ DRUG USED IN TREATMENT OF ANEMIA

Hematinics

Hematinics are compound require in the formation of blood and employed in the treatment of anemias. Hematinics include iron, vitamin B_{12} and folic acid.

Hematopoietic growth factors are also discussed here.

Iron: Iron, vitamin B_{12} and folic acids are essential for normal erythropoiesis. Iron is essential for hemoglobin production. Total body iron is about 2.5–5 g two-third of which is present in hemoglobin.

Doses of Iron is Calculated using a Formula

Iron requirement [mg = 4.4 × body weight (kg) × Hb deficit (g/dL)]

Oral Iron Preparations

Iron preparations are available as ferrous and ferric salts.
- ❖ Ferrous sulfate—200 mg tab
- ❖ Ferrous fumarate—200 mg tab
- ❖ Ferrous gluconate—300 mg tab
- ❖ Ferrous succinate—100 mg
- ❖ Iron calcium complex—5% iron
- ❖ Ferric ammonium citrate—45 mg
    - Expensive preparations of iron with vitamins, liver extract, amino acids, etc., are available but have no obvious benefits.
    - Dose: Ferrous sulfate 200 mg thrice daily. The elemental iron content of different varies. If ferrous sulfate is not well tolerated, may change to ferrous gluconate 300 mg twice daily.
    - Though iron absorption is better when taken on an empty stomach, gastric irritation is more and therefore should be given along with food.

Adverse Effects of Oral Iron

Epigastric pain, nausea, vomiting, gastritis, metallic taste, constipation (due to astringent effect) or diarrhea (irritant effect) is the usual adverse effects. Liquid preparations of iron cause staining of the teeth. Patients should be informed that there would be blackening of stools.

Parenteral Iron

Iron can be administered parenterally as deep IM injection or intravenously.

Indications for parenteral iron are:
- ❖ When oral iron is not tolerated
- ❖ Failure of absorption—as in malabsorption, chronic bowel disease
- ❖ Noncompliance
- ❖ Severe deficiency with bleeding
- ❖ Patients of gastrectomy
- ❖ Patients receiving erythropoietin—oral iron absorption may not be enough.

Preparations

Intramuscular injection of iron is given deep IM in the gluteal region using "z" technique to avoid staining of the skin. Intravenous iron is given slowly over 5-10 minutes or as infusion after a test dose.
- ❖ **Iron dextran** has 50 mg elemental iron/mL (2 mL ampoule). It is the only preparation that can be given intravenously. It can also be given deep IM. Hypersensitivity reactions to iron dextran can be

serious but not very common. A test dose of 0.5 mL of iron dextran is injected slowly over 5-10 minutes. Patients should be constantly monitored for signs of allergy.
- **Iron sucrose and sodium ferric gluconate** can be given IV. Allergy is lower than with iron dextran.
- **Iron-sorbitol-citric acid complex** contains 50 mg elemental iron/mL; given only IM. This preparation should not be given IV because it quickly saturates the transferrin stores. As a result, free iron levels in the plasma rises and can cause toxicity.

Ferric Carboxymaltose and Ferumoxytol

Two parenteral preparations enclosed in a carbohydrate shell have been introduced. Ferumoxytol is an aqueous preparation containing super paramagnetic iron oxide nanoparticle which is coated with a carbohydrate.

Disadvantage: It interfere with MRI for 3 months after the last dose and the patient should be educated to inform the radiologist if any MRI is needed.

Adverse effects of parenteral iron:
- **Local**: Pain at the site of injection, pigmentation of the skin and sterile abscess.
- **Systemic:** Fever, headache, joints pain, palpitation, difficulty in breathing, lymph node enlargement and rarely anaphylaxis.
- **Acute iron poisoning** is common in infant and children in whom about 10 tablets (1-2 can be lethal. Manifestations include vomiting abdominal pain, hematemesis, bloody diarrhea, shock, drowsiness, cyanosis, acidosis, dehydration, cardiovascular collapse and coma. Immediate diagnosis and treatment are important as death may occur in 6-12 hours.

Treatment
- Gastric lavage with sodium bicarbonate solution.
- **Desferrioxamine** is the antidote. It is instilled into the stomach after lavage, to prevent iron absorption; injected IV/IM.
- Correction of acidosis and shock.

Treatment of Anemia

Indications for Iron

Iron-deficiency anemia—both for the prophylaxis and treatment. The cause for iron deficiency should be identified. Based on patients' condition and need, oral or parenteral iron has to be given.

Treatment should be continued depending on the response for 3-6 months to replenish iron store. Prophylactically iron is given in conditions with increased iron requirement as in pregnancy, infancy and professional blood donors.

Treatment of Megaloblastic Anemia

Vitamin B_{12} and Folic Acid

Vitamin B_{12} and folic acid are water soluble vitamins, belonging to the B-complex group. They are essential for normal DNA synthesis. Their deficiency leads to impaired DNA synthesis and abnormal maturation of RBCs and other rapidly dividing cells. This results in megaloblastic anemia, characterized by the presence of red cell precursors in the blood and bone marrow. Vitamin B_{12} and folic acid are therefore called maturation factors. Other manifestations of deficiency include glossitis, stomatitis and malabsorption; neurological manifestations can also result.

Vitamin B_{12}

Vitamin B_{12} (cyanocobalamin) is synthesized by microorganisms. Liver, fish, egg yolk, meat, cheese and pulses are the dietary sources of vitamin B_{12} or extrinsic factor is absorbed with the help of intrinsic factor, a protein secreted by the stomach. It is carried in the plasma by B_{12} binding protein called transcobalamin and is store in the liver.

Functions vitamin B_{12}, and folic acid act as coenzymes for several vital metabolic reactions and are essential for DNA synthesis. Vitamin B_{12} deficiency may be due to:

- ❖ **Addisonian pernicious anemia:** Thomas Addison first described cases of anemia not responding to iron. There is deficiency of intrinsic factor due to destruction of parietal cells resulting in failure of B_{12} absorption.
- ❖ **Other causes:**
  - Gastrectomy
  - Chronic gastritis
  - Malabsorption
  - Fish tapeworm infestation (fish tapeworm consumes B_{12})

Symptoms: Abnormal maturation of RBCs result in megaloblastic anemia, with glossitis, stomatitis, malabsorption, lethargy, palpitation, vertigo, neurological symptoms, such as paresthesia of hands and feet, ataxia, loss of memory, confusion and in more severe cases, hallucination and psychosis.

Preparations: Cyanocobalamin—100 mg/mL injection may be given IM or deep SC—hypersensitivity reactions can occur.
- Hydroxocobalamin—100, 500, 1000 mg/mL injection has longer lasting effect but hydroxocobalamin administration can result in the formation of antibodies.
- Multivitamin preparations contain variable amounts of vitamin B with/without intrinsic factor for oral use.
- Sublingual vitamin B is now available and may be absorbed better.

Uses:
- **Vitamin B deficiency:** Prophylaxis and treatment of megaloblastic anemia due to B deficiency of any cause. If B deficiency is due to lack of intrinsic factor, it is given IM or SC. Pernicious anemia needs lifelong treatment with B. Oral folic acid should be added because B induced brisk hemopoiesis may also increase the demand for folic acid. Prophylactic dose of vitamin B is 3–10 mg daily.
- **B neuropathies,** such as subacute combined degeneration respond to vitamin B.
- **Vitamin B** is also tried in conditions, such as trigeminal neuralgia, multiple sclerosis and some psychiatric disorders and general weakness.

Folic Acid

Folic acid was first isolated from spinach and therefore named as folic acid (from leaf).
- **Dietary source:** Green vegetables, liver, yeast egg, milk and some fruits. Prolonged cooking with spices destroys folic acid.
- **Absorption** takes place in the duodenum and jejunum and is transported in the blood by active and passive transport, widely distributed in the body and is stored in the liver.
- **Functions:** Folic acid is converted to dihydrofolic acid and then to tetrahydrofolic acid which serves as a coenzyme for many vital (one-carbon transfer) reactions necessary for DNA synthesis.
- **Deficiency:** Folate deficiency may be due to dietary folate deficiency, malabsorption and other diseases of the small intestine or drug induced. Phenytoin, phenobarbitone, oral contraceptives, methotrexate and trimethoprim can induce folate deficiency.

ANESTHETICS AGENT

Anesthetics are agents that bring about reversible loss of sensation. They may be general or local.

General Anesthetics

General anesthetics are drugs that bring about reversible loss of sensation and consciousness.

Stages of General Anesthesia

- **Stage of analgesia:** This is from the beginning of inhalation of the anesthetic to loss of consciousness.
- **Stages of delirium:** This stage is from loss of consciousness to beginning of surgical anesthesia.
- **Stage of general anesthesia:** This has four planes. As anesthesia passes to deeper planes, respiratory depression is seen there is gradual loss of reflexes and relaxation of skeletal muscles.
- **Stage of modularly paralysis:** Is seen only with overdose. It is the stage of medullary depression sensation of breathing, circulatory failure of death may follow.

Classification

Inhalational

- **Gases:** Nitrous oxide, cyclopropane, xenon
- **Liquid:** Ether, halothane, enflurane is fluorine methoxyflurane, desflurane, sevoflurane.

Intravenous

- **Inducing agent:** Thiopentone, sodium, methohexital, propofol, etomidate
- **Dissociative anesthesia:** Vitamin
- **Neuroleptanalgesia:** Fentanyl + droperidol
- **Benzodiazepines:** Diazepam, lorazepam, midazolam

Inhalation Anesthetics

Nitrous oxide is a gas with a slightly and wheatish order. It produces light anesthesia without significant depression of respiration or vasomotor center. It has the disadvantage that it produced light anesthesia and therefore, it can be used along with other anesthesia. Long-term exposure to low doses can impair DNA synthesis which may result in fetal abnormalities when such lady staff becomes pregnant.

Ether

Is a colorless volatile liquid. It is a patient of reliable anesthetic good analgesic, muscle relaxant and do not depress cardiovascular respiration of function in therapeutic doses.

Disadvantage
Ether has the disadvantage that it is highly inflammable, vipers are irritant and induction and recovery are slow.

Halothane
Is a colorless volatile liquid with a sweet order, and it is nonirritant and noninflammable.

Advantages:
- Potent, noninflammable anesthetic.
- Induction is smooth of rapid in 2–5 min surgical anesthesia can be produced
- Nonirritant and their force does not payment salary of bronchial secretions
- Recovery is rapid.
- Chances of past per active cause of vomiting are less.

Disadvantage: Halothane is a direct myocardial depressant cardiac output and BP start filling and heart rate may decrease.

Nitrous oxide
- Also called as laughing gas.
- First prepared by Joseph Priestly in 1774.
- Prepared by heating ammonium nitrate to 270°C

Physical properties:
- Colorless, nonirritating and sweet smelling.
- Biology point: 85 critical temperature 36.5°C.
- Stored as liquid and blue cylinders.

Anesthetic properties:
- Noninflammable, nonexplosive
- Good analgesic
- Not a muscle relaxant

Metabolism:
- Highly soluble in plasma.
- Rapidly eliminated, uncharged through the lungs.
- Does not affect hepatic of renal system.

Uses:
- Used with oxygen for anesthesia along with muscle relaxant and analgesia.
- As analgesics in obstetrics, dental pain, burn, dressing, acute trauma.

Contraindications:
- Pneumothorax
- Middle ear surgeries

- ❖ Pneumoperitoneum
- ❖ Eye surgeries

Oxygen
- ❖ First synthesized by Priestly.
- ❖ Medical oxygen is prepared by fraction distillation of air.
- ❖ Medical oxygen is stored in block cylinder at pressure of 2000 (pounds per square inch)
- ❖ **Chemical formula:** Oxygen has two attains forming the formula O_2

Physical properties:
- ❖ Odorless and colorless.
- ❖ **Specific gravity:** 1.527
- ❖ **Boiling points:** 183
- ❖ **Critical temperature:** 119
- ❖ Not inflammable gas.

Uses:
- ❖ Anesthesia is only with nitrous oxide.
- ❖ In hypoxia.
- ❖ A cute respiratory distress.
- ❖ Methods of oxygen therapy

Venturi mask:
- ❖ It is high flow delivery system.
- ❖ Delivery accurate and oxygen can be controlled.
- ❖ The respiratory gas flows should be 3–4 times of minute volume.

Oxygen mask:
- ❖ Very commonly used in words.
- ❖ Maximum concentration of oxygen which can be delivered by this method is 60% at oxygen flow rate 7–8 liters/minutes.

Nasal cannula:
- ❖ The tip of nasal cannula should lie in nasopharynx
- ❖ Maximum oxygen delivered by this method is 44%.

Non-breathing mask: Delivered up to 80% of oxygen.

Re-breathing mask: When tightly fitted can provide approximately 100% oxygen.

Oxygen tents:
- ❖ Used in children.
- ❖ Very comfortable and oxygen can be given for longer periods.

Endotracheal intubation: Done at the time of anesthesia with the help of endotracheal tube by connectivity into the breathing circuit.

Side effect:
- ❖ At high pressure it may lead to long fibrosis.
- ❖ In premature neonates may lead to retrolental fibroplasias.

Intravenous Anesthetics

Thiopentone sodium: Chemically, it is sodium ethyl thiobarbiturate

Advantages
- ❖ Rapid induction and recovery.
- ❖ Nonirritant to respiratory mucosa.

Disadvantages
- ❖ Causes hypotension
- ❖ Respiratory of cardiovascular depression.
- ❖ Causes laryngospasm and burn caspasm.
- ❖ Causes postoperative disorientation

Dose
5 mg/1 kg body out

Uses
- ❖ In induction of anesthesia.
- ❖ As an adjuvant to N_2O.
- ❖ In sport operative procedure.

Contraindication
- ❖ Thin veins
- ❖ Respiratory diseases

Propofol: Chemically consist of fingering with isopropyl group.

Advantages
- ❖ Rapid and smooth recovery.
- ❖ Completely eliminated from body in 4 hours
- ❖ Antiemetic
- ❖ Antipruritic

Disadvantages
- ❖ Server hypotension.
- ❖ Injection is painful.
- ❖ Chances of sepsis with contained solution.
- ❖ Na antianalgesic properties.

Dose: 5 mg/kg body weight.

Uses
- ❖ Induction of anesthesia.
- ❖ In day care surgery.

- ❖ To produce sedation in ICU.
- ❖ In combination combination with inhalant inhalant anesthesia.

Contraindication
- ❖ Obstetrics procedures
- ❖ Children and elderly routes
- ❖ Low BP

Ketamine hydrochloride:
- ❖ Synthesized by stands in 1962 and first—used in humans by domino and larger in 1965.
- ❖ Chemically, it is phencyclidine derivative.
- ❖ Available as solution of 10 mg /mL and 50 mg/mL concentration.

Advantages
- ❖ Rapid induction.
- ❖ Early regain of consciousness.
- ❖ Very good for induction in shock.
- ❖ Patient bronchodilators
- ❖ Good for pediatric patients.

Disadvantages
- ❖ Incidence of hallucinations and emergencies reaction is high.
- ❖ Increases muscle tone.
- ❖ Pharyngeal and respiratory secretion are increased.

Contraindication
- ❖ Head injury.
- ❖ Ischemic heart disease.
- ❖ Vascular aneurysm.
- ❖ Hypertension.
- ❖ Patient with psychiatric diseases.

Opioids drug
Fentanyl:
- ❖ Very commonly used opioid in anesthesia.
- ❖ 100 times more patient than morphine.

Advantages
- ❖ Rapid onset and rapid recovery.
- ❖ Opioid of choice for hepatic and renal diseases.
- ❖ With bupivacaine used epidural for painless labor.

Disadvantages
- ❖ Respiration depression.
- ❖ Chest wall rigidity.
- ❖ Used for induction of anesthesia.

Pentazocine (Fortwin)
- Against at copper and delta receptors and antiaging at mu receptor.
- Mainly act on receptor at spinal level.
- 1/3 as patient as morphine.

Commonly used as:
- Analgesic in moderate to seven pain.
- Preanesthetic medication.
- Pre and postoperative medication.

Doses
- 30-60 mg IM.
- 30 mg IV.
- Maximum dose is 360 mg/day.
- Not recommended in children below year
- Contraindicated in head injury/brain damage.

Side effects:
- Sedation.
- Nausea.
- Constipation.
- Vomiting.
- Dizziness.

Morphine Sulfate
- A potent of narcotic analgesic.
- Produce strange analgesic without loss of memory or motor functions.
- It reduce awareness of anxiety.

Disadvantages
- Causes respiratory dispersion.
- Hypotension due to deserved central sympathetic tone.
- Nausea and vomiting.
- Incompletes anesthesia.
- Muscle rigidity.

Uses
- As analgesic.
- For induction in codpiece patient.
- As an adjunct in general anesthesia.

Pethidine
- An atropine confessor
- One tenth patient than morphine

Advantages
- Effective narcotic analgesic.

- Mild hyponastic action.
- Increases the action of anesthesia is reduced.
- Slight effect on cough and respiration.
- Negligible effect on heart.

Disadvantages
- Dizziness.
- Blurred vision, dryness of mouth sweating.
- Excitement and copulations.
- Used as analgesic and premedication drugs.

Local Anesthetic

The loss of sensation produced by blocking the pain sensation at the site gift origin by injecting the drug into the ensue or in the vicinity of drug is called as local anesthesia.

Methods of Local Anesthesia

Local Infiltration/Infection

- The local anesthetic drug in infiltrated into the skin and subcutaneous tissue at the site of incision.
- For better effect an intradermal wheal should be raised along the site of injection and then the drug should be slowly injected deep to the incisional site and well around it.

Used for:
- Applying superficial skin stitched.
- Reappearing superficial wound.
- Excision of small cysts/lesions.

Topical Anesthesia

Pain sensation in the superficial peripheral nerves is depressed by for endotracheal intubation.

Used for:
- As pain killer spray/ointment/jelly.
- As solution spray on the respiratory passage for endotracheal intubation.
- Laryngoscope.
- Bronchoscope.

Advantages
- Simple and safe.
- Minimum recovery times.

- Normal movement continues after the procedure.
- Patient stays conscious.

Disadvantages
- Needs quality of sedation.
- For desired effect too much dry is required.
- Overdose may cause toxicity.

Contraindication
- Allergy to the dry.
- Apprehensive patient.
- Vicinity of malignancy.

Local Anesthesia

Classification
- Based on chemical structures
- Classified as amino esters and amino amides

Amino Esters
- Procaine
- Benzocaine
- Tetracaine
- Chloroprocaine
- Cocaine

Amino Amides
- Lidocaine
- Bupivacaine
- Mepivacaine
- Etidocaine
- Psilocin
- Ropivacaine

Based on Duration Action and Potency

Short Duration Low Potency
- Chloroprocaine.
- Shortest duration.
- Procaine.

Intermediate Duration into Immediate Potency
- Lignocaine
- Psilocin

- ❖ Mepivacain
- ❖ Cocaine

Long Duration High Potency
- ❖ Bupivacaine
- ❖ Dibucaine
- ❖ Tetracaine
- ❖ Ropivacaine
- ❖ Etidocaine

Commonly used in divided agents:
- ❖ Lignocaine (xylocaine/lidocaine)
- ❖ Most commonly used local anesthesia.
- ❖ First synthesized by Lofgren and first used by Gordh

Duration of Effect
- ❖ **Without adrenaline:** 45-60 minutes
- ❖ **With adrenaline:** 2-3 hours

Maximum Safe Dose
- ❖ **Without adrenaline:** 3 mL/kg (200 mg)
- ❖ **With adrenaline:** 1 mg/kg (500 mg)

Concentration Used
- ❖ **Surface (topical) analgesia:** 4%
- ❖ **Nerve block:** 1-2%
- ❖ **Urethral procedure as jelly:** 2%
- ❖ **Spinal:** 5% (heavy)
- ❖ **Epidural:** 1-2%

Side Effects
- ❖ Allergic reaction
- ❖ Myocardial and circulatory depression due to out dose

Advantages
- ❖ Rapid onset of action
- ❖ Rapid diffusion through tissue
- ❖ Minimal vascular effect.
- ❖ Bupivacaine (sensorcaine, marcaine)
- ❖ Very commonly used drug.
- ❖ Dose: 2 mg/kg body out.

Concentration Used
- **For nerve block:** 0.5%
- **Epidural:** 0.25-0.5%
- **Spinal:** 0.5% (heavy)

Uses
- Local infiltration
- Spinal anesthesia
- Epidural/caudal anesthesia

Side Effects
- Hypotension
- CNS excitation
- Bradycardia
- Cardio toxic.

MUSCLE RELAXANT

Skeletal Muscle Relaxant

Skeletal muscle relaxants act peripherally at the neuromuscular junction or centrally in the cerebrospinal axis to reduce muscle tone.

Classification of Skeletal Muscle Relaxants

I. **Neuromuscular blockers:**
   - D-Tubocurarine
   - Atracurium
   - Pancuronium
   - Vecuronium
   - Succinylcholine
   - Benzoquinonium
   - Dantrolene

II. **Centrally acting muscle relaxants:**
   - Mephenesin
   - Chlorzoxazone (MOBIZOX)
   - Methocarbamol (FLEXINOL)
   - Carisoprodol (CARISOMA)
   - Orphenadrine (ORPHIPAL)
   - Tizanidine (CITANZ)
   - Baclofen (LIORESAL)
   - Metaxalone (FLEXURA)

D-Tubocurarine

It is a dextrorotatory quaternary ammonium alkaloid obtained from chondrodendron tomentosum plant. It initially produced motor weakness followed by flaccid paralysis after parenteral administration. The paralysis occurs in following order e.g., paralysis of fingers, toes, eyes, ears producing diplopia, speech slurring, difficulty in swallowing; the muscles of neck, limb, trunk, paralysis of diaphragm, and death occur due to hypoxia.

In higher doses, D-tubocurarine can produce blockage of autonomic ganglia. It can also produce release of histamine and can cause bronchospasm and increase other body secretions. D-Tubocurarine is not absorbed orally and after intravascular administration, it is widely distributed in tissue. As it does not cross blood in barrier it has no effect on CNS.

Adverse effects include hypoxia, respiratory paralysis, decreased blood pressure; broncho-spasm etc., D-tubocurarine is not used now due to its prominent histamine releasing and ganglion blocking effect.

Pancuronium

Pancuronium is a synthetic steroidal compounds and approximately five times potent than tubocurarine. **Vecuronium** is congener of pancuronium with short duration of action. **Atracurium** is bisquaternary competitive blocker similar to pancuronium in properties and duration of action.

Succinylcholine

It is a quaternary ammonium compound with a structure similar to acetylcholine The common adverse reactions of neuromuscular blockers include bronchospasm, precipitation of asthma, respiratory paralysis, flushing, skin reaction, hypotension, and cardiac arrhythmias.

Therapeutic Uses

- ❖ As adjuvant to general anesthesia (especially in major surgical procedures, e.g., abdominal and thoracic surgery, orthopedic procedures, intubation, etc.).
- ❖ Succinylcholine is used for surgical procedure of brief duration (endotracheal intubation, bronchoscopy, esophagoscopy, laryngoscopy, etc.).
- ❖ Succinylcholine is used to avoid convulsion and coma from electroconvulsive therapy in the treatment of tetanus and emergency or epilepsy (status epilepticus).
- ❖ As a diagnostic tool for myasthenia gravis.

Centrally Acting Muscle Relaxants

These agents reduce skeletal muscle tone by a selective action on cerebrospinal axis without affecting consciousness. Mephenesin was the first drug used as muscle relaxant but due to its serious side effects, e.g., hemolysis, hypotension and thrombophlebitis, it is not clinically used now.

Chlorzoxazone

It is mephenesin related skeletal muscle relaxant. After oral administration, it is rapidly and completely absorbed. It is metabolized in liver and excreted in urine primarily as the glucuronide. Adverse reactions include gastric irritation, nausea, lethargy; headache. It is used in painful skeletal muscle spasm and is used in combination with paracetamol and diclofenac.

Methocarbamol

It causes skeletal muscle relaxation by preferential blockade of polysynaptic spinal reflexes. It is rapidly absorbed from the GI tract, metabolised in the liver and excreted in urine as the glucuronide and sulphate conjugates of its metabolites. Small amount is excreted in feces. Adverse effects include nausea, anorexia, skin rash, vertigo, drowsiness, headache, and fever. It is indicated in skeletal muscle spasm, in surgery, orthopedic procedures, neurological diseases, and tetanus.

Carisoprodol

It is used for the treatment of muscle spasm. It has antipyretic and weak antiadrenergic activity. It is absorbed from the GI tract, metabolized in the liver and excreted in urine as metabolites including meprobamate. It is used in musculoskeletal disorders. Adverse reactions include nausea, rash, headache, drowsiness, constipation, and dizziness.

Orphenadrine

It is a centrally acting, anticholinergic muscle relaxant drug. With administration of 100 mg of orphenadrine, peak plasma concentration is achieved within 2 hours. Half-life is 14 hours for the parent drug and 2 to 25 hours for the metabolites. Excretion is via urine and feces. It is used in musculoskeletal disorders, trauma, sports injuries, low backache, tension headache, sprains and strains, parkinsonism including the drug induced. Adverse effects include dry mouth, blurred vision, nausea, restlessness, dizziness, etc.

Tizanidine

Tizanidine is an O-adrenergic receptor agonist at supraspinal and spinal levels. This effect results in inhibition of spinal polysynaptic reflex activity. It presumably reduces spasticity by increasing presynaptic inhibition of motor neurons. Tizanidine has no direct effect on skeletal muscle, the neuromuscular junction or on monosynaptic reflex activity. In humans, tizanidine reduces pathologically increased muscle tone, including resistance to passive movements and alleviates painful spasms. Adverse effects include nausea, sedation, dry mouth, dizziness, hypotension, headache, palpitation. Other rarely produced side effects include hallucinations, bradycardia etc. It is indicated in spasticity due to neurological disorders, e.g., multiple sclerosis, chronic myelopathy, degenerative diseases of the spinal cord, cerebrovascular accidents and cerebral palsy; painful muscle spasm associated with static and functional disorders of the spine (cervical and lumbar syndromes); painful muscle spasm following surgery, e.g., for herniated intervertebral disc or for osteoarthritis of the hip.

Baclofen

It is beta-4 (chlorophenyl)-gamma aminobutyric acid. It is a powerful neuronal depressant reduces the release of excitatory transmitter and is antinociceptive in animal studies, it inhibits monosynaptic and polysynaptic reflex transmission at spinal level, probably by stimulating the GABA, receptors which in turn inhibit the release of glutamate and aspartate.

After oral administration, it is rapidly completely absorbed and eliminated and the body by kidney in unchanged form.

Adverse effects include weakness, fatigue, dizziness, headache, insomnia, and hypotension confusion, skin rash, constipation, nausea anorexia, dry mouth and taste disturbance etc. It is mainly used in the treatment of spasticity in multiple sclerosis, spastic spinal paralysis etc. It is also used in the treatment of trigeminal neuralgia.

Metaxalone

It is a skeletal muscle relaxant, oxazolidinone derivative used in conjunction with other therapeutic agents to treat and discomfort associated with acute musculoskeletal conditions. Mechanism of action is not known; however, it is thought that the skeletal muscle relaxation is due to its central nervous system depressant action. It probably acts by inhibiting polysynaptic pathways, but has no effect on monosynaptic pathways. It is well absorbed from GIT and mostly metabolized in liver and excreted in urine. Peak plasma levels are reached at 2 hours and action occur within 1 hour.

Adverse effects include blurred or double vision, dizziness, drowsiness, abdominal cramps confusion, headache, hiccups, anemia, etc. it is mainly used to relieve pain and discomfort caused by strains, sprains also painful muscular conditions in which muscles are in spasm, i.e., fibromyalgia, dislocations, and fractures.

PAPER II

Section Outline

3. Surgical Anatomy 225
4. Basics of OT Techniques, CSSD Techniques and Anesthesia Technique 286
5. Hand Hygiene and Prevention of Cross Infection 382
6. Basic Life Support (BLS) and Cardiopulmonary Resuscitation 408

CHAPTER 3

Surgical Anatomy

Chapter Outline

- Structure of Anterior Abdominal Wall Including Clinical Anatomy of Hernia
- Structure of Posterior Abdominal Wall
- Structure of Thoracic Wall
- Meninges and Scalp
- Surface Anatomy and Bony Landmarks
- Concept of Mediastenum
- Skin as Sensory Organ
- Applied Ocular Anatomy
- Major Muscles of Body

STRUCTURE OF ANTERIOR ABDOMINAL WALL INCLUDING CLINICAL ANATOMY OF HERNIA

Introduction

In human anatomy, the body cavity, lying between the chest or thorax above and the pelvis below and from the spine in the back to the wall abdominal muscles in the front. It is the part of the trunk which lies below the thoraco-abdominal diaphragm.

Division of the Abdomen

The regions or quadrants of abdomen are used in clinical context. There are nine abdominal regions **(Fig. 3.1)**.

- **Upper region:**
  - Right hypochondriac
  - Epigastric
  - Left hypochondriac
- **Middle region:**
  - Right lumbar
  - Umbilical
  - Left lumbar

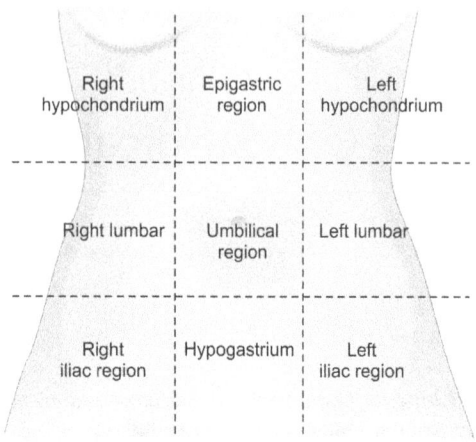

Fig. 3.1: Regions of abdomen.

❖ **Lower region:**
  - Right inguinal
  - Hypogastric or suprapubic
  - Left inguinal region.

They are divided by:
❖ **Two transverse planes:**
  1. Subcostal plane
  2. Transtubercular plane
❖ **Two vertical lines:**
  1. Right midclavicular lines
  2. Left midclavicular lines
❖ **Quadrants:** There are four abdominal quadrants
❖ **Upper quadrant:**
  - Right upper quadrant
  - Left upper quadrant
❖ **Lower quadrant:**
  - Right lower quadrant
  - Left lower quadrant

They are divided by horizontal and vertical imaginary lines that intersect at umbilicus:
❖ Umbilicus
❖ Point where the umbilical cord entered the fetus.
❖ Located midway between the xiphoid process and the pubis symphysis.

Boundaries of Abdomen

Anterior wall: It is musculoaponeurotic and it's formed by three flat muscles namely external and internal oblique and transversus abdominis with their aponeurosis. In the midline it is strengthened by rectus abdominis and pyramidalis is muscles.

Posterior wall: It is osseo musculofascial. It is formed by lumbar vertebrae in midline and the pre and paravertebral muscles on both sides.

Roof: It is formed by the undersurface of thoraco abdominal diaphragm.

Floor: It is formed by pelvic diaphragm posteriorly and the urogenital diaphragm in anterior part.

Anterior Abdominal Wall

The abdominal wall is an anatomically:
- Complex multi-layered structure
- With segmentally derived blood supply and innervations
- Provides structure, protection and support to the abdominal viscera and the peritoneal cavity.

Embryology

- It is mesodermal in origin
- Originate in the paravertebral region
- Develops as bilateral migrating meets and envelope the future abdomen.
- **Superiorly:** Xiphi-sternum, right and costal margin.
- **Inferiorly:** Iliac crest, fold of groin, public tubercle, public crest, symphysis pubis.
- **Each side:** Mid axillary line.

Anterior Abdominal Wall is Made up of Following Eight Layers

1. **Skin:** It is thin and elastic. There is a surface depression present at the level of L3 and L4 known as umbilicus. In females, skin in the lower part of abdominal wall may show white lines called as striae gravidarum **(Fig. 3.2).**
2. **Superficial fascia:** It is a single layer above umbilicus while it splits into two layers in the lower-half and forms the:
   i. *Superficial fatty layer:* Camper's fascia
   ii. *Deep membranous layer:* Scarpa's fascia

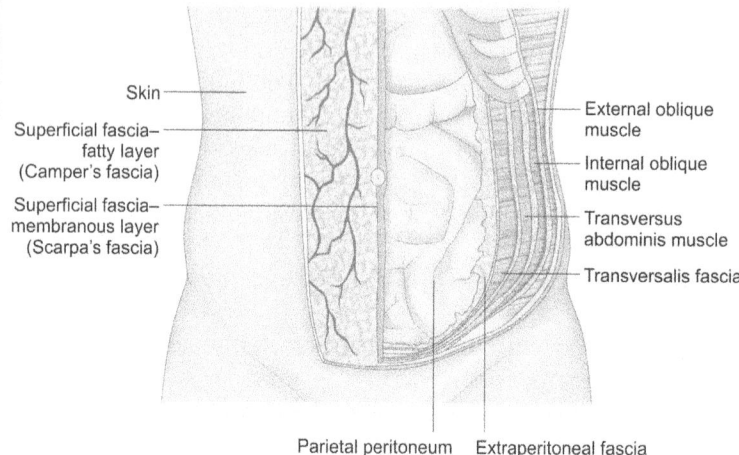

Fig. 3.2: Layers of abdomen.

Extension and modification of fascia scarpa:
- Fundiform ligament of penis
- Colle's fascia of perineum
3. External oblique and its aponeurosis.
4. Internal oblique muscle and its aponeurosis
5. Transversus abdominis muscle and its aponeurosis.
6. **Fascia transversalis:** It forms the endo-abdominal fascia and is made up of areolar tissue which lines the inner surface of trans versus abdominis muscle.
7. **Extra peritoneal tissue:** It is made up of fibro alveolar fatty tissue.
8. **Parietal Peritoneum:** It lines the inner surface of anterior abdominal wall beneath extra peritoneal fat.

Muscles of the Abdominal Wall

Five pair of muscles forms the abdominal wall and from the surface inward they are:
1. External oblique
2. Internal oblique
3. Transverse abdominis
4. Cremaster muscle
5. Rectus abdominis
6. Pyramidalis.

The main function of these paired muscles is to form the strong muscular anterior the abdominal cavity. When the muscle contract together they:
- Compress the abdominal organs

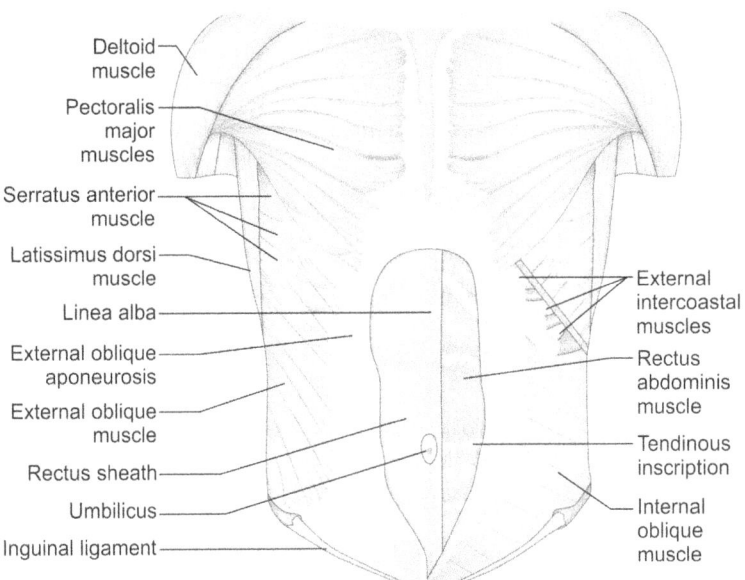

Fig. 3.3: Muscles of abdominal wall.

- ❖ Contraction of the muscle on one side only bends the trunk toward that side.
- ❖ Flex the vertebral column in the lumbar region.
- ❖ Contraction of the oblique muscles on one side rotates the trunk toward that side.

The anterior abdominal wall is divided longitudinally by a very strong midline tendinous cord, the linea alba (meaning white cord) which extends from the xiphoid process of the sternum to the symphysis pubis **(Fig. 3.3)**.

- ❖ **External oblique:** This muscle extends from the lower ribs downward and forward to be inserted into the iliac crest and by an aponeurosis to the linea alba.
- ❖ **Internal oblique:** This muscle lies deep to the external oblique. It's fibers arise from the iliac crest and by broad end processes of lumbar vertebrae. The fibers pass upward toward the midline to be inserted into the lower tiles and by aponeurosis into the linea alba. The fibers are at right angles to those of the external oblique.
- ❖ **Transverse abdominis:** This is the deepest muscle of the abdominal wall. The fibres arise from the iliac crest and the lumbar vertebrae and pass across the abdominal wall to be inserted into the wide area by an aponeurosis. The fibers are at a right angle to those of the rectus abdominis.

- ❖ **Cremaster muscle:** It is middle 1/3rd of the inguinal ligament and to be inserted into scrotum spermatic cord tunica vaginalis. It is in form of loops. It has superficial and deep parts insertion is by four fleshy slips.
- ❖ **Rectus abdominis:** This is the most superficial muscle. It is broad and flat, originating from the transverse part of the pubic bone then passing upward to be inserted into the lower ribs and xiphoid process of the sternum.
- ❖ **Pyramidalis:** It is originated from symphysis pubis and pubic crest and insertion into linea alba. The muscle may not always be present in the body.

Hernia

A hernia happens when an internal organ pushes through a weak spot in your muscles or tissue.

Definition

A hernia occurs when an internal organ for other body part protrudes through. The wall of muscle or tissue that normally contains it. Most hernia occurs within the abdominal cavity between the chest and the hips.

In those affecting the digestive system, a piece of bowel protrudes through a weak point in either the musculature of the anterior abdominal wall or an existing opening **(Fig. 3.4)**.

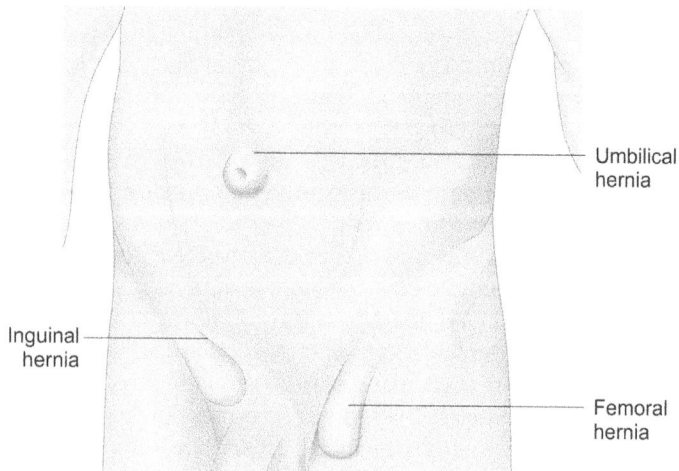

Fig. 3.4: Hernia.

It occurs when there is intermittent increase in intra-abdominal pressure, most commonly in men who lift heavy loads of work.

Outcomes include:
- Spontaneous reduction, i.e., the loop of bowl slips back to its correct place when the intra-abdominal pressure returns to normal.
- Manual reduction, i.e., by applying gentle pressure over the abdominal cavity.
- Strangulation when reduction is not possible and the venous drainage from the herniated loop of bowel is impaired causing congestion ischemia and gangrene.

Common forms of Hernia

- **Inguinal hernia:** In men, the inguinal canal is a passageway for the spermatic cord and blood vessels leading to the testicles. In women, the inguinal canal contains the round ligament that quick support for the womb.

  In an inguinal hernia, fatty tissue or a part of the intestine pokes into the grown at the top of the inner most common type of hernia and affects than women **(Fig. 3.5)**.
- **Femoral hernia:** Fatty tissue or part of the intestine into the groin at the top of the inner thigh. Femoral hernias are much less common than inguinal hernia and mainly affect older women **(Fig. 3.6)**.
- **Umbilical hernia:** Fatty tissue or part of the intestine pushes through the abdomen near the belly **(Fig. 3.7)**.
- **Hiatal (hiatus) hernia:** Part of the stomach pushes up into the chest cavity through an opening in the diaphragm **(Fig. 3.8)**.

Other Types of Hernia Include

- **Incisional hernia:** Tissue protrudes through the sites of an abdominal area from a remote abdominal or pelvic operation.

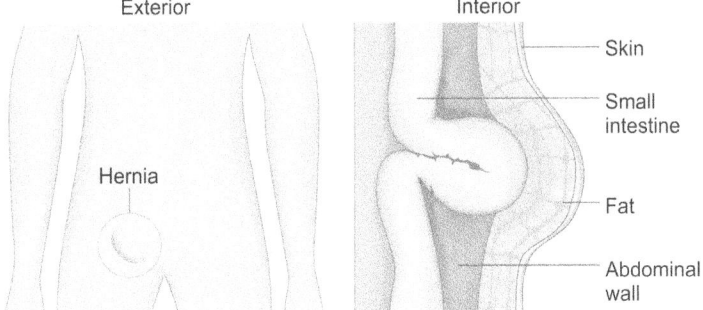

Fig. 3.5: Inguinal hernia.

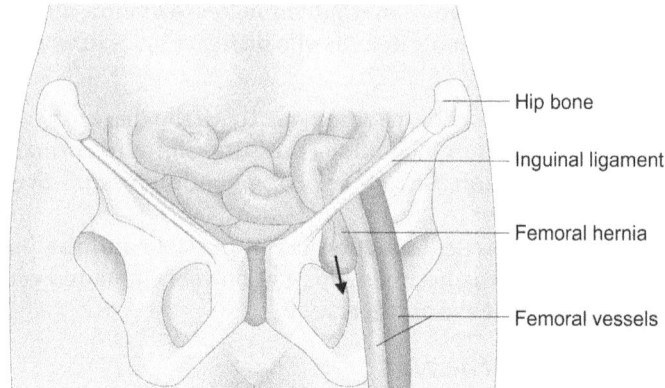

Fig. 3.6: Femoral hernia.

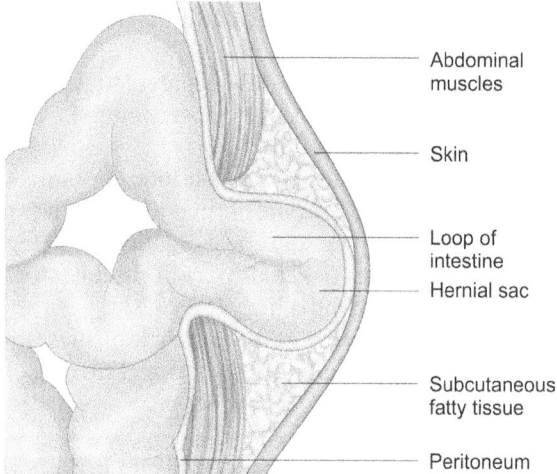

Fig. 3.7: Umbilical hernia.

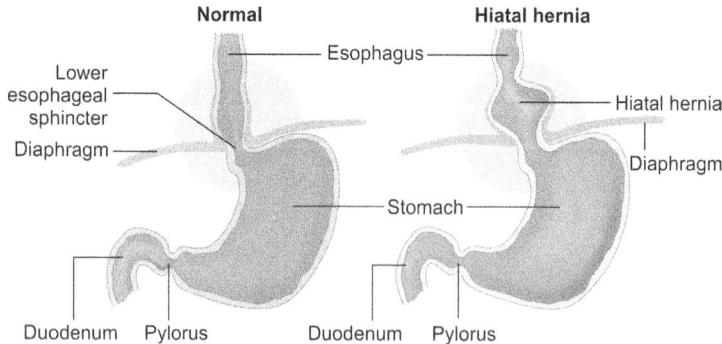

Fig. 3.8: Hiatal hernia.

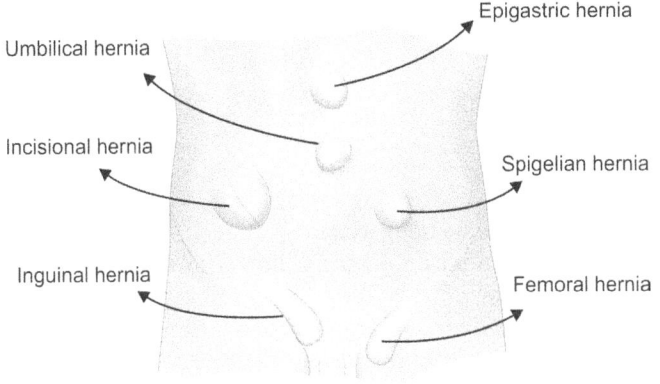

Fig. 3.9: Types of hernia.

- **Epigastric hernia:** Fatty tissue protrudes thorough the abdominal area between the navel belly button lower part of the sternum.
- **Spigelian hernia:** The intestine pushes through the abdomen at the side of the abdominal muscle, below the navel.
- **Diaphragmatic hernia:** Organs in the abdomen move into the chest through an opening in the diaphragm **(Fig. 3.9)**.

Causes of Hernia

- Age
- Smoking
- Chronic coughing
- Family history
- Being constipated
- Damage from injury
- Sudden weight gain
- Being overweight
- Lifting heavy weight
- Pregnancy
- Constipation
- Weakness of the muscles and ligaments

Symptoms of Hernia

Most hernia can be felt. You might notice a lump or bulge (it may be hard or soft) in an area of your body. Not all hernia produces discomfort, but when they do you might experience:

- Burning
- Pulling

- Pain
- Pressure
- Swelling
- Heartburn

Hernia Prevention

- Do not smoke.
- Maintain a moderate body weight.
- Try not to strain while having a bowel movement or during urination.
- Eat enough high fiber foods to prevent constipation.
- Perform exercises that help to strengthen the muscle of your abdomen.
- Avoid lifting weights that are heavy for you.

■ STRUCTURE OF POSTERIOR ABDOMINAL WALL

Introduction

The posterior abdominal wall extends from the 12th rib above the pelvic brim below. It is strong and stable because it is constructed by bones, muscles and fasciae. It is supports retroperitoneal organs, vessels and nerves **(Fig. 3.10)**.

The posterior abdominal wall is constructed:
- **Bony part:** In the median plane, it's created from bodies, intervertebral disc, and transverse processes of the five lumbar vertebrae. Laterally it's divided into upper and lower parts by the iliac crest. The part above the iliac crest is made of inner surfaces the 12th rib and the part below the iliac crest is made iliac fossa.
- **Muscular part:** Above the iliac crest from medial to lateral sides, it's created from psoas major, quadratus lumborum and transversus abdominis muscles. Below the iliac crest on each on each side of the lumbar vertebral column from medial to lateral sides, it's created from psoas major and iliacus muscles. In addition to such muscles, the diaphragm finishes the abdominal wall superiorly.
- **Fasciae (psoas fascia, fascia iliaca and thoracolumbar fascia):** The psoas major and iliacus muscles are covered by fascia iliaca. The quadratus lumborum is enclosed between the anterior and posterior layer of the thoracolumbar fascia.

These and structure can be studied in the posterior abdominal wall.
- Muscles and fasciae of the posterior abdominal call.
- Great vessels of the abdomen [(e.g., abdominal aorta and inferior vena cava (IVC)].

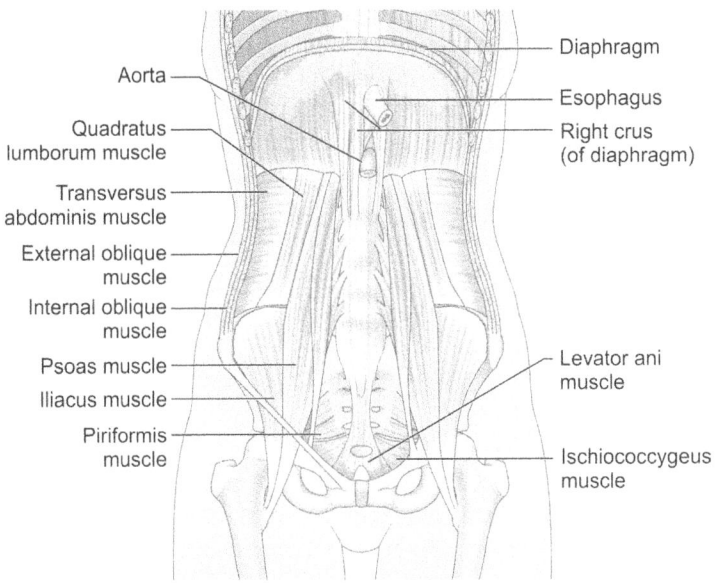

Fig. 3.10: Posterior abdominal wall.

- Azygos and hemiazygos veins.
- Lymph nodes and lymphatics of the posterior abdominal wall.

Muscles of the Posterior Abdominal Wall

Three muscles viz. **Psoas major, iliacus** and **quadratus lumborum**, on every side of the vertebral column create most of the posterior abdominal wall.

Psoas Major Muscles

- **Origin:** The muscle arises from 14 fleshy slips that are as follows:
    - Five slips from intervertebral discs between T12–45 vertebrae and adjoining meninges of the bodies of these vertebrae.
    - Five slips from anterior surfaces and lower borders of the transverse process of five lumbar vertebrae.
    - Floor slip from tendinous arches bridging the contributed sides of the bodies of lumbar vertebrae.
- **Insertion:** Lesser trochanter of femur via iliopsoas tendon.
- **Function:**
    - Action from above, it is the chief flexor of the thigh at the hip joint
    - Action from below, it flexes the trunk on the thigh, as invoicing the from recumbent to sitting position trunk.
- **Innervation:** Ventral Yami L1–L3.

Psoas minor: This muscle is present in about 50% individuals.
- **Origin:** It arise from the side of the intervertebral disc between T12 and 21 vertebrae and adjoining parts of their bodies.
- **Insertion:** The iliopubic eminence.
- **Nerve supply:** It is by a branch of L1 spinal 1 nerve.
- **Action:** It is a weak flexor of the trunk.

Iliacus: It is, a fan-shaped muscle and forms the lateral component of the iliopsoas muscle.
- **Origin:** It arises from the upper two thirds of the floor of iliac fossa, inner lip of iliac crest and upper surface of the lateral, the lateral aspect of the sacrum.
- **Insertion:** Anterior surface of lesser trochanter and an area (2.5 cm long) below it.

Quadratus lumborum
- **Origin:**
  - Posterior one-third of the inner lip of the iliac crest.
  - Lower two to four transverse processor of lumbar vertebrae.
- **Insertion:**
  - The medial part of the anterior surface of the 12th rib.
  - Upper lumbar transverse processes.
- **Nerve supply:** Ventral rami of T12-13/14 lumbar spinal.
- **Actions:** It is a lateral flexor of the lumbar vertebral column. Extend the lumbar vertebral column.

Fasciae of the posterior abdominal wall (Fig. 3.11): The fasciae of posterior abdominal wall are:
- Psoas fascia
- Fascia iliaca

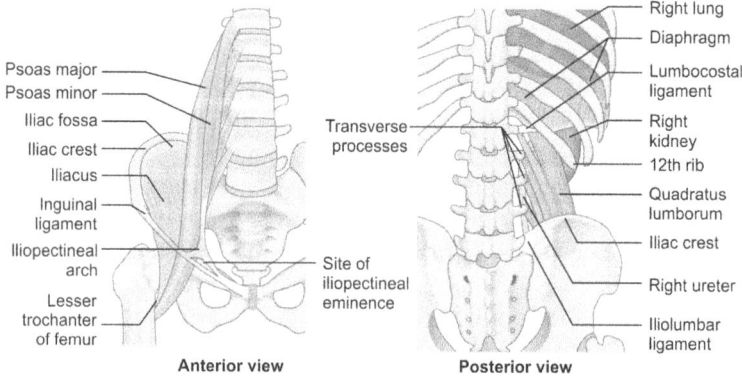

Fig. 3.11: Anterior and posterior view of abdominal wall.

- Thoracolumbar fascia
- **Psoas fascia:**
  - Thick fascial sheath surrounding the psoas muscle.
  - Arises as the muscle enters the abdominal cavity under the medchal arcuate ligament.
  - Ends at the pelvic brim as the muscle leaves the abdomen inferior to the inguinal ligament. (Does not extend into the thigh).
- **Thoracolumbar fascia:**
  - Extends from the back of sacrum
  - Binds erector spinae to vertebral column and encloses the quadratus lumborum spine of the neck.
  - Very strong in the lumbar region.
  - Laterally it gives origin! Muscles to internal oblique and transversus abdominis.
  - Its lumbar part medially splits into three layers.

Psoas abscess
- A focus of pus disc. Pus in the lumbar intervertebral discs can track down track down along the muscle and present as a lump in the groin.
- Tuberculosis of the spine gives rise a psoas abscess.

Lymphatics
The lymph vessels emptying the posterior abdominal wall and mayanti of, the abdominopelvic organs with the exception of part of the liver terminate in the cisterna chyli and thoracic duct. The lymphatic flow is intercepted by a series of lymph node groups before reaching the cisterna chili and the thoracic duct.

Cisterna Chyli
It is an elongated white lymphatic sac about 5-7 cm long and 4 cm wide. It is located on the L 1-2 vertebrae between the aorta and the azygos vein, concealed by the right crus of the diagram. Superiorly it continues as the thoracic duct.

Tributaries
The cisterna chyli gets the following tributaries.
- **Left and right intestinal lymph trunks**—from the preaortic lymph nodes, which open in its middle. These trunks drain the lymph from the small intestine, stomach and liver.
- **Left and right lumbar lymph trunks**—from the para-aortic lymph nodes, which open in it interiorly.
- **A pair of lymph vessels**—from the lower intercostal lymph nodes which open in it superiorly.

Lymph nodes: All these can be found along the external iliac arteries, common in arteries, and abdominal aorta, and consequently called external iliac, common iliac, and aortic lymph nodes.

External iliac nodes: These are 8-10 in number and are located along the external iliac vessels. The medial nodes get the lymph from the pelvic viscera and lower limb, while the lateral nodes get the lymph from the territories of inferior epigastric and deep circumflex iliac vessels. Afferents from these nodes enter the common iliac nodes.

Common iliac nodes: These are 4-6 in number and are located along the common iliac vessels (lateral group) and below the bifurcation of the dorsal (medial group). The lateral group of nodes gets the lymph from the pelvis and lower limb via external and internal iliac nodes, cable the medial group and nodes gets the lymph from the pelvic viscera directly and via internal iliac and sacral nodes.

Aortic lymph nodes: They can be situated along the abdominal aorta and inferior cava, and are ordered into two groups **preaortic** and **para-aortic** vena.

Preaortic nodes: The nodes are situated around a coeliac, superior mesenteric, and inferior mesenteric are levies and are consequently termed as coeliac, superior mesenteric, and inferior mesenteric nodes. They get the lymph from the organs supplied by these arteries.

The efferents from **preaortic** nodes create the intestinal lymph trunk, which drain in the cisterna chyli.

Nerves of the posterior abdominal wall: The nerves of the posterior abdominal wall contain subcostal nerve, ventral sympathetic chains rami of lumbar nerves and lumbar.

STRUCTURE OF THORACIC WALL

The thorax is the body cavity, surrounded by the body ribcage, contains the heart and lungs, the great vessels, the oesophagus and trachea. The thoracic duct and the autonomic innervation for these structures. The inferior boundary of the thoracic cavity is respiratory diaphragm which separates the thoracic and abdominal cavity.

The thoracic wall consists of bony framework that is held together by twelve thoracic vertebrae posteriorly which give rise to ribs that encircle the lateral and anterior thoracic cavity. The first nine ribs curve around the lateral thoracic wall and connect to the manubrium and sternum. Rib 10-12 are relatively short and attach to costal margins of rib just above them. Ribs 10-12 due to their short course, they do not reach the sternum.

The boundaries of thoracic wall are important landmarks used by clinical and surgeons for various procedures including sternotomy pericardiocentesis in patients with cardiac tamponade and thoracentesis for pleural effusion. The thoracic wall is bounded anteriorly by sternum and costal cartilages, laterally by ribs and intercostal space, posteriorly by thoracic vertebrae and intervertebral disc, superiorly by supra pleural membrane, inferiorly by the respiratory diaphragm.

- **Outside:** Skin and by muscles attaching the shoulder girdle to the trunk.
- **Inside:** Lined with parietal pleural.
- **Framework:**
  - *Posteriorly:* The thoracic part of vertebral column
  - *Anteriorly:* The sternum and costal cartilage
  - *Laterally:* The ribs and intercostal space
  - *Superiorly:* The diaphragm.

Position

- Thoracic cavity is situated in upper part of trunk its boundaries are formed by thoracic cage.
- Anteriorly the sternum and costal cartilages of rib and intercostal muscles.
- Posteriorly the thoracic vertebrae.
- Superiorly the structure formed the root of neck.
- Inferiorly the diaphragm dome shaped muscle.

Function

The thoracic cavity subdivides into three compartments, the mediastinum and two pleural cavities one on each sides, the mediastinum is the median compartment containing the heart and great vessels whereas the pleural cavity contains the lungs. The thoracic cage protects the lungs and the heart as well as provide attachment for the muscles of the thorax upper extremities, back and the abdomen. It communicates superiorly with the neck via the thoracic outlet and inferiorly separates the abdomen by the respiratory diaphragm **(Fig. 3.12)**.

Blood Supply and Lymphatic Supply

Three arteries supply each intercoastal spaces, the posterior intercostal artery and two branches of anterior intercoastal arteries. These intercoastal blood innermost intercostal muscles in the groove.

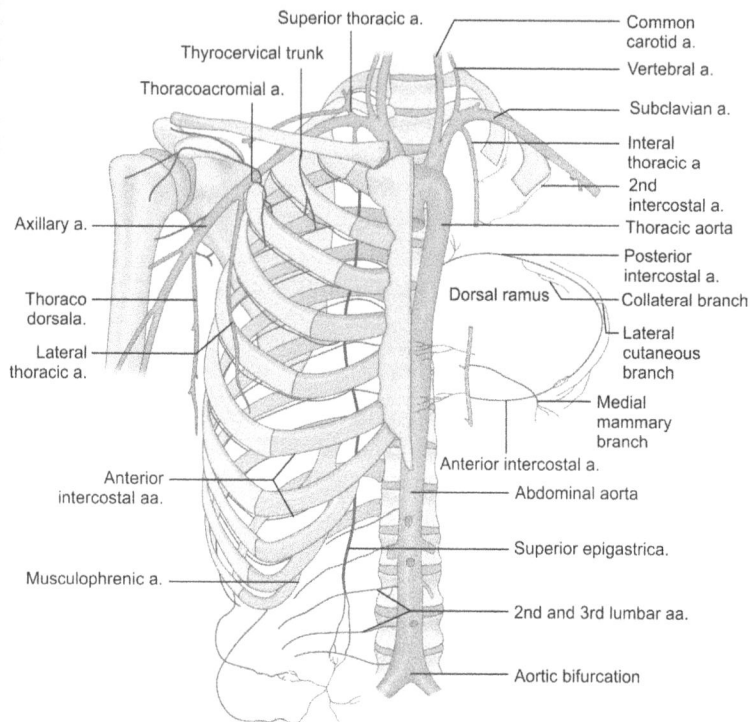

Fig. 3.12: Structure of thorax.

They are arranged in order from superior to inferior vein artery and nerve. The posterior intercoastal artery for the first two intercostal spaces is fed from the superior (supreme) intercoastal artery.

This artery arises from the costocervical trunk other subclavian artery. The remaining pair of posterior intercostal arteries from the 3rd to 11th intercostal space and a pair of subcostal arteries emerges directly descending thoracic aorta.

The anterior intercostal arteries of 1st to 6th intercostal space are branches of the internal thoracic artery which derive from first portion of subclavian artery the anterior intercostal artery of the 7th to 9th intercostal space are branches of the musculophrenic artery which tributary of the intercostal artery. The anterior intercostal artery anastomose laterally in the costal groove.

The corresponding posterior intercostal vein drains into internal thoracic or musculophrenic vein. The lymphatics of the thoracic wall drains into parasternal lymph node and intercostal lymph node from the upper thorax drain into the thoracic duct.

Nerves Supply to the Thoracic Wall

The thoracic wall is primarily innervated by the intercostal nerves, which are the anterior rami of spinal nerves of T1, T11 and the anterior ramus of T12 is a subcostal nerve **(Fig. 3.13)**.

Each intercostal nerve supplies a dermatome and a myotome. Only the anterior nerves of T1 from the lower trunk of the brachial plexus the remanding intercoastal do not from a plexus.

Muscles

There are three intercostal muscles; externally intercostal, internally and innermost intercostal muscles. These muscles are present in the intercostal spaces and the intercostal nerve and blood vessels run between them. The most superficial layer is the external intercostal muscle. The external intercostal muscles extend posteriorly from the rib tubercle to the costochondral junction anteriorly where the anterior (external) intercostal membrane takes the place of muscle fibers **(Fig. 3.14)**.

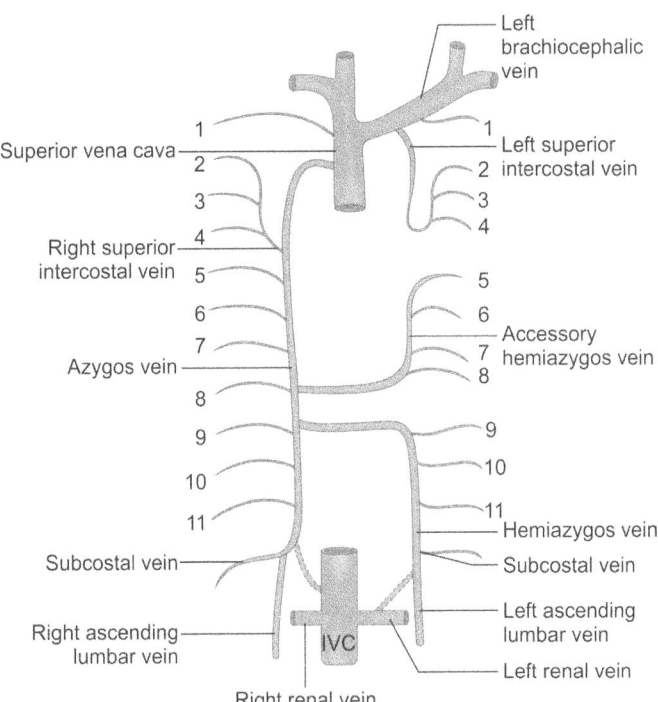

Fig. 3.13: Nerve supply to thoracic wall.

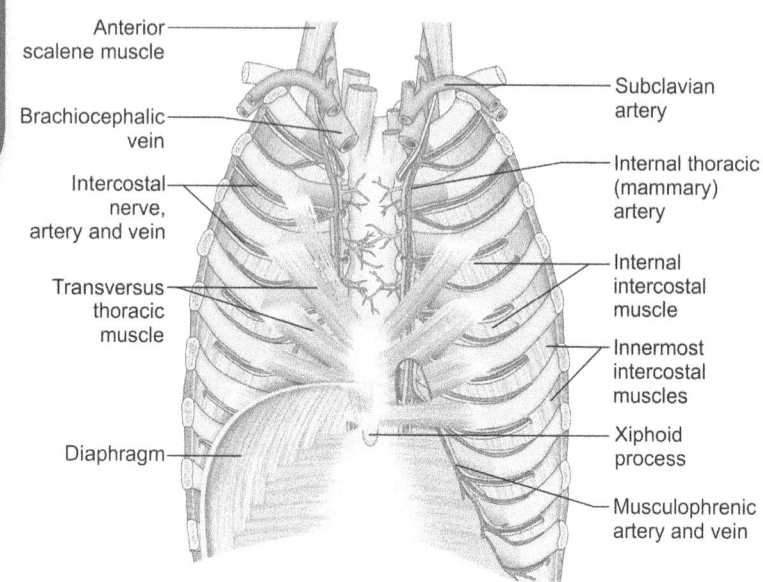

Fig. 3.14: Muscles of thoracic wall.

The Superior Mediastinum

The superior mediastinum is the space behind the manubrium of the sternum. It is bounded by parietal (mediastinal) pleura on each side and the first four thoracic vertebrae behind. It is continuous with the root of the neck at the top of the first ribs and with the inferior mediastinum below the transverse thoracic plane, a horizontal plane that passes from the sternal angle through the space between the T4 and T5 vertebrae. The superior mediastinum contains several important structures including the branches of the aortic arch, the veins that coalesce to form the superior vena cava, the trachea, the esophagus, the vagus and phrenic nerves, the cardiac plexus of autonomic nerves, the thoracic duct, and the thymus **(Fig. 3.15)**.

The internal intercostal muscles from the intermediate layer. This muscle extend anteriorly from the sternum to rib cage posteriorly where the muscle fibers are replaced the posterior (internal) intercostal membrane. The innermost intercostal muscles from the deepest layer and is lined internally by the endothoracic fascia which in turn is lined internally by the parietal pleura.

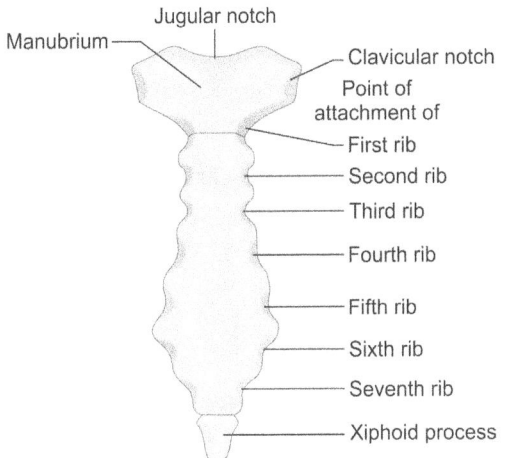

Fig. 3.15: Sternum: anterior view.

Xiphoid Process

The xiphoid process or xiphisternum or metasternum, is a small cartilaginous process (extension) of the inferior (lower) part of the sternum, which is usually ossified in the adult human. It may also be referred to as the ensiform process.

Function

Much the way the first seven ribs articulate with the sternum, the cartilage in the celiac plexus joins on the xiphoid process, reinforcing it, and indirectly attaches the costal cartilage to the sternum. The xiphoid process is involved in the attachment of many muscles, normal breathing. It also anchors the rectus abdominis muscles.

Surgical Consideration

Understanding the anatomy of thorax is vital, as it provides access to the heart, great vessels, lung, diaphragm, and mediastinum.

❖ The intercostal nerve block is a procedure through which local anesthetic agent is injected around the intercostal nerve between the paravertebral line and the area of required anesthesia for different surgical procedures. However, the surgeon needs to anesthetize the adjacent nerve as well as because of considerable overlapping of contiguous dermatomes occurs.

❖ Median sternotomies are the most commonly performed osteotomy in the world and a standard incision for thoracic and

cardiac surgery. The median sternotomy is a critical procedure in which the surgeon splits the sternum in the median plane to gain access to the heart, great vessels, as well as the lungs.
❖ Flail chest is an extremely painful injury affecting the respiration, often caused by blunt chest trauma, resulting in multiple successive rib fractures. The fractured ribs of the anterior and/or lateral chest wall move inward on inspiration and outward on expiration (paradoxical) and may be associated with pneumothorax and/or contusion of the heart and lung. Today, flail chest management is through pain control, pulmonary toilet, and early ambulation. It is not common to surgically repair the ribs.

■ MENINGES AND SCALP

Introduction

The brain and spinal cord are completely surrounded by three layer of tissue. The meninges lie between the skull (scalp) and the brain between the vertebral foramina and the spinal cord.

Named from outside inwards, they are the:
❖ Dura mater
❖ Arachnoid mater
❖ Pia mater

The arachnoid and pia mater are together known as leptomeninges.

The outermost is dura mater, middle layer is delicate cobweb like arachnoid mater and inner one is pia mater.

The subdural space is very narrow while the sub arachnoid space is very big contains very important cerebrospinal fluid, lastly brain and spinal cord with their meninges are securely kept in the body (scalp).

Dura Mater

❖ The cerebral mater consists of two layers of dense fibrous tissue.
❖ The outer layer endosteal layer and an inner meningeal layer.
❖ The outer layer takes the place of the periosteum on the inner surface of the skull bones and the inner layer provides a protective covering for the brain.
❖ There is only a potential space between the two layers except where the inner layer sweeps inwards.
❖ The meningeal layer forms four folds which divides the cranial cavity into intercommunicating compartments for different parts of the brain.
❖ The falx cerebri, which separates the two cerebral hemisphere.

- The flax cerebelli, which separates the two cerebellar Hemisphere.
- The tentorium (meaning 'tent-like') cerebella, which separates the cerebrum and the cerebellum.
- Venous blood from the brain drains into venous sinuses between the two layers of dura mater.
- The Superior sagittal sinus is formed by the flax cerebri and the tentorium cerebella forms the straight and transverse sinuses.
- Spinal dura mater forms a loose sheath round the spinal cord, extending from the foramen magnum to the second sacral vertebra.
- Thereafter it encloses the filum terminate and fuses with the periosteum of the coccyx.
- It is an extension of the inner layer of cerebral dura mater and is separated from the periosteum of the vertebrae and ligament within the neural canal by epidural space.
- Containing blood vessel and areolar connective tissue.
- Different folds of dura mater due to meningeal layer.
- Folds spaces venous sinuses enclosed.
- Falx cerebri its sickle shaped separate the right from left cerebral hemisphere.
- Superior sagittal sinus, inferior sagittal sinus and straight sinus.
- Tentorium cerebelli is tent shaped separate the cerebral hemisphere from hind brain and lower part of the mid brain lift off the weight of occipital lobes from the cerebellum.
- Transverse sinus.
- Falx cerebelli is small sickle shaped fold partly separating two cerebral hemisphere.
- Enclosed occipital sinus.
- Diaphragm sulci is small horizontal fold over hypophyseal fossa.
- Enclosed anterior and posterior inter cavernous sinuses. It is attached to the foramen of magnum and by strands of fibrous tissue of the posterior longitudinal ligaments at interval along its length nerves entry and living spinal cord pass through the epidural space. Dyes, used for diagnostic purposes and local anesthetic or analgesic to relieve pain may be injected into the epidural space.

Arachnoid Mater

The arachnoid (Latin Cobweb-like) mater is a thin transparent membrane that loosely surrounds the brain without dipping into many of the sulci. Thus, its bridges all irregularities of the brain. This is the layer of the fibrous tissue that lie between the dura and pia mater it is separated from the dura mater and pia mater.

It is separated from the dura mater by the subdural space, which contains small amount of serous fluid and from the pia mater by the subarachnoid mater space, which contain CSF. The arachnoid mater passes over the convolution of the brain and accompanies the inner layer of the dura mater in the formation of falx cerebri, tentorium cerebelli and falx cerebella. It continues downward to envelop the spinal cord and ends by margin with the dura mater at the level of second sacral vertebra.

The stem of lateral sulcus where it is pushed by lesser wing of sphenoid. The longitudinal cerebral fissure where its carried by falx cerebella. It surrounds spinal cord and end at sacral second vertebra.

Pia Matter

The pia (Latin words means "loving mother") mater is a thin vascular membrane that closely invests the brain, dipping into various sulci and other irregularities of its surface.

Pia mater is a delicate layer of connective tissue containing many minute blood vessels.

It adheres to the brain, completely covering the convolution and dipping into each fissure.

It continues downward surrounding the spinal cord, blood vessels top nourishes the brain spinal cord pierce it.

It covers spinal cord until the second sacral vertebra arachnoid tube and connect with periosteum of the coccyx. Laterally there are ligamentum denticulate of 21 pairs of teeth like projection which fuse with arachnoid and dura mater. Beyond end of the cord, it continues as the filum terminates, pierces the arachnoid tube goes on, with the dura mater to fuse with the periosteum of the coccyx. Spaces in relation to meninges.

Extradural/Epidural and Subdural Spaces

The extra dural or epidural spaces are potential space between the inner aspect of the skull bone and the endosteal layer of dura mater. Vertebral space is present between the vertebral column and spinal dura mater. The subdural space is transverse by cerebral veins on their path for draining into dural venous sinuses.

Note: The subdural space is also potential space between the dura and arachnoid mater, these become actual space in pathological condition.

Subarachnoid

This is the space between the arachnoid and pia mater. It surrounds the brain and spinal cord, and ends below at lower border of second sacral vertebra. Subarachnoid spaces contain csf, and large vessels of the brain cranial nerves pass through spaces.

The outermost meninx, the dura mater not only separate the right and left cerebral hemisphere but also partitions the cerebrum from cerebellum and hypophysis cerebri. In addition it enclose various venous sinuses.

Function of Meninges

The meninges function primarily to protect and support the central nervous system (CNS).

It connects the brain and spinal cord to the skull and spinal canal. The meninges form a protective barrier that safeguard of the sensitive organ of the CNS against trauma. It also contains ample supply of blood vessels that deliver blood to CNS tissue.

Another important function of the meninges that is produced cerebrospinal fluid. This clear fluid fills the cavities of the cerebral ventricle and surrounds the brain and spinal cord. The CSF fluid protects and nourishes CNS tissue by acting as a shock absorber, by circulating nutrients by getting rid of the waste product. The scalp refers to the layers of skin and subcutaneous tissue that cover the bones of cranial vault.

The scalp is composed of soft tissue layers that cover the cranium. It is an anatomic region bordered anteriorly by the human face, and laterally and posteriorly by the neck. It extends from the superior nuchal lines and occipital turbulences to the supraorbital foramen.

Layers of the Scalp

The scalp consists of five layers. The first three layers are tightly bound together and move as a collective structure.

The mnemonic 'SCALP' can be a useful way to remember the layers of the scalp: skin, dense connective tissue, epicranial aponeurosis, loose areolar connective tissue and periosteum.

- **Skin:** Contains numerous hair follicles and sebaceous glands (thus a common site for sebaceous cysts).
- **Dense connective tissue:** Connects the skin to the epicranial aponeurosis. It is richly vascularized and innervated.
- The blood vessels within the layer are highly adherent to the connective tissue. This renders them unable to constrict fully if lacerated—and so the scalp can be a site of profuse bleeding.

- **Epicranial aponeurosis:** A thin, tendon-like structure that connects the occipitalis and frontalis muscles.
- **Loose areolar connective tissue:** A thin connective tissue layer that separates the periosteum of the skull from the epicranial aponeurosis.
- It contains numerous blood vessels, including emissary veins which connect the veins of the scalp to the diploic veins and intracranial venous sinuses.
- **Periosteum:** The outer layer of the skull bones. It becomes continuous with the endosteum at the suture lines.

Arterial Supply

The scalp receives a rich arterial supply via the external carotid artery and the ophthalmic artery (a branch of the internal carotid). There are three branches of the external carotid artery involved:
1. **Superficial temporal:** Supplies the frontal and temporal regions.
2. **Posterior auricular:** Supplies the area superiorly and posteriorly to the auricle.
3. **Occipital:** Supplies the back of the scalp.

Anteriorly and superiorly, the scalp receives additional supply from two branches of the ophthalmic artery—the supraorbital and supratrochlear arteries. These vessels accompany the supraorbital and supratrochlear nerves respectively.

Venous Drainage

The venous drainage of the scalp can be divided into superficial and deep components.

The superficial drainage follows the arterial supply: superficial temporal, occipital, posterior auricular, supraorbital and supratrochlear veins.

The deep (temporal) region of the skull is drained by the pterygoid venous plexus. This is a large plexus of veins situated between the temporalis and lateral pterygoid muscles, and drains into the maxillary vein.

Importantly, the veins of the scalp connect to the diploic veins of the skull via valveless emissary veins. This establishes a connection between the scalp and the dural venous sinuses.

Innervation

The scalp receives cutaneous innervation from branches of the trigeminal nerve or the cervical nerve roots.

Trigeminal Nerve

- **Supratrochlear nerve:** Branch of the ophthalmic nerve which supplies the anteromedial forehead.
- **Supraorbital nerve:** Branch of the ophthalmic nerve which supplies a large portion of the scalp between the anterolateral forehead and the vertex.
- **Zygomaticotemporal nerve:** Branch of the maxillary nerve, this supplies the temple.
- **Auriculotemporal nerve:** Branch of the mandibular nerve which supplies skin anterosuperior to the auricle.

Cervical Nerves

- **Lesser occipital nerve:** Derived from the anterior ramus (division) of C2 and supplies the skin posterior to the ear.
- **Greater occipital nerve:** Derived from the posterior ramus (division) of C2 and supplies the skin of the occipital region.
- **Great auricular nerve:** Derived from the anterior rami of C2 and C3 and supplies the skin posterior to the ear and over the angle of the mandible.
- **Third occipital nerve:** Derived from the posterior ramus of C3 and supplies the skin of the inferior occipital region.

SURFACE ANATOMY AND BONY LANDMARKS

- Our techniques when examining surface anatomy visual inspection.
- Directly observe the structure and markings of surface features.
- Feeling with firm pressure or perceiving by the sense of touch.
- Precisely locate and identify anatomic features under the skin.
- Tap sharply on specific body sites to detect resonating vibrations.

Listen to Sounds Emitted from Organs

A branch of gross anatomy that examines shapes and markings on the surface of the body as they relate to deeper structures.

"Essential in locating and identifying anatomic structures prior to studying internal gross anatomy."

"Healthcare personnel use surface anatomy to help diagnose medical conditions and to treat patients."

Cranium

- Cranium (cranial region or braincase) is covered by the scalp, which is composed of skin and subcutaneous tissue **(Fig. 3.16)**.

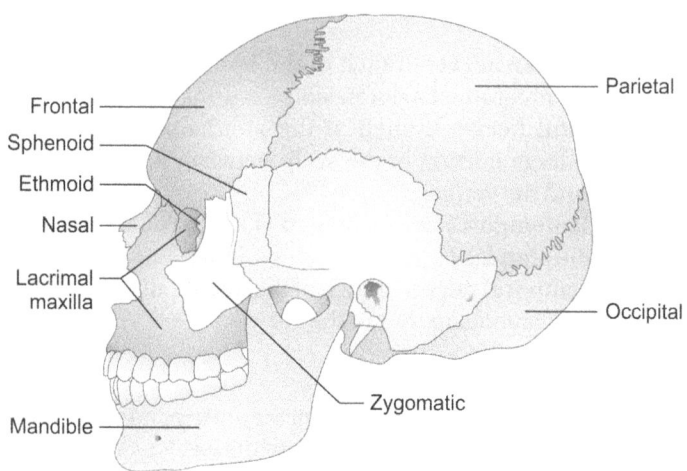

Fig. 3.16: Cranium.

- ❖ Cranium can be subdivided into three regions, each having prominent surface anatomy features.
- ❖ The frontal region of the cranium is the forehead covering the frontal region is the frontalis muscle, which overlies the frontal bone, the frontal region terminates at the superciliary arches.

Face—the Auricular Region

- ❖ Composed of the visible surface structures of the ear as well as the ear's internal organs, which function in hearing and maintaining equilibrium.
- ❖ Auricle, or pinna, is the fleshy part of the external ear. Within the auricle is a tubular opening into the middle ear called the external auditory canal.
- ❖ The mastoid process is posterior and inferior to the auricle.

The Face—Orbital (or Ocular)

Includes the eyeballs and associated structures.

- ❖ Surface features—orbit, eye-lashes, eye-lids, conjuctiva, lacrimal gland help to protect the eyes.
- ❖ Eyebrows protect against sunlight and potential mechanical damage.
  - Eyelids close reflexively to protect against objects moving near the eye.
  - Eyelashes prevent airborne particles from contacting the eyeball.
  - The superior palpebral fissure, or upper eyelid crease.
- ❖ Asians do not have a superior palpebral fissure.

The Face-Nasal Region

The bridge: It is formed by the union of the nasal bones.
The fleshy part of the nose is called the dorsum nasi.
- The tip of the nose is called the apex.
  - Nostrils, or external nares, are the paired openings into the nose.
  - Ala nasi (wing of the nose) forms the flared lateral margin of each nostril. The Face-oral region.
  - Inferior to the nasal region.
- Includes the buccal (cheek) region, the fleshy upper and lower lips (labia), and the structures of the oral cavity (mouth) that can be observed when the mouth is open.
  - The vertical depression between your nose and upper lip is called the philtrum.

The Face—Mental Region

- The mental region contains the mentum, or chin.
- The mentum tends to be pointed and almost triangular in females.
- Males tend to have a "squared-off" mentum.

Triangles of the Neck

- Neck/cervical region/cervix is a complex region that connects the head to the trunk.
  - Spinal cord, nerves, trachea, esophagus, and major vessels traverse this highly flexible area.
  - Neck contains other organs and several important glands.
- Neck can be subdivided into anterior, posterior, and lateral regions.

The Anterior Region of the Neck

- Has several palpable landmarks, including the larynx, trachea, and sternal notch.
  - The larynx—found in the middle of the neck composed of multiple cartilages thyroid cartilage.
- **"Adam's apple:"** Inferior to the larynx are the cricoid cartilage and trachea. Terminates at the sternal (jugular) notch of the manubrium and the left and right clavicles **(Fig. 3.17)**.

The Nuchal Region

- **The posterior neck region**
  - Houses the spinal cord, cervical vertebrae, and associated structures.
  - The bump at the lower boundary of this region is the vertebral prominens.

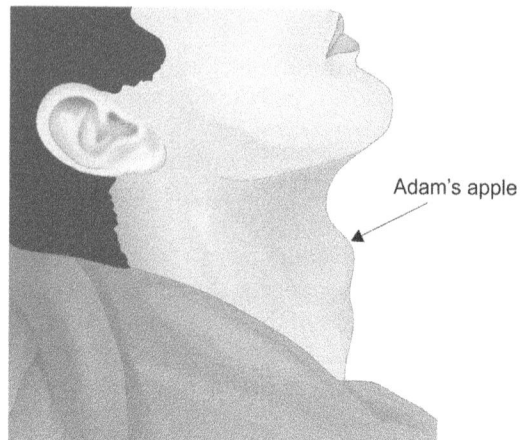

Fig. 3.17: Adam's apple.

- Superiorly along the midline of the neck, is the ligamentum nuchae, a thick ligament that runs from C7 to the nuchal lines of the skull.
- Left and right lateral portions the neck of contain the sternocleidomastoid muscles which partitions the neck into two clinically important triangles, an anterior triangle and a posterior triangle.

❖ Each triangle houses important structures that run through the neck.
❖ Triangles are further subdivided into smaller triangles.
  - Anterior triangle lies anterior to the sternocleidomastoid muscle and inferior to the mandible.
  - Subdivided into four smaller triangles:
    ♦ The submental, submandibular, carotid, and muscular triangles.

The Submental Triangle

The most superiorly placed of the four triangles. Inferior to the chin in the midline of the neck.
❖ Partially bounded by the anterior belly of the digastric muscle.
❖ Contains some cervical lymph nodes and tiny veins, with illness these lymph nodes enlarge and become tender.
❖ Palpation can determine if an infection is present.

The Submandibular Triangle

Inferior to the mandible and lateral to the submental triangle.
❖ Bounded by the mandible and the bellies of the digastric muscle.
❖ The submandibular gland is the bulge under the mandible.

The Carotid Triangle

"Bounded by the sternocleidomastoid, omohyoid, and posterior digastric muscles".
* The strong pulsation is the common carotid artery.
* Contains the internal jugular vein and some cervical lymph nodes.

The Muscular Triangle

Most inferior of the four triangles.
* Contains the sternohyoid and sternothyroid muscles, as well as the lateral edges of the larynx and the thyroid gland.
  * Also contains cervical lymph nodes which are present throughout the neck.

The Posterior Triangle

Lateral region of the neck
* Posterior to the sternocleidomastoid muscle.
* Superior to the clavicle inferiorly.
* Anterior to the trapezius muscle.

Subdivided into two smaller triangles
* The occipital triangle
* Supraclavicular triangle

The Occipital Triangle

Larger and More Posteriorly Placed

Bounded by the omohyoid, trapezius, and sternocleidomastoid muscles. Contains the external jugular vein, the accessory nerve, the brachial plexus, and some lymph nodes.

Supraclavicular Triangle

"Also called omoclavicular and subclavian, bounded by the clavicle, omohyoid, and sternocleidomastoid muscles." Contains part of the subclavian vein and artery as well as some lymph nodes".

Thorax

The superior portion of the trunk sandwiched between the neck superiorly and the abdomen inferiorly.
* Consists of the chest and the 'upper back'.
  * On the anterior surface of the chest are the two dominating surface features of the thorax. The clavicles and the sternum.

The Clavicles

* Paired clavicles and the sternal (jugular) notch represent the border between the thorax and the neck **(Fig. 3.18)**.

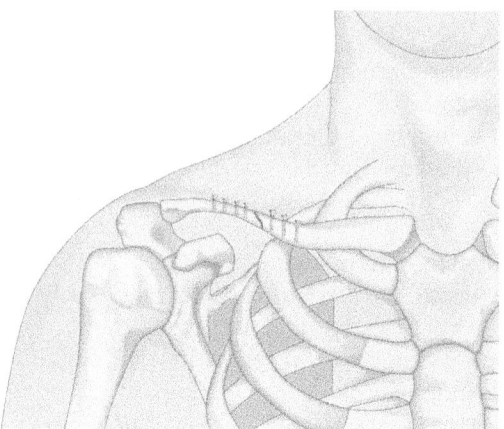

Fig. 3.18: Clavicle bone.

- On the superior anterior surface where they extend between the base of the neck on the right and left sides laterally to the shoulders.
- Left and right costal margins of the rib cage form the inferior boundary of the thorax.
- Costal angle (costal arch) is where the costal margins join to form an inverted V at the xiphoid process.
    - On a thin person, many of the ribs can be seen.
- Most of the ribs (with the exception of the first one) can be palpated.

The Sternum

Palpated readily as the midline bony structure in the thorax.
- The manubrium, the body, and the xiphoid process may also be palpated.
    - Sternal angle can be felt as an elevation between the manubrium and the body.
    - Sternal angle is clinically important because it is at the level of the costal cartilage of the second rib.

It is often used as a landmark for counting the ribs.

The Abdomen

- "On the anterior surface of the abdomen, the umbilicus (navel) is the prominent depression or projection in the midline of the abdominal wall".
- "In the midline of the abdominal anterior surface is the linea alba, a tendinous structure that extends inferiorly from the xiphoid process to the pubic symphysis".
- The left and right rectus abdominis muscles and their tendinous insertions are referred to as "six-pack abs."

- The superior aspect of the ilium (iliac crest) terminates anteriorly at the anterior superior iliac spine.
- Attached to the anterior superior iliac spine is the inguinal ligament, which forms the lower boundary of the abdominal wall.

The Inguinal Ligament

- Terminates on a little anterior bump on the pubis called the pubic tubercle.
- Superior to the medial portion of the inguinal ligament is the superficial inguinal ring.
- A superficial opening in the lower anterior abdominal wall represents a weak spot in the wall can be palpated to detect an inguinal hernia.

Foot and Toes

- The phalanges, metatarsophalangeal joints, PIP and DIP joints, and toenails are obvious surface landmarks readily observed when viewing either the lateral side or the dorsum of the foot.
- The medial surface of the foot clearly illustrates the high, arched medial longitudinal arch.
- At the distal end of the medial longitudinal arch, the head of metatarsal I appears as a prominent bump.

Important Bony Landmark

Bones

Bones are important parts of the skeletal system that make up the framework for the body. Bones are made of connective tissue, of which there are two types. Compact bone tissue which makes up the hard outermost layer of bone; cancellous bone tissue is transformed into thin pieces called trabeculae to form the inner parts of a bone, particularly at the ends of long bones. Bones function as muscle attachment sites to aid in movement, sites for blood cell production, mineral storage, and protection of vital organs.

Describing the Major Landmarks of Bones

Bones come in all shapes and sizes, from the tiny auditory bones in your ear to the large, long bones in your arms and legs. Some look really strange with many shapes that stick out, and some even have holes in them.

Bone may have only a few or many of these landmarks, depending on its size, shape, and function.

Bony Landmarks

When discussing the parts of bones, bony landmarks are important for reference. Anatomically, these landmarks serve primarily as muscle attachment points but can also be passageways for blood vessels and nerves to pass through. There are many terms that are used to describe landmarks which can be applied throughout the skeleton. Learning the landmark terms makes it easier to understand what the bony structure should look like and the function it may serve.

Epiphysis

The term epiphysis can be traced back to its root meaning. The prefix epi- means above or upon. The suffix-physis refers to an area of growth, referencing the growth plate. In a long bone (bones that make up the arms and legs), the epiphysis is the rounded ends of the bone. An example would be the circular ends of the humerus closest to the elbow.

Diaphysis

The term diaphysis can also be traced back to its Latin stems. The prefix dia- means through as in the word diameter. The diaphysis of a long bone is the shaft of the bone which travels "through" both ends of a long bone. An example is the diaphysis of the humerus, the shaft of the upper arm bone.

Tubercle

A tubercle is a small, rounded projection protruding from a bone. Tubercles typically connect tendons to muscles. An example is Gerdy's tubercle that sits to the anterior and lateral surface of the tibia, just below the patella. This tubercle is the insertion for the iliotibial tract (IT band). Other examples of tubercles include the greater and lesser tubercles of the humerus.

Tuberosity

A tuberosity is a small, roughened process on a bone and is typically associated with muscle attachment points. An example is the tibial tuberosity on the anterior and proximal portion of the tibia. The tibial tuberosity is a rough spot that can be felt below the patella and serves as an attachment point for the quadriceps tendon.

Process

A process protrudes from a bone and serves as an attachment point for tendons and ligaments. There are many examples of bony processes, including the spine. The spine has spinous processes which stick out posteriorly and may be noticeable on a person who is undernourished or thin-skinned. The scapula also has many processes, including the acromion process and the coracoid process. These processes are sites of muscle attachment and ligament attachment that bind the scapula to the clavicle.

This image of the shoulder joint shows the acromion process and coracoid process. The coracoid process is a muscle attachment point for the biceps muscle.

Condyle

A condyle is a large, rounded projection. Condyles typically make up the epiphysis of long bones. Examples are the condyles of the tibia, which make up the proximal epiphysis of the bone. These condyles will connect with the femoral condyles, the distal epiphysis, to make up the knee joint.

Trochanter

A trochanter is a large, roughened prominence. A good example is the greater trochanter and lesser trochanter of the femur. Both of these roughened processes serve as muscle attachment points.

Heads

The landmark term "head" refers to a large round prominence. A good example is the head of the humerus which serves as the "ball" part of the shoulder.

Crests

A crest is a raised slender ridge on a bone. Like the crest of a wave or a hill, the crest of a bone is a slender area located at the top of a bone. An example is the iliac crest, a ridge at the top of the ilium.

Foramen

A foramen is a hole or opening through a bone. Typically, blood vessels and/or nerves will pass through a foramen. An example is the foramen magnum of the skull. This is the large opening at the base of the occipital bone in which the spinal cord passes through as it comes from the brain. The spinal cord will continue downward passing through the vertebral foramen of each vertebra.

Sinus

One of the bony landmarks of the skull is the sinus. A sinus is a hollow space within the skull, and there are many sinuses found in the skull. These sinuses are lined with a mucosa that helps trap debris that is inhaled and assists in warming the air. An infection in the sinuses is called sinusitis.

Things that Stick Out

Other terms that describe features of bones can be broken into two general categories—things that stick out, or empty spaces, like holes and pits in the bone. We'll start with the things that stick out.

A process is a prominent projection on a bone. Processes are often locations where bones make connections with ligaments, tendons, and other bones. For example, each vertebra in your back has several processes where tendons connect or where one vertebra connects to another.

Another great example of a process is the mastoid process, which is found on your skull just under ear. They are all prominent projections, so to help you remember what a process looks like, always think a process is a prominent projection!

Processes can be further divided based on their size and shape. Condyles are rounded processes that connect with other bones in a joint. At the base of skull are two condyles known as the occipital condyles. They are the area where the skull connects with the top vertebrae. There are two other big condyles at the front end of femur that connect with the tibia in knee.

A trochanter is another type of large, roughened process where tendons attach. Near the hip on the top of femur, there are two processes known as the greater and lesser trochanters. They are sites where the large muscles in upper leg attach to femur and allow to move hip joint.

Some bones, like the humerus in upper arm, have round enlargements at the end known as heads. These are called heads because they look just like your head—round. Heads always form part of ball and socket joints. The round heads are the balls that fit into a socket on another bone.

■ CONCEPT OF MEDIASTENUM

Introduction

Mediastinum major part of thoracic cavity is occupied by a pair of lungs covered by its serous covering, by its serous covering, the pleura. Mediastinum is the median septum which lies between the two pleural sacs.

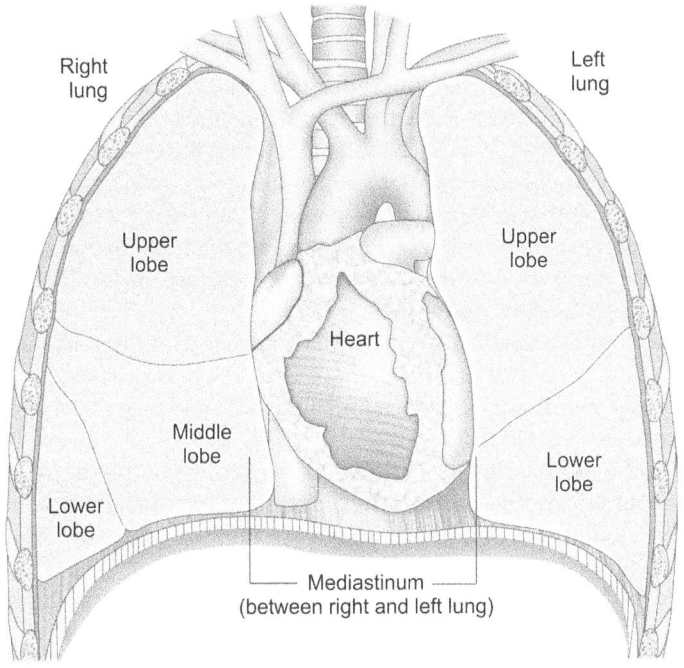

Fig. 3.19: Mediastinum.

The mediastinum lies within the thorax and is enclosed on the right and left by pleurae. It is surrounded by the chest wall in front, the lungs to the sides and the spine at the back. It extends from the sternum in front to the vertebral column behind. It contains all the organs of the thorax except the lungs. It is continuous with the loose connective tissue of the neck **(Fig. 3.19)**.

Definition

The thoracic mediastinum is the compartment that runs the length of the thoracic cavity between the pleural sacs of the lungs. This compartment extends longitudinally from the thoracic inlet to the superior surface of the diaphragm.

It is a partition between the right and left pleural sacs. It includes all the structures which lie in the intermediate compartments of the thoracic cavity.

Structure and Function

Mediastinum

The mediastinum is divided compartmentally and consists of subdivisions that house and support vital structures within the thorax. Below are the borders of each region of the mediastinum.

- **Superior mediastinum:** Bordered by the thoracic outlet superiorly, transverse thoracic plane (the plane of Ludwig) or sternal angle inferiorly, medial border of the pleural sacs laterally, dorsal surface of the sternum anteriorly, and ventral surface of the first four thoracic vertebral bodies posteriorly.
- **Anterior mediastinum:** Bordered by the pericardium posteriorly, medial border of the pleural sacs laterally, and the sternum, transversus thoracis muscles, and fifth, sixth, and seventh left costal cartilages anteriorly.
- **Middle mediastinum:** Formed by the borders of the pericardial sac anteriorly and posteriorly, reflected to the medial borders of the pleural sacs bilaterally, transverse thoracic plane superiorly, and thoracic surface of the diaphragm inferiorly.
- **Posterior mediastinum:** Bordered by the pericardium anteriorly, the thoracic surface of the diaphragm inferiorly, the transverse thoracic plane superiorly, the bodies of the fifth to the twelfth thoracic vertebrae posteriorly, and the pleural sacs laterally.

Function

- **Serving as a "house":** For heart and the roots of great vessels. These are the blood vessels that attach directly to the heart to carry blood into or out of heart.
- **Protecting thymus:** Heart and other structures. Fatty tissue and connective tissue in mediastinum provide cushioning. Mediastinum sits behind sternum, or "breastbone," which provides additional protection to this important area.
- **Providing a passageway:** For structures to travel between your neck and chest, and between chest and belly. It contains body structures that act as railroad tracks, transporting cargo (like food or air) where it needs to go. For example, esophagus carries foods and liquids through mediastinum to get from throat to stomach.

Organ in your mediastinum include:
- **Esophagus:** Esophagus (food tube) passes through mediastinum as it travels from throat to stomach.
- **Heart:** Heart is a muscular organ that pumps blood throughout body. It is located in the middle of mediastinum. Heart is surrounded by a protective sac called pericardium.

- **Thymus:** Thymus supports your immune system and is most active before puberty. It is located in the front, upper part of mediastinum.
- **Trachea:** Trachea (windpipe) helps to breathe. It is located just in front of esophagus. It travels from lower neck into chest, before branching in two and traveling into each of pleural cavities.

Parts of Meadiastinum

Superior Mediastinum

- **Organs:** Thymus, trachea, esophagus.
- **Arteries:** aortic arch, brachiocephalic trunk, left common carotid artery, left subclavian artery.
- **Veins and lymphatics:** Superior vena cava, brachiocephalic veins, the arch of the azygos, thoracic duct.
- **Nerves:** Left and right vagus, recurrent laryngeal, cardiac, left and right phrenic nerves.

Anterior Mediastinum

- **Organs:** Thymus
- **Arteries:** Internal thoracic branches
  - *Veins and lymphatics:* Internal thoracic branches, parasternal lymph nodes.
  - *Nerves:* None.

Middle Mediastinum

- **Organs:** The heart and its great vessel roots, trachea and main bronchi.
- **Arteries:** Ascending aorta, pulmonary trunk, pericardiacophrenic arteries
  - *Veins and lymphatics:* Superior vena cava, pulmonary veins, pericardiacophrenic veins.
- **Nerves:** Phrenic, vagus, sympathetic.

Posterior Mediastinum

- **Organs:** Esophagus
- **Arteries:** Descending thoracic aorta
- **Veins and lymphatics:** Azygos hemiazygos veins, thoracic duct.
- **Nerves:** Vagus, splanchnic, sympathetic chain.

The superior mediastinum is essentially a conduit space allowing structures to pass between the head, neck, and thorax. The anterior mediastinum is protective in nature and filled with connective and fatty tissue that cushions and supports the thymus as well as the vital cardiac structures just posterior to it. The middle mediastinum houses the heart and the roots of the great vessels. The posterior mediastinum, which can be thought of as a continuation of the superior mediastinum, also serves as a conduit. It provides space for the passage of structures between the thoracic and abdominal cavities.

Blood Supply and Lymphatics

The thoracic mediastinum houses the heart and the great vessels. Due to this anatomical configuration, the thoracic mediastinum has many blood vessels travelling through it. Since the lymphatic system closely integrates into the cardiovascular system, there is also a significant presence of lymphatics in this area.

The superior mediastinum contains the arch of the aorta and its three associated major branches: the brachiocephalic trunk, the left common carotid, and the left subclavian arteries. In addition to these large arteries, some smaller branches of the aorta are present within the superior mediastinum including the thymic branches of the internal thoracic arteries, the proximal portions of the pericardiophrenic arteries, and the third and fourth posterior intercostal arteries. The majority of lymphatic drainage in this region coalesces at the thoracic duct, which empties into the bloodstream at the left subclavian vein.

The internal thoracic arteries descend inferiorly and deep to the lateral borders of the sternum. These arteries exit the anterior thoracic mediastinum inferiorly and branch into the musculophrenic arteries and superior epigastric arteries. Lymphatics in this region include the parasternal, pericardial and superior diaphragmatic lymph nodes. The middle thoracic mediastinum, bounded by the pericardium, contains the coronary arteries and its associated branches. The lymphatics within the pericardium are a complex network of vessels that penetrate all layers of the cardiac tissue. These vessels ultimately drain posteriorly towards the pretracheal lymph nodes that lie between the aorta and the trachea.

The posterior thoracic mediastinum contains the descending aorta as it courses slightly left of midline down towards the diaphragm. The most notable arterial branches in this region are the proximal portions of the intercostal arteries. The lymphatics of this region include the thoracic duct, retrocardiac lymph nodes, diaphragmatic lymph nodes, posterior mediastinal lymph nodes, and prevertebral lymph nodes.

Nerve

In the superior mediastinum, there are two broad categories of nerves passing within the region, nerves that originate superior to the thorax and nerves that originate within the thorax. The superior thoracic mediastinum contains the left and right phrenic nerves (C3-C5), the left and right vagus nerves, and other associated vagal branches including the esophageal plexus, the inferior cervical cardiac branches, the thoracic cardiac branches, and the recurrent laryngeal nerves. As for the nerves originating from within the thorax, there is the superior portion of the sympathetic trunk (T1 through T4) and its associated sympathetic branches such as the thoracic cardiac and pulmonary branches.

The anterior mediastinum does not contain any major named nerves.

The middle mediastinum is densely innervated by the autonomic nervous system and somatically innervated by the phrenic nerves.

The sympathetic innervation arises from branches of the sympathetic trunk around the T2 through T4 levels while parasympathetic innervation derives from branches of the left and right vagus nerves. Branches of the left and right phrenic nerves provide somatic innervation to the fibrous and parietal pericardial layers. Because the boundaries of the middle mediastinum are the borders of the pericardium itself, only a small portion of the nerves mentioned truly reside within the middle mediastinum.

The posterior mediastinum contains many autonomic and somatic nerves. Sympathetic nerves arise from the sympathetic chain at the T5 to T12 levels and parasympathetic innervation is provided by the left and right vagus nerves which form of the esophageal plexus. The somatic nerves in the posterior mediastinum are the intercostal nerves.

Muscle

Although often overlooked, there are many critical muscular structures within the thoracic mediastinum. For example, the superior thoracic mediastinum contains the skeletal and smooth muscle of the esophagus and the left and right inferior oblique portion of longus colli muscle which assists in mobilizing the cervical spine. The anterior thoracic mediastinum contains the transversus thoracis muscles, an accessory muscle of expiration. The transversus thoracis muscles originate on the posterolateral area of the sternum and aid in depressing the ribs during active expiration. The middle thoracic mediastinum houses one of the most important muscles of the body, the heart. The posterior thoracic mediastinum contains the distal smooth muscular portion of the esophagus. Many of the large blood vessels in the mediastinum comprise numerous layers of smooth muscle that allow for cardiovascular homeostasis.

Clinical Siginificance

The thoracic mediastinum is a significant region of the human body that includes vital cardiopulmonary structures. The mediastinum is involved in a variety of clinical abnormalities at all ages. Below is an abbreviated list of clinical correlations organized by subdivision.

The superior thoracic mediastinum is clinically relevant due to its large vessels and nerves. Penetrating wounds to this area have a high likelihood of affecting important vessels or nerves resulting in critical damage on impact, as well as during extraction. The arch of the aorta, the site of a potential aneurysm, runs through the center of the superior thoracic mediastinum. It carries the entirety of the cardiac output before its distribution throughout the body. An aneurysm in the arch of the aorta is dangerous and if untreated for long enough can dissect and result in near-instant death. The superior thoracic mediastinum also houses parts of the esophagus and trachea, which are both conduits that commonly are obstructed and injured by ingestion and inhalation of foreign substances.

The anterior mediastinum may appear clinically benign, but it is responsible for many clinical considerations. The thymus, located in the superior portion of the anterior mediastinum, is notorious for its role in diseases such as myasthenia gravis, pure red cell aplasia, and thymus cancer. Additionally, the anterior mediastinum is located directly posterior to the sternum and is therefore vulnerable to trauma to the anterior thorax which can result in an intrathoracic or thymic hematoma.

The middle mediastinum is arguably the most important subdivision of the region as it contains the pericardium, heart, and great vessel roots. Myocardial infarction, pericardial effusion, cardiac tamponade, tetralogy of Fallot, and cardiomegaly are just a few examples of pathologies that manifest in the middle thoracic mediastinum.

The posterior mediastinum a large amount of its clinical importance from the structures descending from the superior thoracic mediastinum. The descending aorta, autonomic nervous networks, extensive lymphatics, and esophagus are all capable of causing vast systemic dysfunction in the presence of pathology. Descending thoracic aortic aneurysm, thoracic duct obstruction, and distal esophageal related dysphagia are problems that can quickly evolve into life-threatening situations.

These examples are just a few of the many pathologies involved in the thoracic mediastinum. These compartments and their structures are often involved in diseases from acute to chronic, infectious to traumatic, and congenital to neoplastic. Therefore, understanding the distinct regions of the thoracic mediastinum, the contained structures, landmarks, and physiologic variants, is essential to clinicians at all levels.

Common conditions affect the mediastinum: Many different conditions can affect the organs and tissues in your mediastinum. Some conditions begin in the mediastinum, such as primary tumors or cysts. Other times, a disease (like cancer) spreads to your mediastinum from somewhere else in your body. Infections that affect your whole body (systemic) can also impact your mediastinum.

Some conditions that may affect your mediastinum:
- Aortic dissection.
- Cardiac tamponade.
- Esophageal cancer.
- Goiter.
- Heart disease.
- Lymphoma.
- Mediastinal tumors.
- Mediastinitis (swelling or infection).
- Myasthenia gravis.
- Thoracic aortic aneurysm.

Tests check the health of the mediastinum:
- Chest X-ray.
- Computed tomography (CT) scan.
- Magnetic resonance imaging (MRI) scan.
- Mediastinoscopy.
- Ultrasound.

Ways to keep mediastinum healthy:
- Avoid smoking and all tobacco products. Ask your provider for resources to help you quit.
- Eat a heart-healthy diet.
- Exercise regularly.
- Check with your provider before starting a new exercise plan.
- Limit alcohol intake.
- Take your medications as prescribed.
- Visit your provider for yearly.

SKIN AS SENSORY ORGAN

Introduction

Skin is the general covering of the entire external surface of the body. It is continuous with the mucous membrane at the orifices of the body. It has sensory nerve ending that helps in perceiving pain, touch, hot or cold, etc., because of the presence of sweat glands, it helps the body in temperature regulation. It protects the underlying structures from injury and from invasion by microbes.

It is made up of three layers, the epidermis, dermis and the hypodermis, all three of which vary significantly in their anatomy and function. Skin (including cutaneous and sub cutaneous tissues) plays a crucial role in the formation, structure and function of extra-skeleton apparatus such as a mammal.

Definition

The skin is the largest organ of the human body and has a range of vital functions in supporting survival. The primary function of the skin is to form a physical barrier between the internal environment of an organism and the outside world.

The skin also helps to maintain homeostasis by preventing water and regulating body temperature. It protects the organism from the damaging effects of UV lights and helps to produce vitamin D when exposed to the sun.

Structure of the Skin

In adults the skin is the largest organ and has a surface area of about 1.5–2 m^2 (average 1.7 m^2). It contains accessory structure glands, hair and nails.

Layers of the skin:
- Epidermis
- Dermis
- Hypodermis

Epidermis

It is the superficial, avascular layer of the stratified squamous epithelium. It is ectodermal in origin and gives rise to appendages of the skin. Namely hair, nail, sweat gland and sebaceous gland. Structurally the epidermis is made up of deep germinative zone comprising **(Fig. 3.20)**.
- Stratum basale
- Stratum spinosum

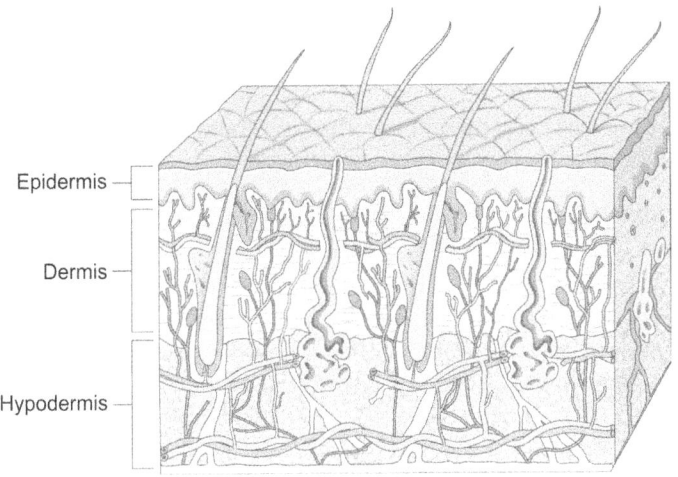

Fig. 3.20: Layers of skin.

- Stratum granulosum
- Stratum lucidum
- Stratum corneum

Stratum Basale

It is the deepest basal layer of the epidermis made of a single layer of columnar cell that rest on basal lamina these cells undergo mitotic division and give off cells keratinocytes which form superficial layer of epidermis. Therefore, the basale layer is also known as the germinal layer or stratum germinativum.

Stratum Spinosum

It consists of several layers of the polygonal keratinocytes. These cells appear to have a number of spines that is why this layer is called as stratum spinosum.

Stratum Granulosum

It consists of 1–5 layers of flattened cells, containing deeply staining granules in their cytoplasm. The granules consist of protein called keratohyalin.

Stratum Lucidum

This layer appears clear, homogenous, with distinct cells boundaries.

Stratum Cornium

Most superficial layer of the epidermis. The cells or corneocytes are dead. These have lost their nuclei and organelle. They are extremely flattened. These are scale like (squamous). These cells contain keratin. They are held together by a layer of lipid, which makes the layer "waterproof".

Dermis

The dermis is tough and elastic. It is form from connective tissue and the matrix contains collagen interlaced with the elastic fibers, rupture of elastic fibers occurs the skin is over stretched, resulting in permanent striae, or stretch marks, which are typically formed in pregnancy and obesity. Collagen fibers bind water and give the skin its tensile strength, but as this ability declines with age, wrinkles develop. Fibroblasts, macrophages and mast cells are the main cells found in the dermis. The subcutaneous layer, containing areolar tissue and varying amount of adipose (fat) tissues, lies under the dermis. Structure found in the dermis are:
- Small blood and lymph vessels
- Sensory nerves ending
- Sweat gland and their ducts
- Hair, arrector-pili muscles and sebaceous glands.

Hypodermis

The hypodermis is the bottom layer of the skin. Also known as subcutaneous tissue. The hypoderm is insulates and protects the body, store energy (fat), help to regulates the body temperature, and connects the skin to muscles and bone. The hypodermis contains collagen fibres, adipose tissue, connective tissue, larger nerves and blood vessels. It also includes the macrophages cells that are the part of immune system and help keep your body free of introduces.

Pigmentation of Skin

The color of the skin is determined by at least five pigments present in it:
1. Melanin (brown), presented in the germinative zone of the epidermis.
2. Melanoid (resembles melanin present diffusely throughout the epidermis).
3. Carotene (orange and yellow), present in the stratum cornium and fat cells of the dermis and superficial fascia.
4. Hemoglobin (purple)
5. Oxyhemoglobin (red), present in the cutaneous vessels.

Types of Skin

There are two types of skin:
1. **Thick skin or glabrous skin:** In this type of skin epidermis is very thick with a thick layer of stratum corneum. It is found in palm hands and soles of feet. It has no hair.
2. **Thin or hairy skin:** In this type of skin epidermis is very thin. It contains hair and found in other parts of body except palm and soles.

- ❖ **Blood supply:** Skin is a highly vascular organ. It drives its arterial blood from a number of plexuses. One plexus of arteries is present over the deep fascia; another plexus, just below the dermis is called reticular plexus, the papillary plexus lies just below the dermal papilla. Capillary loops arising from the plexus pass into each dermal papilla.

  The epidermis has no blood supply. It derives its nutrition entirely by diffusion from the capillary loops of the dermal papillae. There are numerous arteriovenous anastomoses in the skin, which have an important role in temperature regulation.
- ❖ **Nerve supply:** There are motor and sensory nerves
  - The motor nerve fibers are autonomic nerve fibers which are sudomotor, pilomotor and vasomotor. The sensory nerve ending in the skin are of the following type:
    - ♦ Free nerve ending, Merkel's disc, Meissner's corpuscles
    - ♦ Pacinian corpuscles, Ruffini's ending, Krause bulbs.

Appendages of Skin

Nails

Nails are hardened keratin plates (cornified zone) on the dorsal surface of the tips of finger and toes. Each nails have following parts:
- ❖ Root is the proximal hidden part which buried into the nail grove and is overlapped by the nail fold of the skin.
- ❖ Body is the exposed part of the nail which is adherent to the underlying skin, root and body together form nails plate.
- ❖ Free boarder is the distal part free form the skin it is attach to the undersurface by hyponychium.

The proximal part of the body present white opaque crescent called lunula. Each lateral border of the nail body is over lapped by a fold of skin, termed the nail fold and the groove between nail body and nail fold which is called nail groove.

The skin (germinative zone + dermis) of the nail bed beneath the root and lunula is thick proliferative (germinal matrix), and is responsible for the growth of the nail. The rest of the nail bed is thin (sterile matrix) over which the growing nail glide. Under the translucent body (except lunula) of the nail, the corium is very vascular. This accounts for their pink color.

The nail of middle finger grows the fastest.

Hair

Hairs are keratinous filaments derived from invaginations of the germinative layer of epidermis into the dermis. These are peculiar to mammals and help in conservation of their body heat. Hairs are distributed all over the body, except for the palm, soles, dorsal aspect of distal phalanges, umbilicus, glans penis, inner surface of prepuce, the labia minora and inner surface of labia minora, and inner surface of labia majora.

Structure of hair: Each hair has an implanted part called the root, a bulb and a projecting part, called the shaft.

Layers of shaft: Innermost is the medulla, cortex is the middle one and cuticle is a single outer layer:

- The root is surrounded by a hair follicle (a sheath of epidermis and dermis), and is expanded at its proximal end to form the hair bulb. Each hair bulb is invaginated at its end or from nails by hair papilla (vascular connective tissue) which forms the neurovascular hilum of the hair and its sheath.
- Hair follicle surrounds the hair. Wall of the follicle comprises:
  - Inner root sheath
  - Outer root sheath
  - Connective tissue sheath

The arrectores pilorum muscles (smooth muscles supplied by sympathetic nerve) connect the undersurface of the follicles to the superficial part of the dermis. Arrector pili muscles are absent in a few regions like hair of face, axilla eyelashes, eyebrows, hair of anterior nares and of external auditory meatus.

Growth of hair: The hairs grow at the rate of about 1.5–2.2 mm/week.

Color of hair: Color of hair depends upon the amount and type of melanin pigment.

Sweat Glands

Sudoriferous or sweat glands are distributed all over the skin, except for the lips, glans penis, and nail bed. These glands are of two types; eccrine and apocrine.

Eccrine Glands

The eccrine glands are much more abundant and distributed in almost every part of the skin.

The coiled part, called the body of the gland, lies in the deeper part of corium or in the subcutaneous tissue. The straight part, called the duct, traverses the dermis and epidermis and opens on the surface of the skin.

- **Location**: The glands are large in the axilla and groin, most numerous in the palms and soles. The eccrine glands are merocrine in nature, i.e., produce thin watery secretion without any disintegration of the epithelial cells.
- **Functions**: The glands help in regulation of the body temperature by evaporation of sweat, and also help in excreting the body salts.

Apocrine Glands

Apocrine glands are confined to axilla, eyelids (Moll's glands), nipple and areola of the breast, perianal region and the external genitalia.

- **Structure:** They are larger than eccrine glands and produce a thicker secretion having a characteristic odor. They develop in close association with hair. Ceruminous glands of the external auditory meatus are modified apocrine sweat glands.
- **Nervous control:** The apocrine glands also are merocrine in nature, but are regulated by a dual autonomic control.
- **Functions:** In animals, they produce chemical signals or pheromones, which are important in courtship and social behavior.

Sebaceous Gland

- **Location:** Sebaceous glands, producing an oily secretion, are widely distributed all over the dermis of the skin.
- **Structure:** Sebaceous glands are small and sacculated in appearance, made up of a cluster of about 2-5 piriform alveoli. Most of their ducts open into the hair follicles. Sebaceous glands are holocrine in nature.
- **Nervous control:** The secretion is under hormonal control, especially the androgens.
- **Functions**: It lubricates skin and protects it from moisture. Sebum also lubricates hair and prevent thems from becoming brittle.

Functions of Skin

- **Protection:** Skin protects the body from mechanical injuries.

- **Physical barrier:** Due to stratum corneum, skin acts as a barrier against bacterial infections, heat and cold, wet and drought, acid and alkali.
- **Immune properties:** Langerhans cells phagocytose antigen and take it to T lymphocytes.
- **Reflex action:** Sensory nerve endings start reflex action against painful stimuli and prevent it from damage.

Regulation of body temperature: The internal body temperature is maintained in a normal range by homeostatic mechanisms despite wide fluctuations in environmental temperature. Humans and mammals are homeothermic, i.e., they maintain constant body temperature. Body temperature is least at 5 AM and is highest in afternoon. If the rate of body heat production equals the rate of heat loss, the body maintains a constant core temperature near 98.6°F (37°C). Core temperature is the temperature in body structures that lie deep to the skin and subcutaneous layer. Shell temperature is the temperature near the body surface in the skin and the subcutaneous layer. Normally, shell temperature is lower than core temperature by 1–6°C depending on environmental temperature.

- **Heat production:** The production of body heat is proportional to metabolic rate. Factors affecting the metabolic rate are:
  - *Body temperature:* Higher the body temperature, higher is the metabolic rate. For each 1°C rise in core temperature, metabolic rate increases by 10%.
  - *Exercise:* During strenuous exercise metabolic rate may increase up to 20 times the basal metabolic rate (BMR) due to contraction of skeletal muscles.
  - *Nervous system:* Stimulation of sympathetic division of autonomic nervous system releases norepinephrine and epinephrine, both of which increase the metabolic rate.
  - *Hormones:* Thyroid hormones are the main regulators of BMR. BMR increases as blood levels of thyroid hormones rise. Growth hormones, testosterone and insulin also increase the BMR.
  - *Ingestion of food:* This activity raises the metabolic rate by 10–20% due to the increase in metabolic rate during the process of digestion, absorption and storage of nutrients. This food induced increase in heat production is maximally seen after eating a high protein diet. Metabolic rate is also affected by gender (lower in females except during pregnancy and lactation), sleep (lower), and age (higher in children).
- **Heat loss:** Normal body temperature is maintained when heat is lost to the environment at the same rate as it is produced by metabolic reactions. Heat from the body can be lost by only.

- *Conduction:* It is the exchange of heat that occurs between molecules of two materials that are in direct contact with each other. At rest, about 3% of body heat is lost via conduction to solid materials in contact with body such as chair and clothing. If a body is submerged in cold or hot water, heat loss or gain via conduction is much greater because water conducts heat 20 times more effectively than air.
- *Convection:* It is the transfer of heat by movement of a gas/liquid between areas of different temperature. Contact of air/water with human body results in heat transfer by both conduction and convection. When cool air comes in contact with body, it warms and become less dense; and is carried away by convection currents created as less dense air rises. At rest, about 15% of body heat is lost to air via conduction and convection.
- *Radiation:* It is the transfer of heat in the form of infrared rays between a warmer object and a cooler one without physical contact. About 60% heat loss occurs via radiation in a resting room at 21°C.
- *Evaporation:* It is the conversion of liquid to a vapor. Every milliliter of water evaporates taking with it about 0.58 calories of heat. At rest, about 22% of heat is lost through evaporation of about 700 mL water per day (300 mL in exhaled air and 400 mL from skin surface).

Heat is also lost through respiratory tract, urine and via feces.

❖ **Hypothalamic thermostatic**: The control center that regulates the temperature is the preoptic area in the anterior hypothalamus. Nerve signals from preoptic area are transmitted to the heat losing center and heat promoting center of the hypothalamus send nerve impulses to control centers in hypothalamus, which in turn sends impulses to heat promoting center.

These impulses also cause release of thyroid-stimulating hormone (TSH). These impulses help to raise the core temperature by:

❖ **Constriction of blood vessels of the skin:** Decreases heat loss through skin by decreasing flow of blood to skin. Piloerection, i.e., contraction of arrector pili muscles, which causes skin hair to stand up. These form an insulating layer to conserve heat.
❖ **Increased release of hormones by adrenal medulla:** These hormones bring about an increase in cellular metabolism, which increases heat production.
❖ **Increased TSH releases:** Increased secretion of thyroid hormones from thyroid gland, which in turn increases metabolic rate.

Impulses from the brain cause shivering (skeletal muscles contract in a repetitive cycle), increasing the metabolic rate.

APPLIED OCULAR ANATOMY

Introduction

The eye is the organ of sight. it is situated in the orbital cavity, a bony socket built into the bones of the face and supplied by the optic nerve (2nd cranial nerve). It is almost spherical in shape and about 2.5 cm in diameter. The space between the eye and the orbital cavity is occupied by adipose tissue. The bony walls of the orbit and the fat within it protect the eye from injury.

Structurally, the two eyes are separate but, unlike the ears, some of their activities are coordinated so that they normally function as pair. It is possible to see with only one eye (monocular vision) but three-dimensional vision is impaired when only one eye is used, especially in relation to the judgment of speed and distance.

Definition

The human eye is a sensory organ, part of sensory nervous system that react to the visible light and allows human to use visual information for various purposes including seeing things, keeping balance.

Structure

Internally, the eye is divided into the chambers the anterior and the posterior chambers, with the lens of the eye, the ciliary body and the suspensory ligaments separating them.

The anterior chamber is filled with clear, watery fluid called aqueous humor, and the posterior chamber is filled with a jelly like substance called vitreous humor (vitreous body).

There are 3 layers of the tissue in the walls of the eye:
1. **The outer fibrous layer:** Sclera and cornea.
2. **The middle vascular layer:** The choroids, ciliary body and iris.
3. **The inner nervous tissue layer:** The retina.

Sclera

The sclera, or white of the eye, forms the outermost layer of the posterior and the lateral aspects of the eyeball and is continuous anteriorly with the cornea. It is a firm fibrous membrane that

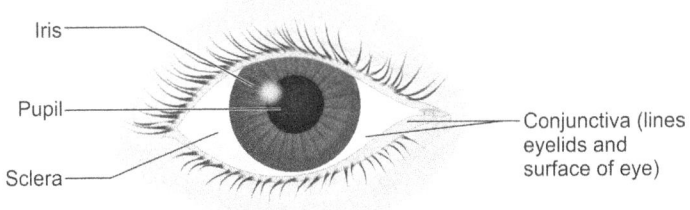

Fig. 3.21: Sclera.

maintains the shape of the eye and gives attachment to the extrinsic muscle of the eye (**Fig. 3.21**).

The anterior part of the external surface of the sclera is covered by the ocular conjunctiva. The rest of the sclera is in contact with a fascial sheath which surrounds the eyeball.

The sclera provides a smooth external surface that facilitates the movement of the eyeball.

This surface also provide attachment to the extrinsic muscles of the eyeball. Anteriorly the sclera becomes continuous with the cornea at the sclerocorneal junction.

Cornea

As the cornea is more convex than the sclera the junction to the marked, on the exterior of the eyeball, by a groove called the sulcus sclerae. The cornea is made up of five layers:
1. Corneal epithelium
2. Anterior limiting lamina
3. Substantia propria
4. Posterior limiting lamina
5. Endothelium of anterior chamber

Light rays pass through the cornea to reach the retina, the cornea is convex anteriorly and is involved in refracting (bending) light rays to focus them on the retina.

Choroid

The choroid consists of networks of blood vessels supported by connective tissue containing many pigmented cells that give it a dark brown color.

It is the dark color of the choroids that darkens the interior of the eyeball. It also prevents reflection of light within the eyeball.

Both these factors are necessary for formation of sharp image on the retina. Light enters the eye through the pupil, stimulate the sensory receptors in the retina (see below) and is then absorbed by the choroids.

Ciliary Body

The ciliary body is the anterior continuation of the choroid, consisting of ciliary muscle (circular smooth muscle fibers) and secretory epithelial cells. The lens is attached to the ciliary body by radiating suspensory ligaments like the spokes of a wheel. Contraction and the relaxation of the ciliary muscle fibers, which are attached to these ligaments, determine the size and the thickness of the lens. The ciliary body is supplied by parasympathetic branches of the oculomotor nerve (3rd cranial nerves).

Iris

The iris is the visible colored ring at the front of the eye and extends anteriorly from the ciliary body, lying behind the cornea and in front of the lens. It divides the anterior chamber of the eye into anterior and posterior cavities, which contains humor secreted by the ciliary body. The iris is composed of pigment cells and two layers of smooth muscle fibers, one circular and the other radiating in the center is an aperture called the pupil. The iris is supplied by parasympathetic and sympathetic nerves. Parasympathetic stimulation constricts the pupil and the sympathetic stimulation dilated it. The colors of the iris are genetically determined and depend on the number of the pigment's cells present. Albinos have no pigment cells and people with blue eyes have fewer than those with brown eyes.

Lens

The lens is a highly elastic circular biconvex body, lying immediately behind the pupil.

It consists of fibers enclosed within a capsule and is suspended from the ciliary body by the suspensory ligament. The lens bends (refracts) light rays reflected into the eye from objects in the visual field. When the ciliary muscle contracts, it releases its pull on the lens increasing its thickness. The nearer the object viewed, the thicker the lens becomes to allow focusing.

Retina

The retina is the innermost lining of the eye. It is an extremely delicate structure composed of several layers of nerve cell bodies and their axons, lying on the pigmented layer of epithelial cells. The retina lines about three quarters of the eyeball and is thickest at the back.

It thins out anteriorly to end just behind the ciliary body. Near the center of the posterior part is the macula lutea or yellow spot.

In the center of the yellow spot is a little depression called the fovea centralis, consisting only of cones. Toward the anterior part of the retina there are fewer cones than rods. About 0.5 cm to the nasal side of the macula lutea all the retinal nerve fibers converse to form the optic nerve. The small of retina where the optic nerve leaves the eye is the optic disc or blind spot. It has no light-sensitive cells.

Arterial Supply

Arterial supply is from the ciliary arteries and the central retinal artery. This are the branches of the ophthalmic artery, a branch of the internal carotid artery.

Venous drainage is by a number of veins including the central retinal veins, which eventually empty into a deep venous sinus. The central retinal artery and vein are encased in the optic nerve, which enters the eye at the optic disc.

Anterior of the Eye

The anterior chamber of the eye, i.e., the space between the cornea and the lens, is incompletely divided into anterior and posterior cavities by the iris. Both cavities contain a clear aqueous fluid, aqueous humor, secreted into the posterior cavity by the ciliary glands. It circulates in front of the lens, through the pupil into the anterior cavity and returns through scleral venous sinuous (canal of Schlemm) in the angle between the iris and the cornea the intraocular pressure remains fairly constant between 1.3 and 2.6 kPa (10-20 mm Hg), as production and drainage rates of aqueous humor are equal, an increase in the pressure causes glaucoma.

Aqueous humor supplies nutrients and removes waste from the transparent structures in the form of the eye that have no blood supply that is the cornea, lens and lens capsule. Behind the lens and filling the posterior chamber of the eyeball is the vitreous body. This is a soft colorless transparent jelly like substance composed of 99% water, mineral salt, mucoprotein, it maintains sufficient intraocular pressure to support the retina against the choroid and prevent the eyeball from collapsing.

The eye keeps its shape because of the intraocular pressure excreted by the vitreous body and the aqueous humor.

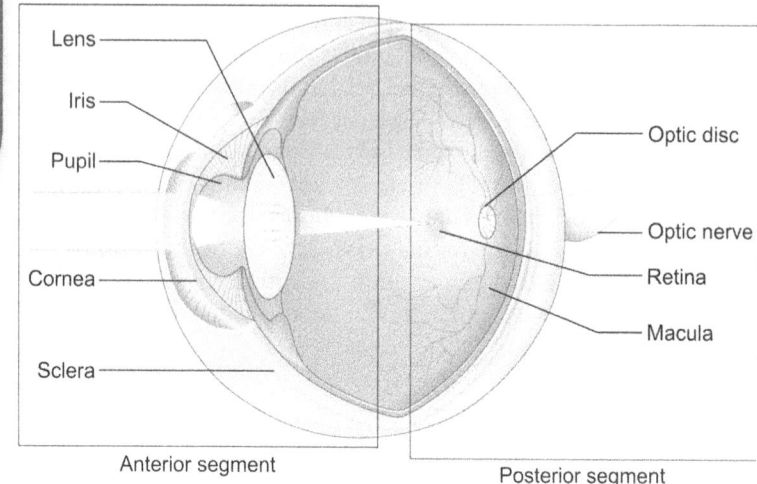

Fig. 3.22: Segment of eye.

Optic Nerves (Second Cranial Nerve)

The fibers of the optic nerve originate in the retina and converge to form the optic nerve about 0.5 cm to the nasal side of the macula lutea at the optic disc. It the passes through the optic foramen of the sphenoid bone, backward and medially to meets it counterpart from the outer eye at the optic chiasma **(Fig. 3.22)**.

Optic Chiasma

This is situated immediately in front of an above the pituitary gland which lies in the hypophyseal fossa of the sphenoid bone in the optic chiasma. The nerve fibers of the optic nerve from the nasal side of each retina cross over to the opposite side. The fibers from the temporal side do not cross but continue backward at the same side. This crossing over provides both cerebral hemispheres with sensory input from each eye.

Optic Tracts

These are the pathways of the optic nerves, posterior to the optic chiasma. Each tract consists of the nasal fibers from the retina of one eye and the temporal fibers from the retina of other. The optic tracts pass backward to synapse with the nerve's cells of the lateral geniculate bodies of the thalamus. From there nerves fibers proceed backwards a medially as the optic radiation, to terminate in the visual area of the cerebral cortex in the occipital lobes of the cerebrum. Other neurons originating in the lateral geniculate bodies transmit impulses from the eyes to cerebellum, where, together with impulses from the semicircular canal of the inner ears and from the skeletal muscles and joints, they contribute to the maintenance posture and balance.

MAJOR MUSCLES OF BODY

Myology: It is the term which is used to describe the study of muscles.

Muscles of the Face

There are many muscles involved in changing the facial expression and with movement of the lower jaw during chewing and speaking.

- **Occipitofrontalis (unpaired):** This consists of a posterior muscular part over the occipital bone, an interior part over the frontal bone and an extensive flat tendon that stretches over the dome of the skull and joins the two muscular parts.
- **Levator palpebrae superioris:** This muscle extends from the posterior part of the orbital cavity to the upper eyelid.
- **Orbicularis oculi:** This muscle surrounds the eye, eyelid and orbital cavity. It closes the eye and when strongly contracted 'screws up' the eyes.
- **Buccinator:** This flat muscle of the cheek draws the cheeks towards the teeth in chewing and in forcible expulsion of arc from the mouth.
- **Orbicularis oris (unpaired):** It surrounds the mouth and blends with the muscles of the cheeks. It closes the lips and strongly contracted the shapes of mouth for whistling.
- **Masseter:** This is a broad muscle extending from the zygomatic arch to the angle of the jaw.
- **Temporalis:** This muscle covers the squamous part of the temporal bone. It passes behind zygomatic arch to be inserted into the coronoid process of the mandible. It closes the mouth and assists with chewing.
- **Pterygoid:** This muscle extends from the sphenoid bone to the mandible. It closes the mouth and parts of the lower jaw forward.

Muscles of the Neck

The region of the neck is divided into two main triangles—anterior and posterior by the sternomastoid muscle which running obliquely from the mastoid process of the temporal bone to the front of the clavicle which is palpable in its entire length.

The posterior of the neck is bounded infront by the sternomastoid muscle and behind by the anterior border of trapezius; it contains portions of the cervical and brachial plexuses of nerves—a chain of lymphatic glands which lie posterior to the sternomastoid and nerves and blood vessels. At the base of this, lies the first rib cover in which the subclavian artery passes. It is here that digital pressure can be applied to the subclavian artery.

Muscles of the Pelvic Floor

- **Levator ani:** This is a part of broad flat muscles, forming the anterior part of the pelvic floor.
- **Coccygeus:** This is a paired triangular sheet of muscle and tendinous fibers situated behind the levator ani.

Muscles of the Shoulder and Upper Limb

- These muscles stabilize the association between the appendicular and axial skeletons at the pectoral girdle and stabilize and allow movement of the shoulders and upper arms.
- **Deltoid:** These muscles fiber originate from the clavicle, acromion process and spine of scapula and radiate over the shoulder joint to be inserted into the deltoid tuberosity of the humerus.
- **Pectoralis major:** This lies on the anterior thoracic wall. The fibers originate from the middle third of the clavicle and from the sternum and are inserted into the lip of the intertubercular groove of the humerus.
- **Coracobrachialis:** This lies on the upper medial aspect of the arm.

Muscles of the Thorax

The main muscles used in normal breathing are the intercostal and the diaphragm.

- **Intercostal muscles:** There are 11 pairs of intercostal muscles that occupy the spaces between the 12 pairs of ribs. They are arranged in two layer—the external and internal intercostal muscles.
    1. *The external intercostal muscle fibers:* These extent downwards and forwards from the lower border of the rib above to the upper border of the rib below.
    2. *The internal intercostal muscle fibers:* These extend downwards and backwards from the lower border of the rib above to the upper border of the rib below, crossing the external intercostal muscle fibers and right angles.
- **Diaphragm:** The diaphragm is dome shaped muscular structure separating the thoracic and abdominal cavities. It forms the floor of the thoracic cavity and the roof the abdominal cavity and consists of a central tendon from which muscle fibers radiate to be attached to the lower ribs and sternum and to the vertebral column by two crura.

Muscles of the Trunk

These muscles stabilize the association between the appendicular and axial skeletons at the pectoral girdle and stabilize and allow movement of the shoulder's upper arms.

Muscles of the Back

The arrangement of these muscles is the same on each side of the vertebral column.
- **Trapezius:** This muscle covers the shoulder and the back of the neck.
- **Latissimus dorsi:** This arises from the posterior part of the iliac crest and the spinous processes of the lumbar and the lower thoracic vertebrae.
- **Teres major:** This originates from the inferior angle of the scapula and is inserted into the humerus just below the shoulder joint.
- **Quadratus lumborum:** This muscle originates from the iliac crest, and then it passes upwards, parallel and close to the vertebral column and it is inserted into the 12th rib.
- **Sacrospinalis:** This is a group of muscles lying between the spinous and transverse processes of the vertebrae. They originate from the sacrum and are finally inserted into the occipital bone.

Muscles of the Abdominal Wall

Four parts of muscles from the abdominal wall are:
1. **Rectus abdominis:** It is the most superficial muscle. It originating from the transverse part of pubic bone then passing upwards to be inserted into the lower ribs and the xiphoid process of the sternum.
2. **Transverse abdominis:** The fiber arises from the iliac crest and the lumbar vertebrae and pass across the abdominal wall to be inserted into the linea alba by an aponeurosis. This is the deepest muscle of the abdominal wall.
3. **External oblique:** This muscle extends from the lower ribs downwards and forward to be inserted into the iliac crest.
4. **Internal oblique:** This muscle lies deep to the external oblique. Its fibers arise from the iliac crest and by a broadband of fascia from the spinous processes of the lumbar vertebrae.

Muscles of Arm

- **Biceps:** This lies on the anterior aspect of the upper arm. At its proximal end, it is divided into two parts each of which has its own tendon. The short head rises from the coracoid process of the scapula and passes in front of the shoulder joint to the arm.

- **Brachialis:** This lies on the anterior aspect of the upper arm deep to the biceps. It originates from the shaft of the humerus, extends across the elbow joint.
- **Triceps:** This lies on the posterior aspect of the humerus. It arises from three heads, one from the scapula and two from the posterior surface of the humerus.
- **Brachioradialis:** The brachioradialis spans the elbow joint, originating on the distal end of the humerus and inserts on the lateral epicondyle of the radius.
- **Pronator quadratus:** This square-shaped muscle is the main muscle causing pronation of the hand and has attachments on the lower sections of both the radius and the ulna.
- **Pronator teres:** This lies obliquely across the upper third of the front of the forearm. It arises from the medial epicondyle of the humerus and the coronoid process of the ulna and passes obliquely across forearm which to be inserted into the lateral surface of the shaft of the radius.
- **Supinator:** This lies obliquely across the posterior and lateral aspects of the forearm.
- **Flexor carpi radialis:** This lies on the medial aspect of the forearm.
- **Extensor carpi radialis longus and brevis:** These lies on the posterior aspect of the forearm. The fibers originate from the lateral epicondyle of the humerus and are inserted by a long tendon into the second and third metacarpal bones.
- **Extensor carpi ulnaris:** This lies on the posterior surface of the forearm. It originates from the lateral epicondyle of the humerus and is inserted into the fifth metacarpal bone.
- **Palmaris longus:** This muscle resists shearing forces that might pull the skin and fascia of the palm away from the underlying structures, flexes and wrist.
- **Extensor digitorum:** This muscle originates on the lateral epicondyle of the humerus and spans both the elbow and wrist joints; in the wrist, it divides into four tendons, one for each finger.

Muscle that Control Finger Movements

Large muscles in the forearm that extend to the hand give power to the hand and fingers but not to the delicacy of movement needed for fine and dexterous finger control.

Muscles of the Hip and Lower Limb

- **Psoas:** The upper part of the psoas lies behind the diaphragm in the lower part of the media sternum. It also lies in relation to the quadratus lumborum. The lumbar plexus lies in the substance of this muscle and the abdominal aorta, the inferior vena cava and the receptaculum chyli and many lymphatic glands lie infront of it.

- ❖ **Iliacus:** This lies in the iliac fossa of the innominate bone. It originates from the iliac crest passes over the iliac fossa and joins the tendon of the psoas muscle, to be inserted into the lesser trochanter of the femur.
- ❖ **Quadriceps femoris:** This is a group of four muscles lying in the front and sides of the thigh. They are rectus femoris and three vastus: lateralis, medialis and intermedius.
- ❖ **Obturators:** These are the deep muscles of the buttock, have their origins in the rim of the obturator foramen of the pelvis and insert into the proximal femur.
- ❖ **Glutes:** These consist of the gluteus maximus, medius and minimus which together form the flesh part of the buttock.
- ❖ **Sartorius:** This is the longest muscle in the body and crosses both the hip and knee joints.
- ❖ **Adductor group:** This lies on the medial aspect of the thigh. They originate from the pubic bone and are inserted into the linea aspera of the femur.
- ❖ **Hamstrings:** These lie on the posterior aspect of the thigh. They originate from the ischium and are inserted into the upper end of the tibia.
- ❖ **Gastrocnemius:** This forms the bulk of the calf of the leg. It arises by two heads, one from each condyle of the femur and passes down behind the tibia to be inserted into the calcaneus by the calcaneal tendon.
- ❖ **Anterior tibialis:** This originates from the upper end of the tibia, lies on the anterior surface of the leg and is inserted into the middle uniform bone by a long tendon.
- ❖ **Soleus:** This is one of the main muscles of the calf of the leg, lying immediately deep to the gastrocnemius.

CHAPTER 4

Basics of OT Techniques, CSSD Techniques and Anesthesia Technique

Chapter Outline

- Handwashing and Surgical Scrubbing
- Preoperative Preparation of Patient Including Surgery Site
- Postoperative Care Including Dressing
- Methods of Sterilization and Basic Functioning of CSSD
- Central Sterile Supply Department
- Various Positions Used in Different Surgeries
- Anesthesia, Boyle's Machine and Anesthesia Work Station
- Gases Used in Anesthesia
- Triage of Patients
- Details of Hand Instruments Used in Common Surgeries
- Preanesthesia Checkup
- Infection Control in OT
- Basic Ideas of Different IV Fluids
- Needles, Sutures and Knots
- Cauterization (Cautery)

■ HANDWASHING AND SURGICAL SCRUBBING

Hand washing is important in every setting, including hospitals. It is an effective infection control measure, as it prevents the spread of microorganisms. For routine client care, the center for disease control (CDC) recommends vigorous hand washing under a stream of water for at least 10 seconds using soap **(Fig. 4.1)**.

Hand washing should be done:
- When there are known multiple resistant bacteria.
- Before invasive procedures.
- In special care units, such as nurseries, ICUs and OTs.

Purpose
- To remove transient and resident bacteria from fingers, hands and forearms.
- To prevent the risk of transmission of infection to patients.

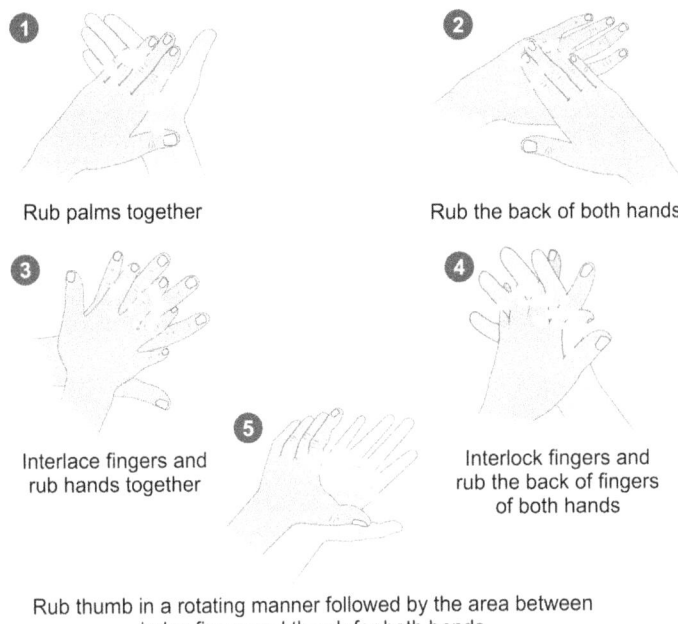

Fig. 4.1: Steps of handwashing.

- To reduce the risk of transmission of infection organisms to oneself.
- To prevent cross infection among clients.

Equipment/Articles

Articles	Rationale
Soap in a soap dish	Soap contains antibacterial agents and has a lasting bacteria static effect
Nail brush	To clean nails
Running water	To rinse soap and thoroughly wash hands
Towel	To dry hands

Steps of Procedure

Steps	Rationale
File the nails short; ensure that nails are free of nail polish	Short nails are less likely to harbor resident and transient microorganisms
Remove all jewelry and wrist watch	Microorganisms can be inside the settings of jewelry and under rings. Removal facilitates proper cleaning of hands and arms
Turn on the water to adjust the flow so that water is lukewarm.	Warm water removes less of the protective oil of the skin than hot water
• **Medical asepsis:** Wet the hands thoroughly by holding the hands lower than the elbows so that water flows from arms to fingertips	It allows water to flow from the least contaminated area (elbow) to the most contaminated area (hands)
• **Surgical hand washing:** Wet hands and forearms liberally, keeping arms and hands above elbow level during the entire procedure	Water runs by gravity from fingertips to elbows. Keeping hands elevated allows water to flow from least to the most contaminated area
Apply liberal amounts of soap into hands and later hands and arms using hand brushes	Soap emulsifies the oil and lowers the surface tension of water, facilitates the removal of micro-organisms, dust and oils. Brushes are used to enhance mechanical friction during hand washing
Thoroughly wash and rinse the hand using firm rubbing and circular movements to wash the palm, back and wrist of each hand. Interlace the fingers during hand washing	The circular action helps to remove micro-organisms mechanically. Running water and friction used in cleaning are the mechanical action of cleaning
Dry arms and hands thoroughly from fingers to wrists and forearms. Discard the towel in a proper container	Drying helps in removing moisture, prevents chapping and roughening of skin. Drying from cleaner to least clean area prevents contamination
Turn off the water tap using a paper towel or using an elbow	The handle is contaminated. Use of a paper towel or washed hands

Gowning

Clean or disposable gowns or plastic aprons are worn during procedures when the nurse's uniform is likely to become soiled. Sterile gowns may be indicated when the nurse changes the dressings of a client with extensive wounds, burns, etc. (**Fig. 4.2**).

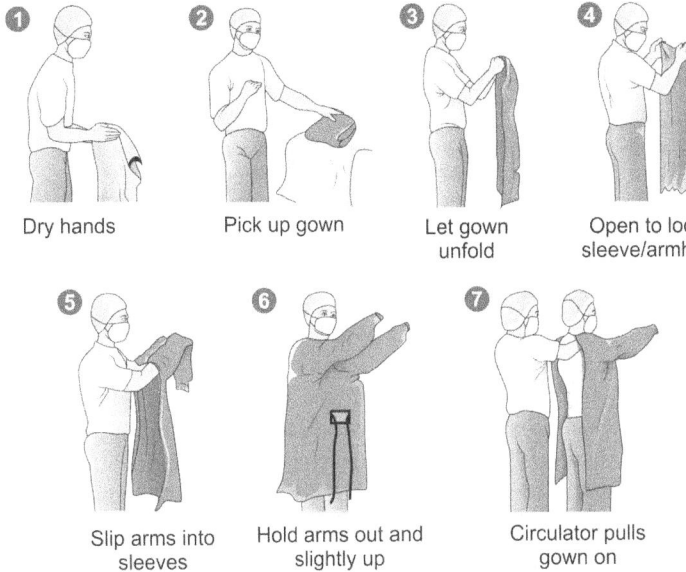

Fig. 4.2: Steps of gowning.

Procedure

Gowning technique (sterile).

Purpose

- To prevent soiling of clothes during contact with the patient.
- To protect health care personnel from coming in contact with infected material.

Steps of Procedure

Steps	Rationale
Pick up a sterile gown and allow it to unfold keeping inside of the gown towards the body without allowing the outside of the gown to touch any area	To prevent soiling/contamination of the gown
With hands at shoulder level, slip both arms into armholes simultaneously. Ask the circulating nurse to bring the gown over shoulders	It prevents contamination of the sterile gown
The circulating nurse fastens the ties at neck. Overlap the gown at the back as much as possible and fasten the waist, ties or belt	It keeps the gown at place and covers the uniform at the back

Contd...

Contd...

Steps	Rationale
Prevent the gown from becoming wet	Moisture allows organisms to travel through the gown to the uniform
While removing avoid touching soiled parts on the outside of the gown. Roll up the gown with the soiled part inside and discard in the appropriate container	It prevents contamination of the uniform. It prevents cross-inflection

Gloving

Gloves are worn to protect hands when the nurse is likely to handle any body substances, e.g., blood, urine, fasces, sputum, mucous membranes and nonintact skin. Gloves also reduce the likelihood of the nurse's transmitting their own endogenous microorganisms to individuals receiving care. For most activities, disposable clean gloves are used. Sterile gloves are used when the hands will come in contact with an open wound or when the hands might introduce microorganisms into a body orifice (**Fig. 4.3**).

Procedure: Wearing and Removing Disposable Gloves

Gloving	Rationale
Thoroughly wash hands	Removes bacteria from skin surfaces and reduces transmission of infection
Open a sterile glove packet of proper size on a flat surface above waist level	A sterile object held below waist gets contaminated
If gloves are not powdered, take a packet of powder and apply lightly to hands	Powder allows gloves to slip on easily
Identify right and left hand. Glove dominant hand first	Proper identification of gloves prevents contamination by improper fit
With thumb and the first two fingers of the nondominant hand, grasp and edge of the glove's cuff. For dominant hand, touch only the glove's inside surface (Step 1)	Inner edge of the cuff will lie against skin and thus is not sterile
Carefully pull the glove over the dominant hand. Ensure the thumb and fingers are in proper spaces (Step 2)	Proper fitting of gloves on fingers
With gloved dominant hand, slip fingers underneath the second glove's cuff (Step 3)	This prevents glove contamination

Contd...

Contd...

Gloving	Rationale
Carefully pull the second glove over the nondominant hand. Do not allow fingers of the thumb of the gloved dominant hand to touch any part of the exposed nondominant hand (Step 4)	Contact of the gloved hand with the exposed hand results in contamination
After the second glove is on interlock hands together (Step 5)	Ensures smooth fit over fingers

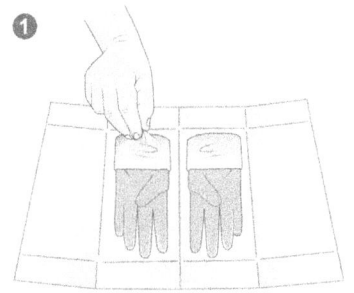

Pick up one glove with thumb and forefinger

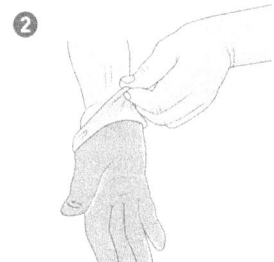

Pull glove on hand

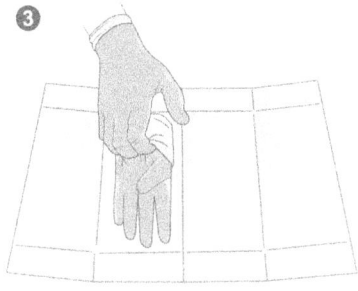

Slip partially the gloved hand under cuff of second glove

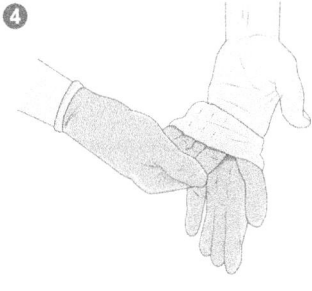

Pull second glove over other hand and pull the glove up to gowned wrist

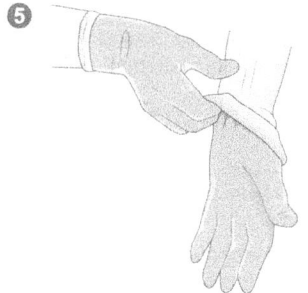

Slip fingers of completely gloved hand under cuff of first hand, pull glove to gowned wrist

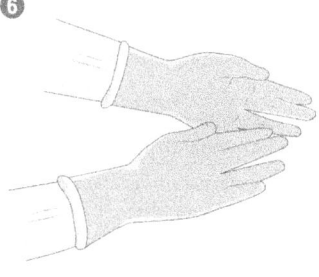

Gloving procedure completed

Fig. 4.3: Steps of gloving.

Removing Disposable Gloves

Remove the first glove by grasping it on its palmar surface just below the cuff, taking care to touch only glove to glove. Pull the first glove completely off by inverting or rolling the glove inside out	This keeps the soiled parts of the used gloves from touching the skin of the wrist or hand
Place the first two fingers of the bare hand inside the glove and remove the second contaminated glove	To prevent touching the outside of the second soiled glove with the bare hand
Dispose them of in the appropriate container	To prevent cross infection

Wearing Masks

Masks are worn to reduce the risk for transmission of organisms by the droplet contact, air borne routes, and splatters of body substances. The CDC recommends that masks should be worn:

❖ By personnel who work close to the client if the infection is transmitted by large particle aerosols, e.g., measles, mumps, acute respiratory diseases in children.

❖ By all personnel entering the room if the infection is transmitted by small particle aerosols (droplet nuclei); e.g., pulmonary tuberculosis.

Procedure

Using disposable mask:

Putting of mask	Rationale
Hold mask by top two strings. Tie two top ties at the top of the back of the head with ties above ears	Position of ties at the top of the head provides a tight fit. Ties over ears may cause irritation
Tie two lower ties snugly around the neck with the mask well under the chin	Prevents escape of micro-organisms through sides of the mask
Ensure that the mask covers the mouth and the nose adequately	Prevents (inhalation and escape of) microorganism from and into the air
If glasses are worn, fit the upper edge of the mask under the glasses	To prevent glasses from clouding
Avoid unnecessary talking and, if possible, sneezing or coughing	To prevent the mask from getting moist
When removing a mask with strings, first untie the lower strings of the mask	To prevent the top part of the mask from falling on to the chest

Contd...

Contd...

Putting of mask	Rationale
Discard a disposable mask in the waste container	To prevent cross infection
Wash the hands if they have become contaminated by accidentally touching the soiled part of the mask	To prevent infection

Principles of Surgical Asepsis

Principles	Reasons
Always face the sterile field. Do not turn your back or side on a sterile field	Sterile objects, which are out of vision, are considered questionable and their sterility cannot be guaranteed
Keep sterile equipment above your waist level or above table level	Because waist level and table level are considered margins of safety and will promote a maximum sterile field
Do not speak or cough over a sterile field. If it is necessary to do so, turn your head from the sterile field	To prevent droplet infection
Never search or cross a sterile field	When a nonsterile object crosses the sterile field, gravity causes the microorganisms to fall into the sterile field
Prevent excessive air currents around sterile areas. Air current can be caused by moving fast, flapping the cloth sand drapes and by closing the doors etc.	Microorganisms are present in the air and they travel in air current
Keep the wet unsterile object away from the sterile field	Microorganisms may be transferred whenever a nonsterile wet object touches a sterile field. The microorganisms may be transferred consequently. The sterile area becomes unsterile by capillary action
Keep the sterile field dry	Microorganisms do not pass easily through a dry surface
Handle liquids cautiously near the sterile field or prevent drapes or wrappers from becoming wet	When a liquid comes in contact with a notsterile field, the microorganisms may be transferred. Consequently, the sterile area becomes unsterile by capillary action
The edge of the sterile field is considered unsterile	Proximity to a contaminated area makes sterility doubtful

Contd...

Contd...

Principles	Reasons
Each sterile supply should be clearly labelled as to its contents, time and date of sterilization	To ensure sterility
Never assume that an object is sterile. Always check the expiry date of sterility	Sterility of an object wrapped in paper or cloth becomes doubtful after four weeks and those sealed in polythene bags become doubtful after one year
Avoid sweeping and dusting when sterile objects are opened	Microorganisms travel in dust particles
Wash hands, put on gowns, gloves and mask before handling the sterile supplies	To prevent contamination
Open the sterile package in such a way that the edges of the wrapper are directed away from the worker	To avoid the possibility of a sterile surface touching the uniform
Hold the transfer forceps pointing downwards	To prevent the solution from flowing into the contaminated areas (the handle of the forceps) and then back to the sterile area (the tip of the forceps)
When removing the forceps from the container lift it without touching the sides and the rim of the container	The tip of the forceps becomes contaminated when touching the container that is not in direct contact with the disinfectant solution
Keep the prongs together directly over the container to remove the excess solution	To prevent the solution from dribbling onto the sterile field and wet it
Transfer forceps and the container should be sterilized daily	There is a great possibility of these articles becoming contaminated because of the frequency and varied use

Use of the Container: With Sterile Supplies

Remove the cover from the container when necessary and only for a short period	Air currents can contaminate the cover
Leave the cover of the container in such a way that the inside of the lid is pointing downwards	Air currents can contaminate the inside of the cover
Invert the cover only when it is necessary to place it downwards	Contact with the unsterile surface contaminates sterile objects

Contd...

Contd...

Consider the rim of the cover and the container to be contaminated	Proximity to a contaminated area makes the sterility doubtful
Do not return the unused sterile objects to the container, once they have been taken out	It is considered to be contaminated by air currents

PREOPERATIVE PREPARATION OF PATIENT INCLUDING SURGERY SITE

Introduction

- ❖ To obtain satisfactory results in general surgery requires a careful approach to preoperative preparation of patients.
- ❖ Specific patient groups have specific needs
- ❖ High-risk patients should be identified early and appropriate measures taken to reduce complications.

Preoperative Preparation for Surgery

- ❖ Prior to consideration of surgical intervention, it is necessary to prepare the patient as fully as possible so as to optimize him according to his comorbidities.
- ❖ The extent of preoperative preparation will depend on:
  - Nature of surgery (minor or major)
  - Facilities available
  - Preoperative preparation for surgery
- ❖ **Situation:**
  - *Emergency:* Life-threatening condition requiring immediate action (e.g., ruptured aneurysm, penetrating trauma, peritonitis).
  - *Urgent:* Surgery required within few hours (e.g., intestinal obstruction, appendicitis, wound debridement).
  - *Elective:* For example, hernia, varicose vein, colorectal malignancies, breast malignancy)

Complication

Elective Urgent Emergency

- ❖ The rational for preoperative preparation is to: anticipate difficulties.
  - Make advanced preparation and organize facilities, equipment and expertise.
  - Enhance patient safety and minimize chances of errors.

- Relieve any relevant fear/anxiety perceived by patient.
- Routine preparation for surgery

❖ History
❖ Physical examination
❖ Special investigation
❖ Informed consent
❖ Marking the site/side of operation
❖ Thromboembolic prophylaxis
❖ Antibiotic prophylaxis

Preparing for Surgery

Preparations for surgery depend on your diagnosis. Your physician will discuss with you how to prepare for your surgery. However, if you will undergo general anesthesia, you may be asked to do the following:

❖ Stop drinking and eating for a certain period of time before the time of surgery.
❖ Bathe or clean, and possibly shave the area to be operated on.
❖ Undergo various blood tests, X-rays, electrocardiograms, or other procedures necessary for surgery.
❖ Sometimes a patient may be asked to take an enema the evening before surgery, to empty the bowels. Please check with your physician.
❖ Do not wear makeup the day of surgery
❖ Do not wear nail polish
❖ Do not wear your eye contacts
❖ Leave valuables and jewelry at home
❖ Advise the medical staff of dentures or other prosthetic devices you may be wearing.

Often, to make their experience more comfortable and efficient, patients are advised to bring the following:

❖ Loose-fitting clothes to wear
❖ Social security card number
❖ Insurance information
❖ Medicare or medicaid card

Surgical Site Preparation

Important to consider the best surgical site preparation routine:

❖ Hair removal
❖ Preoperative and intraoperative skin preparation solutions
❖ Sterile draping

Preparation is extended well beyond the surgical margins to ensure that the areas surrounding the incisions are properly sterilized.

Iodine, alcohol, and chlorhexidine-based preparations have been shown to reduce bacterial burden at various surgical sites.

Awareness of the recommended skin preparation solution based on anatomic location of surgery is warranted due to local microbiome and skin flora (i.e., shoulder area higher bacterial burden of *Cutibacterium acnes* which chlorhexidine solution is recommended.)

Surgeon Tools/Recommendations

Hair Removal

- Remove hair with a dedicated clipping device with a prepackaged razor in the preoperative area the same day as surgery before entrance into the sterile operating room setting.
- Proper disposal of the razor after each patient is advised.

Preoperative/Preadmission Skin Preparation

- Recommend patients' perform specific cleanses of surgical site while at home the day before and morning of surgery.
  - Includes shower with chlorhexidine solution or using wipes at home.
- On the day of surgery, gently wipe the skin with either an alcohol or chlorhexidine-based solution (i.e., 70% isopropyl alcohol, chlorhexidine gluconate) in the preoperative area or in the operating room to provide a preliminary cleanse of the entire surgical field.
- Consider the fire risk associated with isopropyl alcohol in the operating room.
  - May be required to isolate surgical field with clear drapes to ensure that the alcohol-based solutions do not saturate cloth or fabric to reduce the risk of fire.
- Allow optimal drying time for specific initial preparatory solution to maximize adhesion and technique or proper sterile draping.

Intraoperative Skin Preparation

- Iodine, alcohol, and chlorhexidine-based solutions are used after the surgical site has been appropriately isolated, marked and the team has appropriate visualization and working area to successfully complete the procedure.
- Allow each of the skin preparation solutions adequate time to dry
  - Follow manufacture's recommendations for drying time.
- Be aware that some surgical skin preparation solutions have been shown to have a greater propensity for erasing surgical markings than others.

Sterile Draping
- Once the solution of choice is dry, drape the sterile field.
- Often, surgeons will choose to use iodine impregnated sticky drapes or incise drapes either along the edges of the sterile drapes or over the entire surgical field.

Evidence shows that iodine impregnated sticky drapes adhere better to certain skin preparation solutions than others.

■ POSTOPERATIVE CARE INCLUDING DRESSING

Introduction

The postoperative period begins from the time the patient leaves the operating room and ends with the follow-up visit by the surgeon.

Definition

Postoperative care is the care that the patient receives after a surgical procedure. The type of postoperative care that the patient needs depends on the type of surgery as well as the patient's history. It often depends upon pain management and wound care.

Phases

- Immediate (postanesthetic) Phase (1)
- Intermediate (hospital stay) Phase (2)
- Convalescent (after discharge to full recovery)

Purposes

- To enable a successful and faster recovery of the patient postoperatively.
- To reduce postoperative mortality rate.
- To reduce the length of hospital, stay of the patient.
- To provide quality care service.
- To reduce hospital and patent cost during postoperative period.

Postoperative Care Unit or PACU

PACU should be:
- Soundproof
- Painted in soft color
- Isolated

These features will help the patient to reduce anxiety and promote comfort.

Phase 1: Immediate (Postanesthetic)

- It is the immediate recovery phase and requires intensive nursing care to detect early signs of complications.
- Receive a complete patient record from the operating room which to plan postoperative care.
- It is designed for the care of surgical patients immediately after surgery and patient requiring close monitoring.

Nursing Management in Postoperative Care Unit

Assessing the Patient

Frequent assessment of the patient for: Oxygen saturation, pulse volume and regularity depth and nature of respiration, skin color depth of consciousness.

Maintaining a Patent Airway

- The primary objectives are to maintain pulmonary ventilation and prevent hypoxia and hypercapnia.
- Provide oxygen, and assesses respiratory rate and depth, oxygen saturation.

Maintaining Cardiovascular Stability

- Assess the patient's mental status, vital signs, cardiac rhythm, skin temperature, color and urine output, central venous pressure, arterial lines and pulmonary artery pressure.
- The primary cardiovascular complications include hypotension, shock, hemorrhage, hypertension and dysrhythmias.

Relieving Pain and Anxiety

Opioid analgesic.

Assessing and Managing the Surgical Site

The surgical site is observed for bleeding, type and integrity of dressing and drains.

Assessing and Managing Gastrointestinal Function

- Nausea and vomiting are common after anesthesia.
- Check of peristalsis movement.

Assessing and Managing Voluntary Bonding

- Urine retention after surgery can occur for a verity of reasons.
- Opioids and anesthesia interfere with the perception of bladder fullness.

Encourage Activity

- Most surgical are encouraged to be out of bed as soon as possible.
- Early ambulation reduces the incidence of postoperative complication as atelectasis, pneumonia, gastrointestinal discomfort and circulatory problem.

Complications

- **Shock:** It is the response of the body to a decrease in the circulating volume of blood, tissue perfusion impaired, cellular hypoxia and death.
- **Hemorrhage:** It is the escape of blood from a blood vessel.
- **Deep vein thrombosis (DVT):** Occur in pelvic vein or in lower extremities, and it's common after hip surgery.
- **Pulmonary embolism:** It is the obstruction of one or more pulmonary arterioles by an embolus originating somewhere in the venous system or in the right side of heart.
- **Urinary retention:** Condition in which urine cannot empty from the bladder.
- **Intestinal obstruction:** Result in partial or complete impairment to the forward flow of intestinal content.

Causes of Complications and Death

- Acute pulmonary problems
- Cardiovascular problems
- Fluid derangements

Preventions

Recovery Room

- Anesthetist responsibilities towards cardiopulmonary functions.
- Surgeon's responsibilities towards the operation site.

Trained Nursing Staff

- To handle instruction.
- Continuous monitoring of patient, (vital signs etc.)

Dressing

A dressing is a sterile pad, compress that is applied directly over a wound to promote healing.

Purpose

- To protect the wound

- To control/stop bleeding
- To apply medication
- To absorb excess moisture/discharge from the wound
- To prevent infection
- To prevent further injury
- To promote healing
- Provide comfort

Points to be Considered (Dressing in First Aid)
- If the situation permits, wash hands with soap and water.
- Wear gloves if available
- Control bleeding before applying dressing
- Apply the sterile pad without touching the part that comes in contact with the wound.
- Avoid touching the wound, coughing/sneezing into the wound.
- Use dressing that is large enough to cover the whole area of the wound.
- In case of bleeding, more pads may be added on top of previous pads and apply adhesive tape with pressure.
- Bandage may be necessary to hold it in position.

Types
1. **Adhesive dressing:** A sterile pad of absorbent gauze/cellulose is held in place by a layer of adhesive material.
2. **Nonadhesive dressing:** This type of dressing does not contain an adhesive material with it to fix the dressing. It includes sterile readymade dressing or gauge-piece dressing. The dressing material has to be held in place by using a bandage or an improves material like scarf or towel.

Method of Dressing
- Wash hands and wear gloves if possible.
- In case of contaminated wounds clean the antiseptic solution. If antiseptic solution is unable wash the wound with soap and water.
- Dry the sides of the wound.
- Open the dressing by removing the wrappings.
- Place the dressing directly over the wound.
- Bandage formulae using triangular bandage and secure it by trying the two ends together by reef knot.
- Gauge-piece taken in layers may be used instead of dressing.
- A piece of cloth cut in the shape of bandage may be used instead of bandage.

- Plastic bag maybe used instead of gloves.
- Wash hands with soap and water after dressing.

METHODS OF STERILIZATION AND BASIC FUNCTIONING OF CSSD

Heat is the reliable and short period process of sterilization. Proteins of bacteria coagulate at high temperature resulting in death of bacteria. The majority of bacteria die in moist heat at 50–70°C in 2–3 minutes. *Streptococcus faecalis* is destroyed on high temperature. Vegetative forms are killed at low temperature, but spores required high temperature. High temperature required less period. Two types of heat are used:
1. Dry heat
2. Moist heat

Dry Heat

It is used to sterilize metal made instruments such as needles, syringes, test tubes, etc. Scalpel, forceps, needle, glass slide, cover slip are placed directly on flame and sterilized without becoming red. Bunsen burner is used in this method. Platinum loop and vaccinating instruments are also sterilized by this procedure. Test tube, pipette, petal dish are kept in hot air oven wrapped in paper. These instruments operated by electricity and controlled by heat regulator.

Moist Heat

Three manners are adopted for sterilization by moist heat.
1. **Heating:** Heating liquid on 100°C
2. **Boiling:** Instruments are kept in water contained by sterilizer which is boiled at 100°C. Syringes, needles, knives or other surgical instruments are sterilized by the procedure.
3. **Vapor sterilization:**
   - Sterilization by vapor at 100°C is an effective method. It is done with the help of a steamer. Broth or agar is retained in vapor for one- and half-hours.
   - Vapor is used several times on short intervals in intermittent vapor sterilization. Vapor at 100°C is used for 3 days continuously at an interval of 20–20 minutes. Sugar and gelatin are sterilized by this method. Twice sterilization kills vegetative bacteria and spores completely.

- Sterilization is done at above 100°C in pressure cooker or autoclave. Water boils at 121°C temperature in presence of 15 lbs (pounds) vapor pressure.

Chemical Sterilization (Tables 4.1 and 4.2)

- **Glutaraldehyde:** Endoscope is sterilized by 2% liquid.
- **Formaldehyde gas:** Sterilizes endoscope.
- **Ethylene gas:** It sterilizes heart lung machine, respirator, and dental instruments. These are retained in gas for 2–4 hours. It is also used in fumigating atmosphere.
- **Beta propiolactone:** Its 0.2% gas is also used for sterilization.

Ultraviolet Radiation

- Low pressure mercury vapor lamp is used to destroy gram-negative and gram-positive bacteria.
- Sun-ray has capacity to kill bacteria due to presence of ultraviolet ray. TB 'causing bacteria are killed on exposure to sunlight (by sitting in sunlight).
- Besides these, disposable medical materials are sterilized by X-ray, Beta-rays and Y-rays. Filtration is also a process for sterilizing liquid materials. An apparatus, namely, seitz filter is used for sterilization of medium components, preparation of vaccine and separation of bacteria from toxic liquid.

Table 4.1: Classification of chemical sterilizing agents.

Chemical disinfectant	Examples
• **Interfere with membrane functions:** ➤ Surface acting agents ➤ Phenols ➤ Organic solvent ➤ Acids and alkalis	• Quaternary ammonium compounds • Tween 80 • Soaps and fatty acids • Phenol, cresol, hexylresorcinol • Chloroform, alcohol • Organic acids • Hydrochloric acids, sulfuric acids
• **Destroy functional groups of properties** ➤ Heavy metals ➤ Oxidizing agents ➤ Dyes ➤ Alkylating agents	• Copper, silver, mercury • Iodine, chlorine, hydrogen peroxide • Acridine orange, acriflavine • Formaldehyde, ethylene oxide

Table 4.2: Applications and in-use dilution of chemical disinfectants.

Agent	Common use	Use dilution (%)
• Alcohols	• Skin antiseptic • Surface disinfectant	70
• Mercurials	• Skin antiseptics • Surface disinfectant	0.1
• Silver nitrate	• Antiseptics (eyes and burns)	1
• Phenolic compounds	• Antiseptics skin washes	5
• Iodine	• Disinfect inanimate object • Skin antiseptic	2
• Chlorine compounds	• Water treatment • Disinfect inanimate object	5
• Quaternary ammonium compounds	• Skin antiseptic • Disinfects inanimate object	<1
• Glutaraldehyde	• Heat sensitive instruments	1–2

Preferred methods of sterilization for the sterilization of a small and closed common use articles are given **(Table 4.3)**.

Table 4.3: Preferred method of sterilization of commonly use articles.

Autoclaving	Hot air oven	Ethylene oxide	Autoclaving	Ethylene oxide
Animal cages	Glassware	Fabric	Test tubes	Plastics
Sugar tubes	Beakers	Bedding	Enamel metal trays	Flasks
Lab coats	Flasks	Blanket	Wire baskets	Petri dish
Cotton	Petri dish	Clothing	Wood	Tubes
Filters	Pipette	Mattresses	Tongue depressor	Tubing
Instruments	Slides	Pillows	Applicator	Rubber
Culture media	Syringes	Disposable Instruments	Endodontic Instruments	Drains
Rubber	Test tubes	Blades	Catheters	Special items
Gloves	Glycerin	Knives	Orthodontic kits	Bronchoscope
Stopper	Needles	Scalpels	Saliva ejector	Gloves
Tubing	Scissors	Scissors	Hand pieces	Heart lung machine
Oils	Paper	Talcum power	Cavitron heads	
Slides	Matrix band	Books	Steel burs	
Syringe	Saliva ejector	Cups, plates	Steel tumbler	
Wax needles			Hand instruments	

■ CENTRAL STERILE SUPPLY DEPARTMENT

The central sterile supply department (CSSD) comprises that service within a hospital which receives, stores; processes, distributes and controls professional supplies and equipment, both sterile and non-sterile to and from all departments of the hospital for the care and safety of patients

Ideally, CSSD is an independent department with facilities to receive, clean, pack, disinfect, sterilizes, store and distribute instruments and supplies as per well-delineated protocols.

By custom diets, medicines, laundry, supply of blood and crystalloid are not included in activities of CSSD.

Objective and Functions

- To provide sterilized material.
- Contributing to a reduction in the incidence of hospital infection.
- To avoid duplication of costly equipment.
- To maintain record of effectiveness of cleaning, disinfection and sterilization process.
- To monitor and enforce controls necessary to prevent cross infection.
- To maintain an inventory of supplies and equipment.
- To stay updated regarding developments in the field.
- To provide a safe environment for the patients and staff.

Designing of a CSSD

- Size and location of CSSD varies
- 7-10 square feet per bed is recommended.
- It should be located as close as possible to operation theatres, accidents and emergency department and wards.

The CSSD layout should be designed for a unidirectional flow. CSSD should have four zones for a smooth work flow:
1. The unclean and washing area
2. The assembly and packing area
3. The sterilization area
4. The sterile area

Planning of CSSD

- The materials/items from contaminated and sterile areas should not get mixed.
- There should be a physical barrier between clean and dirty areas.
- The floor should be smooth, impervious, nonskid and robust.
- Relative humidity should be maintained at 45 ± 5%.
- The clean area should be maintained at positive pressures.
- The minimum ventilation rate should be 6-10 air changes/hour.

- The work area should be made of marble/granite/stainless steel.
- The sterilization must be planned for autoclaving by steam as well as by gas.
- Location—the CSSD should be close to the casualty, operation theatre and wards which are the largest consumer of the sterilized material.
- In multi-storied buildings, CSSD may be planned in the lower floor right under the operation theatre, where vertical movement will be the quickest possible movement of the material.
- Floor space serial beds available floor space required for CSSD:
  - 75-99 10 sq feet per bed
  - 100-149 9 sq feet per bed
  - 150-199 8.5 sq feet per bed
  - 200-249 8 sq feet per bed
  - 250-299 7.5 sq feet per bed
  - 300 or more 7 sq feet per bed

Layout of CSSD

	Physical facility and Equipment Availability at CSSD		
Sl. No.	Rooms in the CSSD	Nature of the work	Provision of the space %
1.	Wash rooms	Dirty	10
2.	Work room (packing room)	Clean	26
3.	Syringe and needle processing	Clean	9
4.	Unsterile pack store	Clean	4
5.	Bulk store	Clean	11
6.	Sterile store	Sterile	16
7.	Miscellaneous: a. Gloves room b. Office room	Clean	19

Distributing to User Departments

- Storing (temporary)
- Sterilizing
- Packing
- Cleaning
- Receiving the used items from user departments
- Major activities in a CSSD: Workflow

Workflow of CSSD

Receiving Area

- Used items from various departments of the hospital are shifted to CSSD for cleaning and sterilization.
- Ideally, the items that get soiled with blood or body fluid should be decontaminated with sodium hypochlorite solution in the user department itself before sending to CSSD.
- The receiving area of CSSD should have access to the outside through a window with a counter the items (especially for instruments in trays) are counted and received.
- Thereafter, the instruments are inspected and blunt/unsuitable instruments are segregated/discarded.
- Necessary entries are made for records.
- Thereafter, the items are shifted to cleaning area.

Cleaning Area

- Here the instruments are washed either manually or by machines.
- For manual washing, sinks with water supply and working counters are organized. Detergents and brushes of various sizes and shapes are required in this area.
- Ultrasonic washer is a machine used for cleaning surgical instruments. It converts high frequency sound waves into mechanical vibration that produces small bubbles that burst on the internal surfaces of instruments and dislodge the waste particles.
- Tunnel washer' is a highly sophisticated and expensive machine that allows totally hand-off processing. Instruments in perforate or mesh bottom trays coming from operating room or other departments are placed into the tunnel washer without any further handling. The instruments are subjected to cycles of washing, rinsing, ultrasonic cleaning and drying.
- After the instruments are washed, they are dried in oven dryer and shifted to packing area.

Packing Area

Clean and dry instruments are packed before sterilization, so that they are not contaminated while handling after they are sterilized. Most of the instruments are packed in trays (tray assembly) that are wrapped with double layer of cotton cloth. Paper envelopes are also available for packing the instruments. These are equally effective but expensive. Plastic bags (ETO bags) are used for packing the items for ETO sterilization. The packs are labelled indicating date of sterilization and date of expiry (wherever possible)—sealing machine is used for the sealing the plastic bags in which instruments are packed. After packing and sealing, the instruments are shifted for sterilization.

Flash Sterilizer

This is a special type of autoclave that has a very short sterilization cycle of about 3–5 minutes because of its ability to raise the temperature to 132°C.

- **Autoclave:** Steam under pressure is the most cost-effective method of sterilization; "autoclave" generates steam at a temperature of 121°C under 15 pounds of pressure. An exposure of 20 minutes is required for sterilization.
- Gas sterilization by ETO (ethylene oxide) machines:
  - Steam sterilization by autoclaves
  - *Sterilizing area:* Sterilization is done by either of the two methods in CSSD:
    1. ETO sterilizer: The items like cardiac catheters are thermo sensitive and therefore cannot be sterilized by steam. Such items are sterilized by ethylene oxide (ETO) gas sterilization. The ETO is an expensive and toxic gas. It is absolutely necessary to ensure that these items are made free of gas molecules before using them on a patient. This is achieved by subjecting the items to forced ventilation. The entire cycle may take about 8–12 hours.
    2. Store after sterilization: The items are temporarily stored in a clean store (on racks) from where they are distributed to user departments.

Distribution Area

It should be away from the receiving area and may comprise of a window with a counter.

In modern hospitals, there may be a separate lift for transporting the sterile materials to user departments.

Transport to OT used materials: Transport cleaning disinfection inspection tray assembly packaging sterilization sterile storage CSSD.

Staffing of CSSD

CSSD is usually manned by following staffs:
- **CSSD incharge/manager:** Supervises activities of CSSD.
- **CSSD technicians:** Operate the autoclave and ETO machines.
- **CSSD assistants:** Perform the cleaning and packing, gauge cutting and cotton ball making.
- **Clerk or storekeeper:** To manage the inventory and sterile stores—housekeeping staff.
- **Staffing should be planned based on the following factors:**
  - Average two technicians for 100 beds and 01 technical supervisors.

- One clerk for keeping records, accounting and supply per shift.
- Average four attendants per 100 beds in all shifts.
- Adequate number of cleaning attendants and transporters.
- One technician and two attendants should be stationed in each zone.
- ❖ Organogram—CSSD supervisor, CSSD attendant, CSSD technician, messengers, boiler attendant, clerks, cleaners.

Quality Assurance

Mechanical indicators: Monitoring record time, temperature, humidity and pressure during the sterilization cycle.
Chemical indicators: Devices with a sensitive chemical or dye to monitor one or more parameters of a sterilization cycle.
Biological indicators: Employ the principle of inhibition of growth of microorganism of high resistance.

Role of CSSD Manager

- ❖ Maintenance and repair of equipment
- ❖ Inventory management of supplies and consumable
- ❖ Ensure quality of sterilization
- ❖ Ensure proper distribution and transport
- ❖ Cost control measure, to analyze and reduce the number of cycle
- ❖ Record keeping and data analysis
- ❖ Optimal utilization of manpower and equipment
- ❖ Motivation of staff and training inter departmental coordination.

Conclusion

In most healthcare facilities, the central sterile supply department (CSSD) plays a key role in providing the items required to deliver quality patient care. A well-planned, well-managed and well-staffed CSSD can ensure an infection free environment of hospital and save valuable life and money.

VARIOUS POSITIONS USED IN DIFFERENT SURGERIES

Introduction

Positions used for comfort are one of the important aspects in nursing interventions. Different positions are used for physical examinations so that the body parts are accessible and the client's stay is comfortable.

Purpose

- ❖ To promote comfort and safety.
- ❖ To protect from pressure, abrasion, injuries, etc.
- ❖ To prevent muscle stretches and muscle strains.
- ❖ To provide adequate circulatory and respiratory function.

Common Comfort Positions

Recumbent or Supine and Dorsal Position

In the recumbent position, the patient lies on his back with one pillow at the head end. Legs can be extended or slightly flexed with a small pillow under the knee. Cotton rings/pillows can be placed under the elbow, heel and an air cushion under the buttocks. Foot support is used for to prevent foot drop in bed ridden patients.

Semi-recumbent Position/Elevated

In this position the patient lies in the bed with two or more pillows, semi-recumbent which may be arranged in armchair fashion to support the shoulders, arms and elbows. This is used as convalescence/bedridden, and in patients with minor respiratory diseases.

Prone Position

In the prone position the patient lies flat in bed with face downwards or sideways with one pillow under the waist and one under the ankles, to take the weight off the toes.

Uses

- ❖ This is used for patients with a spinal injury, surgery spine, and back injuries, burnt over back.
- ❖ This is used for patient after anesthesia to prevent aspiration of saliva and mucus, in such a situation no pillow is used under the head.

Lateral or Side Lying Position: Right or Left

In the side lying position the patient lies on his side with both knees slightly flexed towards the abdomen, one knee more acutely than the other. Pillow can be placed at the head, back and at the sides for support. One pillow can be placed between the knees to take the weight off the under leg and prevent friction.

Uses

- ❖ The left lateral position is used for giving enema or suppositories.
- ❖ The left lateral position is also used for taking temperature and doing recital examination.

Fowler's Position

Fowler's position is a semi-sitting position with head elevated to 30 with the support of back rest and pillows. The comfort devices like air cushion, foot rest, elbow rings can be used to provide comfort to the patient, under the arms and knees extra pillows to be placed.

Uses

- ❖ Fowler's bed can also be used for giving this position.
- ❖ This position is used in chest and abdominal operation to promote drainage also used in patients with dyspnea, as this position expands the thoracic cavity by pushing the diaphragm down. It relieves tension to the abdominal sutures and relaxes the large muscles of back and thigh. It gives a sense of well-being and it enables the patient to take part in self-core.
- ❖ This position is used whenever; the drainage of abdominal cavity is desired to localize infection (e.g., peritonitis).
  - To relieve breathing difficulty. (dyspnea)
  - To relieve tension on abdominal sutures and to release the large muscles of back and higher.

Cardiac Position

In the cardiac position the patient is in high Fowler's position, a cardiac table is placed in front of the patient with a pillow for him to lean on it. It relieves dyspnoea, and adds to the comfort of the patient

Uses

- ❖ This position is used for patient with cardiac disease who cannot breath easily in lying down position.
- ❖ Change in essential to relieve fatigue and to prevent embolism.

Positions Used for Physical Examination

Dorsal or horizontal position: It is a back lying position with legs extended or knees flexed according to the need. A small pillow is placed under the head.

Uses

This position is used for the examination of head and neck, axillary, anterior thorax, lungs, breast, heart, abdomen, vagina, etc.

Erect Position or Standing

This is a normal standing position with both feet on the floor.

Uses

In this position the patient is examined for orthopedic and neurological disorders or for hernia.

Sim's or Left Lateral Position

In Sim's position the patient lies on his left side with one pillow under the head and left cheek resting on it. The left arm is drawn behind the back and the right arm in any position comfortable for the patient. The right thigh is flexed against the abdomen.

Uses

This position is used for rectal and vaginal examination.

Knee Chest Position

In the knee chest position the patient rests on the knees and the chest. The head is turned to one side with the cheek on a pillow. A small pillow may be placed under the chest. The arms are placed at the sides of the head. The weight is resting on chest and knees. The knees are flexed in a kneeling position and the thighs are at right angles to the legs.

Uses

This position is used for rectal, vaginal examination and management of prolapsed uterus.

Trendelenburg Position

In the trendelenburg position the patient lies on his back, the foot of the bed is elevated at 45° angle. The head is low and the body is on inclined plane. This position is used in surgery of pelvic organs as this position displaces the intestines.

Lithotomy Position

Lithotomy position is a back lying position with feet supported in stirrups. The hips should be in line with the edge of the table. This position is used for rectal, vaginal and urethral examination, catheterization and during vaginal deliveries.

ANESTHESIA, BOYLE'S MACHINE AND ANESTHESIA WORK STATION

Anesthesia is a way to control pain during a surgery or procedure by using medicine called anesthetics. It can help control your breathing, blood pressure, blood flow, and heart rate and rhythm.

Anesthesia may be used to relax you, block pain, make you sleepy or forgetful and make you unconscious for your surgery. Besides general anesthesia, other forms of anesthesia may provide only light sedation or use injections to numb only a small area (local anesthesia) or a larger region (regional anesthesia) of your body.

What are the risks and complications of anesthesia?

- Major side effects and other problems of anesthesia aren't common, especially in people who are in good health. But all anesthesia has some risk.
  - **For example:** After general anesthesia heart problems, pneumonia, sore throat, over vomiting can occur. With high doses of local anesthesia, the anesthetic can go into the rest of the body and affect your brain or heart. After spinal anesthesia some people get headaches your risk depends on the type of anesthesia
- Some health problems, such as heart or lung disease, increase your chances of problems from anesthesia. Taking certain medicines, smoking, drinking alcohol, and using illegal drugs can also increase your chance of problems.

Stages of Anesthesia

- **Stage 1:** Induction, also known as voluntary excitement is the period between the initial administration of the induction agents and loss of consciousness. During this stage, the patient progresses from analgesia without amnesia to analgesia with amnesia. Patients can carry on a conversation at this time.
- **Stage 2:** Delirium, involuntary excitement is the period following loss of consciousness and marked by excited and delirious activity. During this stage, respirations and heart rate may become irregular. In addition, there may be uncontrolled movements, vomiting, breath holding, and papillary dilation.
- Since the combination of spastic movements, vomiting, and irregular respirations may lead to airway compromise, rapidly acting drugs are used to minimize time in this stage and reach stage 3 as fast as possible.
- **Stage 3 (surgical anesthesia):** During this stage, the skeletal muscles relax, vomiting stops, and respiratory depression occurs. Eye movements slow, then stop, the patient is unconscious and ready for surgery. It has been divided into 4 planes: (1) eyes initially rolling, then becoming fixed, (2) loss of corneal and laryngeal reflexes, (3) pupils dilate and loss of light reflex, (4) intercostals paralysis, shallow abdominal respiration.

- **Stage 4 (overdose):** It is the stage where too much medication has been given relative to the amount of surgical stimulation and the patient has severe brain stem or medullary depression. This results in a cessation of respiration and potential cardiovascular collapse. This stage is lethal without cardiovascular and respiratory support.

Types of Anesthesia

- General Anesthesia
- Regional Anesthesia
- Local Anesthesia

General Anesthesia

General anesthesia acts primarily on the brain and central nervous system to make the patient unconscious and unaware.

It is administered via the patient's circulatory system by a combination of inhaled gas and injected drugs. After the initial injection, anesthesia is maintained with inhaled gas anesthetics and additional drugs through an intravenous line (IV).

Local Anesthesia

It is medicine given to temporarily stop the sense of pain in a particular area of the body. A patient remains conscious during a local anesthetic. For minor surgery, a local anesthetic can be administered via injection to the site.

However, when a large area needs to be numbed, or if a local anesthetic injection will not penetrate deep enough, physicians may resort to regional anesthetics.

Regional Anesthesia

Involves injection of a local anesthetic (numbing agent) around major nerves or the spinal cord to block pain from a larger but still limited part of the body. You will likely receive medicine to help you relax or sleep during surgery. Major types of regional anesthesia include:

- **Spinal:** Often used for lower abdominal, pelvic, rectal, or lower extremity surgery. This type of anesthetic involves injecting a single dose of the anesthetic agent directly into the spinal cord in the lower back, causing numbness in the lower body.
- **Epidural, and caudal anesthesia:** This anesthetic is similar to a spinal anesthetic and also is commonly used for surgery of the lower limbs and during labor and childbirth.

This type of anesthesia involves continually infusing drugs through a thin catheter that has been placed into the space that surrounds the spinal cord in the lower back, causing numbness in the lower body.

Nerve Blocks

- A local anesthetic is injected near a specific nerve or group of nerves to block pain from the area of the body supplied by the nerve.
- Nerve blocks are most commonly used for procedures on the hands, arms, feet, legs, or face. For example, a brachial plexus block may be used by your anesthesiologist to provide anesthesia to your entire arm and shoulder.

Drugs for General Anesthesia

- **Atracurium** is a neuromuscular-blocking agent, used as an adjuvant in anesthesia. This medication provides relaxation of skeletal muscles during surgery.
- **Cisatracurium besylate** is a neuromuscular blocking agent, used as an adjunct to general anesthesia.
- **Desflurane** is a general anesthetic, prescribed for induction of anesthesia during surgery.
- **Enflurane** is a structural isomer of isoflurane, prescribed for induction and maintenance of general anesthesia.
- **Halothane** is an inhalational general anesthetic, prescribed for the induction and maintenance of general anesthesia.
- **Ketamine** is a hydrochloride salt, used as an anesthetic.
- **Hyoscyamine** is an anticholinergic agent, used as pain killer (belladonna alkaloid). It blocks cardiac vagal inhibitory reflexes during anesthesia induction and intubation, used to relax muscles.
- **Methohexital** is a barbiturate anesthetic, prescribed for inducing anesthesia before surgery.
- **Propofol** is a general anesthetic, prescribed for induction and maintenance of general anesthesia.
- **Rapacuronium** is a neuromuscular blocker, prescribed as an adjunct to general anesthesia to facilitate tracheal intubations.
- **Rocuronium** is a neuromuscular blocker, prescribed as an adjunct to general anesthesia for muscle relaxation and to provide skeletal muscle relaxation during surgery or external breathing.
- **Sevoflurane** is a halogenated hydrocarbon, acts as a general anesthetic during surgery either alone or combined with other medications. It is given by inhalation. This helps to produce more effective anesthesia in some patients.
- **Succinylcholine** is a depolarizing muscle relaxant, used for induction and maintenance of general anesthesia.

Drugs for Local Anesthesia

- **Articaine HCl and epinephrine:** Injection is a local dental anesthetic, used as an anesthesia for dental procedures.
- **Benzocaine** is a local anesthetic used to treat painful conditions such as mouth ulcers, sore throat, before inserting instruments into the rectum or vagina for examination.
- **Bupivacaine** is a local anesthetic, used for surgery and for obstetrical procedures.
- **Lidocaine** is a local anesthetic, indicated for local or regional anesthesia.
- **Lidocaine and prilocaine** is a dermal anesthesia, prescribed for tingling, pricking or numbness of a person's skin.
- **Mepivacaine** is a local anesthetic, prescribed for inducing local or regional analgesia and anesthesia during surgical procedures, labor, or delivery.
- **Oxethazaine** is a potent local anesthetic, prescribed for rapid and effective relief in gastritis, esophagitis, hiatus hernia, heartburn of pregnancy and peptic ulcer.
- **Bupivacaine** is a local anesthetic, used for surgery and for obstetrical procedures. Spinal and epidural anesthesia.

Anesthesia Machine

- First Boyle's machine was made by Edmund Gaskin Boyle in 1917. The Boyle's machine is a continuous flow type of machine used for administration of anesthesia.
- These gases mix in a common manifold at the top of the flow meter.
- From where they pass through the vaporizer containing inhalational agent, the vapors get mix with gaseous mixture and finally reaches to the machine outlet at a pressure of 5–8.

Mechanism of Gas Flow

- Gases in cylinders are at high pressure (2,000 psi) for oxygen and 760 psi for nitrous oxide. Which are reduced to 45–60 psi by pressure regulator 1st some machines have 2nd pressure reducing valve which further decrease the pressure to 15–20 psi.
- Gases from pressure reducing valve reach flow meters where flow is controlled by flow control knobs.

Anesthesia Machine is Divided into three Parts

1. High flow system
2. Intermediate flow system
3. Low flow system

High flow system includes:
- Cylinders
- Pressure regulator (1st pressure reducing valve)
- Yoke assembly
- Oxygen flush

Cylinders
- Made of molybdenum steel
- Aluminum cylinders are also used
- Smallest size available is AA type
- Biggest is H
- Commonly used of anesthesia machines are of E type.

Oxygen cylinder: Black body white shoulders pressure is 2,000 psi.
- **Nitrous oxide:** Blue color, filled as a liquid, pressure is 760 psi.
- **Cyclopropane:** Orange color, pressure 75 psi, filled in the form of liquid.
- **Carbon dioxide:** Grey in color, pressure 750 psi, stores as liquid.

Pressure regulator
- It converts high variable pressure in cylinders to constant working pressure 45–60 psi.
- In most of the machines it is set at 60 psi

Oxygen flush
Bypass system:
- It bypasses the intermediate and low flow system and oxygen reaches directly to the machine outlet.
- It delivers 36 liters of oxygen.
- Pressure is 60 psi.

Yoke assembly
- It is the portion of machine where cylinders get fitted.
- It Consists of:
  - Pin index
  - Bodok seal or washer or gas seal

Pin index safety system (PISS)
- Safety mechanism so that one cylinder cannot be fitted at others position.
- Consists of 2 pins 4 mm and 6 mm long on the yoke of the anesthesia machine.
- These pins are so positioned that the cylinder with corresponding holes can only be fitted.

Bodok seal: To prevent leak between cylinder and yoke and a filter.

Diameter index safety system (DISS)
- Like PISS which prevents wrong fitting of cylinders to machine.
- DISS is to prevent wrong fitting of central supply pipes to machine.
- **Second pressure reducing valve:** Reduces pressure further 15-20 psi.
- **Oxygen failure alarm:** Alarm will set up of when O_2 pressure falls below 30 psi.
- It is pressure dependent not flow dependent
- **Fail safe valve:** It prevents the delivery of hypoxic mixtures.
- If oxygen falls nitrous falls proportionally
- If oxygen falls, nitrous will shut off
- Usually shuts off if oxygen pressure falls become less than 25 psi.

Low pressure system
Consists of:
- Rotameter
- Vaporizers
- One way check valve
- **Rotameter:** Most important component of low flow system
  - It contains flow meters Thorpe tube
  - Bobbin
  - Flow control knob
  - Florescent back panel
- **Vaporizers:** Device used to deliver inhalational agents
  - Inhalational agents are liquid form in vaporizer
  - Made of copper

Safety Features
- Inter locking mechanism of vaporizers
- Antistatic rubber tyres
- Pin index system
- One way valve
- Oxygen flush
- Oxygen failure alarm
- Different physical appearance of oxygen knob
- Pressure reducing valve
- Color coding of flow control knobs
- Fail safe valve
- Oxygen–nitrous proportional device
- Fluorescent back panel of rotameter
- Oxygen flow meter tube placed mostly downstreams
- Pressure relief valve
- DISS

One way check valve:
- It is placed just before the machine outlet
- Prevents back flow

GASES USED IN ANESTHESIA

Anesthetic Agents

I. Inhalational

- **Nitrous oxide:** Traditionally advantageous because of its low solubility in blood and lipids. Therefore, it has a fast onset/offset and can decrease the required amount of a longer acting volatile agent administered in conjunction, promoting a faster wakeup. Because of its preference for the gaseous phase, nitrous oxide will expand the volume of closed internal cavities. It is therefore contraindicated for such situations as patients with a pneumothorax, middle ear surgery (increased pain and dislodgement of prosthetic devices), retinal reattachments (repeat detachment), and intra-abdominal surgery (bowel expansion with obscured surgical field this is controversial). It does support combustion.
- **Volatile agents:** Desflurane, isoflurane, sevoflurane, halothane. All decrease cardiac output by decreasing chronotropy, inotropy, or vasodilation to varying degrees. Isoflurane causes the most vasodilation. Halothane sensitizes myocardium to catecholamines which increases the risk of arrhythmias. Sevoflurane has been implicated in renal failure (in mice) when used at low ventilator gas flows. Sevoflurane is the only agent that cannot cause volatile agent hepatitis (autoimmune response to hepatic metabolites) as it undergoes only minimal, renal metabolism. Desflurane has a low blood/lipid solubility approaching that of nitrous oxide, but can cause tachycardia. All support combustion at supraclinical concentrations. All volatile agents can cause malignant hyperthermia. All inhalational agents increase the risk of postoperative nausea and vomiting.

II. Induction

- **Lipophilic:** It has a large volume of distribution and short-context sensitive half-life. Wears off within 10-15 minutes unless supraclinical doses saturate its volume of distribution. Has the least incidence of postop nausea and vomiting of induction agents and can be used in treatment of nausea. Alcohol used to emulsify propofol in solution burns upon injection (lidocaine in IV first). Causes the most hypotension of all induction agents through

vasodilation and myocardial depression (controversial). Does not have preservatives and supports bacterial growth after 6 hours from opening.
- **Barbiturates:** Thiopental and methohexital. Thiopental has a longer half life (10 hours vs. 4 hours). Both can cause hypotension from vasodilation. Can cause acute porphyric state in patients with porphyric disease (metabolism upregulates porphyria production hepatically).
- **Etomidate:** Causes the least amount of hypotension of the induction agents via minimal vasodilation. Lipophilic, packaged with alcohol (burning) like propofol.
- **Ketamine:** Mediates "dissociative anesthesia" (profound separation of consciousness from body and its vital processes resulting in a cataleptic-like state). Causes the least respiratory depression (unless induction dose given) of induction agents. Only induction agent providing analgesia. Only induction agent that supports cardiovascular system by increasing sympathetic tone. Increases intracranial pressure. Only induction agent that works by antagonizing NMDA receptors (excitatory). All others have effect by upregulating GABA-receptor (inhibitory) function.
- **Benzodiazepines:** Midazolam, lorazepam. Best agents at producing amnesia (lasting 30-45 minutes for midazolam). Have mild muscle relaxant ability. Only induction agent with reversal agent.

III. Muscle Relaxants

Depolarizing

- **Succinylcholine:** Fasting-acting relaxant (within 30-60 seconds). Contraindicated in denervating muscular disease/injury including CVA, 3rd-degree bums, myopathies). Can cause malignant hyperthermia.

Nondepolarizing

- **Short acting:** Atracurium, rocuronium—can cause hypotension due to histamine release and is metabolized by hydrolysis in plasma.
- **Intermediate acting (45 minutes):** Vecuronium—most cardiovascularly stable.
- **Long acting (1 hour):** Pancuronium—can cause tachycardia.

Opioids

- **Morphine:** Can cause hypotension from histamine release.

- **Fentanyls:** Alfentanyl, fentanyl, sufentanil, remifentanil—can cause bradycardia. Remifentanil has shortest half-life (4 minutes).
- **Hydromorphone (dilaudid):** Seven times as potent as morphine.
- **Meperidine (demerol):** Treatment for anesthetic induced shivering. Normeperidine metabolite can cause seizures.

TRIAGE OF PATIENTS

The word triage is derived from the French word trier, which means, "to sort out or choose" the Baron Dominique Jean Larrey, who was the chief surgeon Nepoleon, is credited with organizing the first triage system.

Triage is the process of determining the priority of patient treatments based on the severity of their condition. Triage is the process of sorting people based on their need for immediate medical treatment as compared to their chance of benefiting from such care.

Triage is a process which places the right patient in the right place at the right time to receive the right level of care (Rice and Abel, 1992).

Triage is the process of prioritizing which patients are to be treated first and is the cornerstone of good disaster management in terms of judicious use of resources (Auf der Heide, 2000).

Need of the Triage

- Inadequate resource to meet immediate needs
- Infrastructure limitations
- Inadequate hazard preparation
- Limited transport capabilities
- Multiple agencies responding
- Hospital resources overwhelmed

Aims of Triage

- To sort patients based on need for immediate care
- To recognize futility
- Medical needs will outstrip the immediately available resources
- Additional resources will become available given enough time.

Principles of Triage

The main principles of triage are as follows:
- Every patient should receive and triaged by appropriate skilled healthcare professionals.
- Triage is a clinic-managerial decision and must involve collaborative planning.

- The triage process should not cause a delay in the delivery of effective clinical care.

Advantages of Triage

- Helps to bring order and organization to a chaotic scene.
- It identifies and provides care to those who are in greatest need.
- Helps make the difficult decisions easier.
- Assure that resources are used in the most effective manner.
- May take some of the emotional burden away from those doing triage.

Types of Triage

Simple Triage

Simple triage is used in a scene of mass casualty, in order to sort patients into those who need critical attention and immediate transport to the hospital and those with less serious injuries. This step can be started before transportation becomes available. The categorization of patients based on the severity of their injuries can be aided with the use of printed triage tags or colored flagging.

S.TA.R.T. (**S**imple **T**riage **a**nd **R**apid **T**reatment) is a simple triage system that can be performed by lightly trained lay and emergency personnel in emergencies. Triage separates the injured into four groups:

0: The deceased who are beyond help
1: The injured who can be helped by immediate transportation
2: The injured whose transport can be delayed
3: Those with minor injuries, who need help less urgently.

Advanced Triage

In advanced triage, doctors may decide that some seriously injured people should not receive advanced care because they are unlikely to survive. Advanced care will be used on patients with less severe injuries. Because treatment is intentionally withheld from patients with certain injuries, advanced triage has an ethical implication. It is used to the chances of survival of others who are more likely to survive.

Principles of advanced triage is:
- Do the greatest good for the greatest number
- Preservation of life takes precedence over preservation of limbs
- Immediate threats to life: Hemorrhage.

DETAILS OF HAND INSTRUMENTS USED IN COMMON SURGERIES

The operating room contains a multitude of instruments fit for accomplishing a number of procedures. Note that this is not an exhaustive list of instruments, but rather some that you will encounter frequently.

Scalpel

Used for initial incision and cutting tissue. Consists of a blade and a handle. Surgeons often refer to the instrument by its blade number.

#10 Blade (Fig. 4.4)

Used primarily for making large skin incisions, e.g., in laparotomy.

Fig. 4.4: Scalpel blade 10.

#11 Blade (Fig. 4.5)

Used for making precise or sharply angled incisions.

Fig. 4.5: Scalpel blades 11.

#15 Blade (Fig. 4.6)

Smaller version of #10 blade used for making finer incisions.

Fig. 4.6: Scalpel blade 15.

Scissors

Used for cutting tissue, suture, or for dissection. Scissors can be straight or curved and may be used for cutting heavy or finer structures.

Mayo Scissors (Fig. 4.7)

Heavy scissors are available in multiple varieties. Straight scissors are used for cutting suture ("suture scissors"), while curved scissors are used for cutting heavy tissue (e.g., fascia).

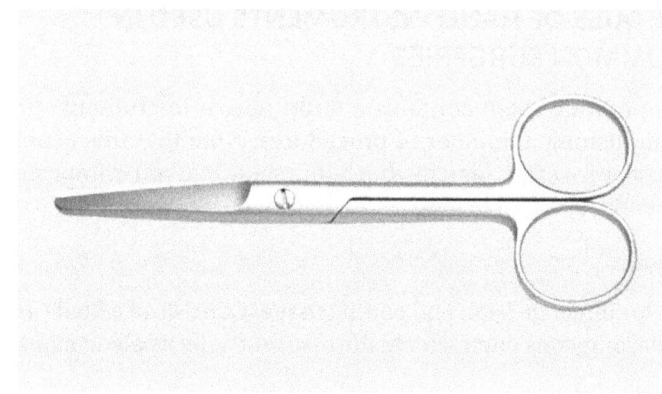

Fig. 4.7: Mayo Scissors.

Metzenbaum Scissors (Fig. 4.8)

Lighter scissors are used for cutting delicate tissue (e.g., heart) and for blunt dissection. Also called "Metz" in practice.

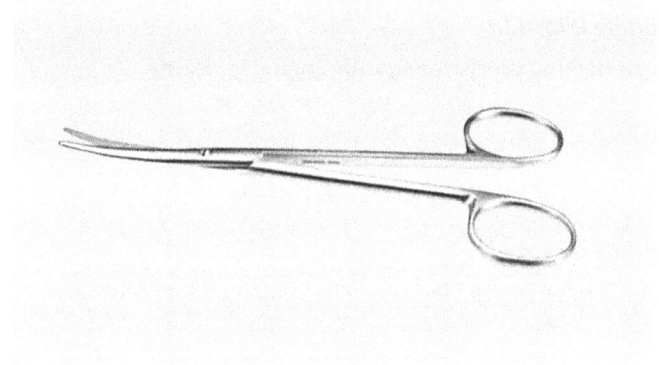

Fig. 4.8: Metzenbaum scissors.

Pott's Scissors (Fig. 4.9)

Fine scissors are used for creating incisions in blood vessels.

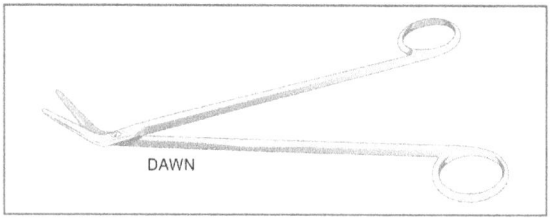

Fig. 4.9: Pott's scissors.

Iris Scissors (Fig. 4.10)

Used for fine dissection and cutting fine suture. Originally for ophthalmic procedures, but now serves multipurpose role.

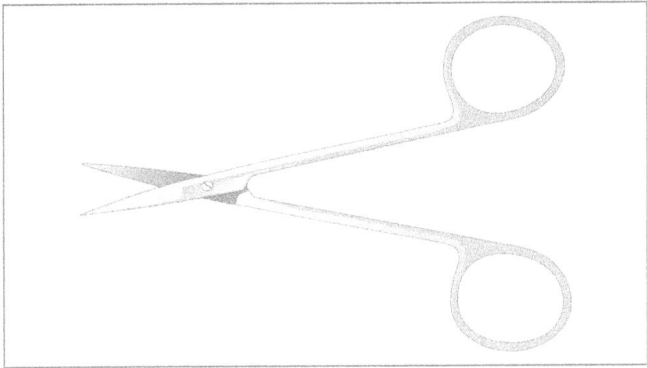

Fig. 4.10: Iris scissors.

Forceps

Also known as nonlocking forceps, grasping forceps, thumb forceps, or pick-ups. Used for grasping tissue or objects. Can be toothed (serrated) or nontoothed at the tip.

Tissue Forceps (Fig. 4.11)

Nontoothed forceps used for fine handling of tissue and traction during dissection.

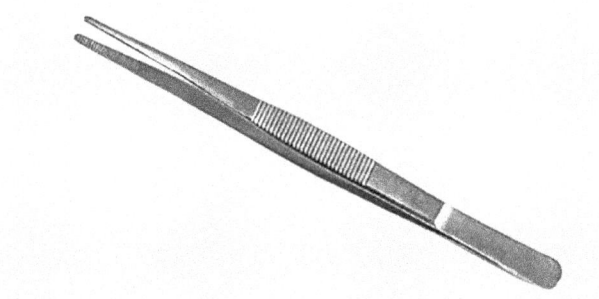

Fig. 4.11: Tissue forceps.

Adson: Toothed Forceps (Fig. 4.12)

Forceps toothed at the tip used for handling dense tissue, such as in skin closures.

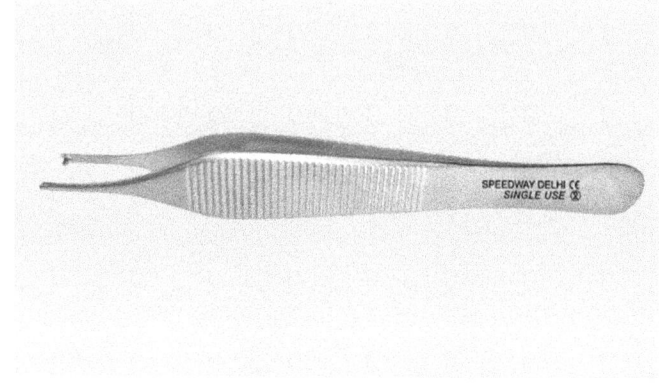

Fig. 4.12: Adson forceps.

Adson: Non-toothed Forceps (Fig. 4.13)

Heavy forceps used for holding thick tissue (e.g., fascial closure).

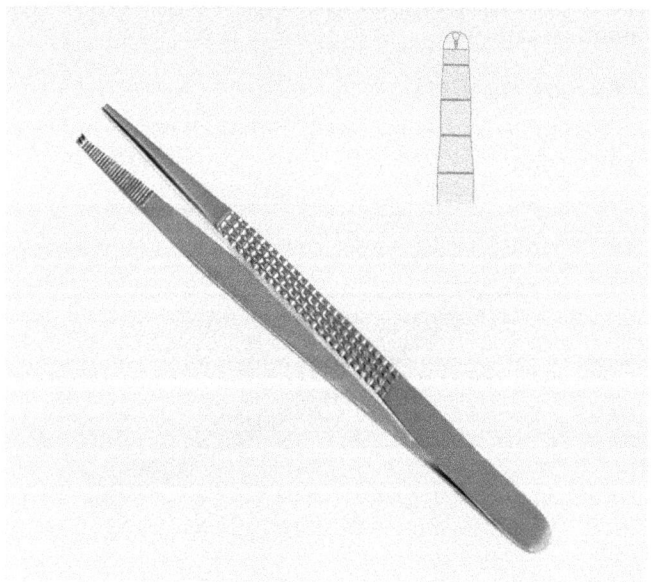

Fig. 4.13: Adson forceps.

DeBakey Forceps (Fig. 4.14)
Used for atraumatic tissue grasping during dissection.

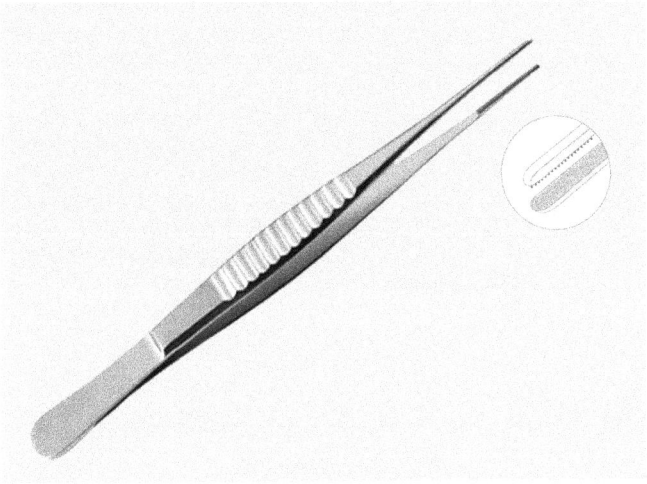

Fig. 4.14: DeBakey forceps.

Russian Forceps (Fig. 4.15)
Used for atraumatic tissue grasping during dissection.

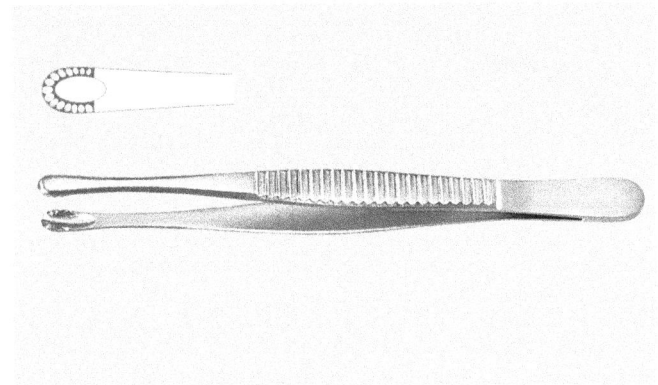

Fig. 4.15: Russian forceps.

Clamps
Also called locking forceps, these are ratcheted instruments used to hold tissue or objects, or provide hemostasis. Can be traumatic or atraumatic.

Crile Hemostat (Fig. 4.16)

Also known as "snap," atraumatic and nontoothed clamp used to grasp tissue or vessels that will be tied off. Also used in blunt dissection.

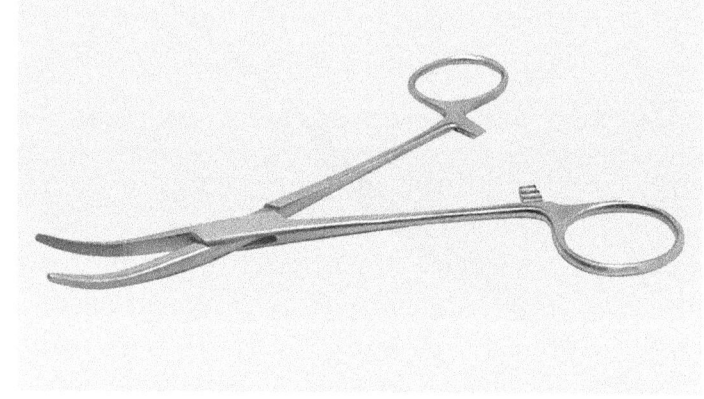

Fig. 4.16: Crile hemostat.

Kelly Clamp (Fig. 4.17)

Larger size variation of hemostat with similar function for grasping larger tissues or vessels.

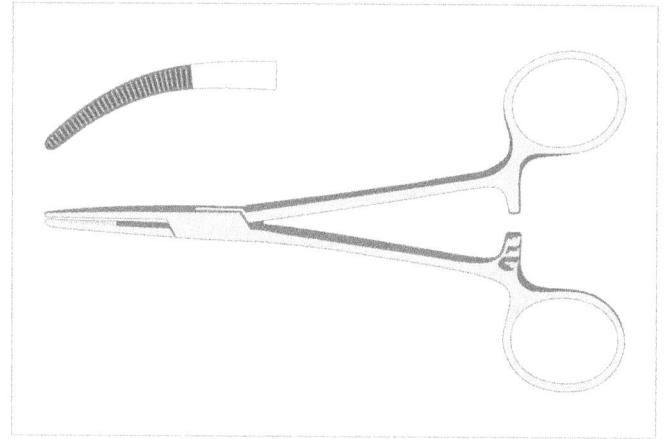

Fig. 4.17: Kelly clamp.

Kocher Clamp (Fig. 4.18)

A traumatic toothed clamp used to hold tissue that will be removed.

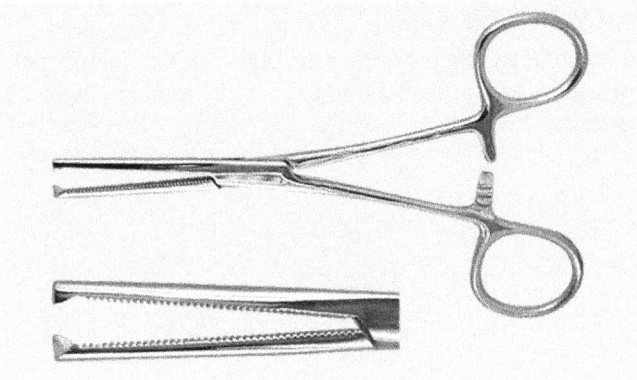

Fig. 4.18: Kocher clamp.

Allis and Babcock Clamps (Fig. 4.19)
Slightly rounded jaws, both are used for grasping intestine.

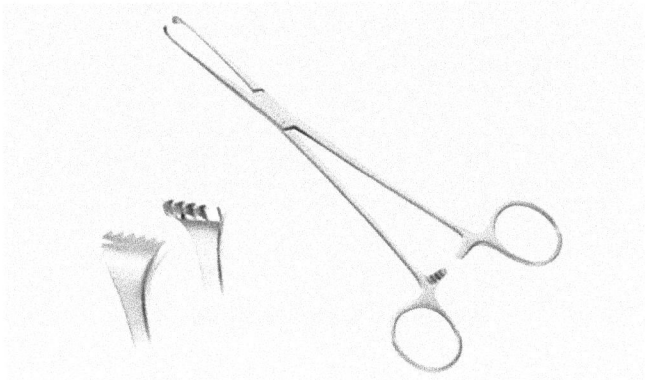

Fig. 4.19: Allis and Babcock clamps.

Needles and Suture
Needles come in many shapes and cutting edges for various applications. Suture can be absorbable, nonabsorbable, and is available in different sizes.

Needle Types
Needles must dissect through tissue to pass suture. They come in various sizes, types, and shapes depending on the application. Here are a few (though not all) examples:

Tapered Needle (Fig. 4.20)

Needle is round and tapers to a simple point. Most commonly used in softer tissue such as intestine but may also be used in tougher tissue such as muscle.

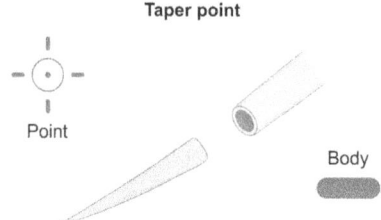

Fig. 4.20: Tapered needles.

Conventional Cutting Needle (Fig. 4.21)

Needle is triangular with sharp edges, and one edge faces the inside of the curved needle. Used for tougher tissues such as skin.

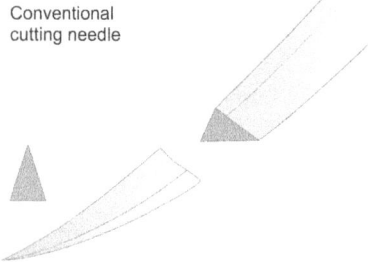

Fig. 4.21: Conventional cutting needle.

Suture Sizing

Available in sizes between #5 and #11-0. Higher numbers indicate larger suture diameter (e.g., #3 is larger than #2), and more zeros indicate smaller suture diameter (e.g., #4-0, or #0000, is smaller than #3-0, or #000).

Suture Types

There are two main types of suture:
1. The first is braided and nonbraided, or monofilament.
2. The second is absorbable and nonabsorbable. Additionally, suture can be made with natural or synthetic materials. Some (brand) names and uses are given in **Table 4.4**.

Table 4.4: Types of sutures.

Suture Types			
Absorbable		Nonabsorbable	
Braided	Monofilament	Braided	Monofilament
Vicryl® Polysorb®	Monocryl® Maxon® PDS® Chromic gut	Silk	Prolene® Surgipro® Monosof® Nylon
Internal anastomosis	Fascial closure Subcuticular skin closure	Vessel ligation	Skin closure Reapproximate lacerations

Needle Shape

The shape of the needle is also important. The curvature of the needle allows for use in specialized applications. Curved needles are used in most general surgical procedures, while straight needles are used for skin and subcuticular suturing **(Fig. 4.22)**.

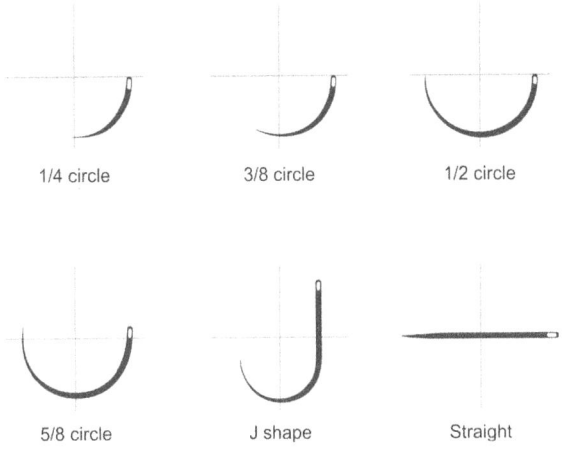

Fig. 4.22: Shapes of needles.

Skin Glue and Staplers (Fig. 4.23)

For skin closures, in particular, staplers and skin glue may be used in lieu of suture. This is usually based on cosmetic outcome and surgeon preference.

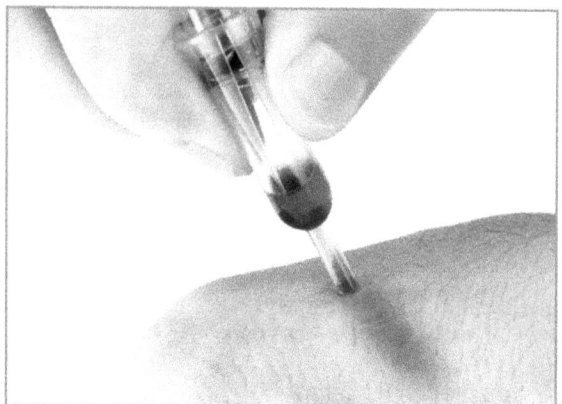

Fig. 4.23: Skin glue.

Retractors

In varying forms, retractors are used to hold an incision open, hold back tissues or other objects to maintain a clear surgical field, or reach other structures. They can either be hand-held or self-retaining via a ratcheting mechanism.

Deaver Retractor (Fig. 4.24)

Used to hold back the abdominal wall.

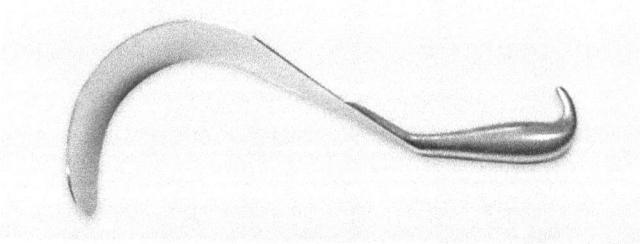

Fig. 4.24: Deaver retractor.

Army-Navy Retractor (Fig. 4.25)

Used to gain exposure of skin layers.

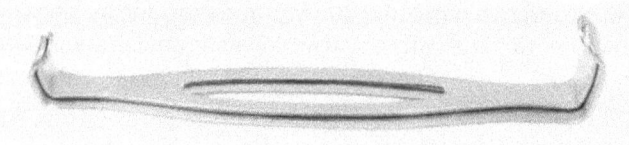

Fig. 4.25: Army-Navy retractor.

Weitlaner Retractor (Fig. 4.26)
Self retaining for exposing deep or smaller surgical sites. Also called "Wheaty."

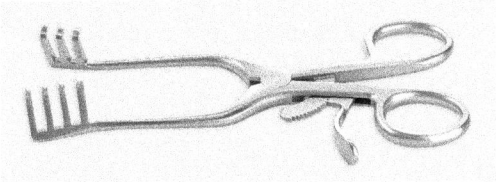

Fig. 4.26: Weitlaner retractor.

Richardson Retractor (Fig. 4.27)
Used to hold back deep tissue structures. Also called "Rich."

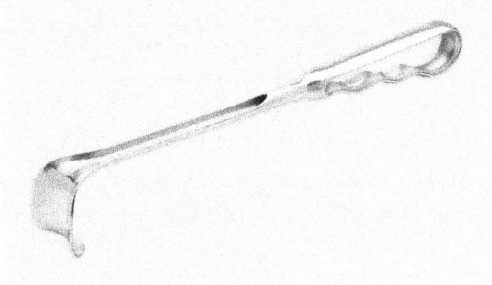

Fig. 4.27: Richardson retractor.

Bookwalter Retractor (Fig. 4.28)
Self-retaining retractor system that is anchored to the operating table.

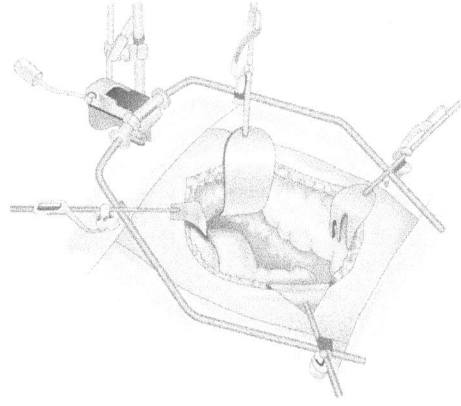

Fig. 4.28: Bookwalter retractor.

Bookwalter Retractor (Fig. 4.29)

Used primarily for surface suction and some intra-abdominal suction.

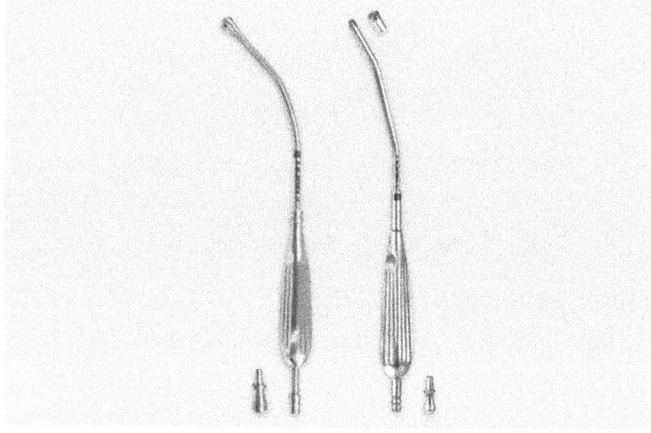

Fig. 4.29: Bookwalter retractor.

Suction

Suction tips, combined with a suction source, help to remove debris and fluid from the surgical field. It can also be used to clear surgical smoke.

Poole Suction Tube (Fig. 4.30)

Used to remove large amounts of fluid from the surgical field, as well as intra-abdominal suction.

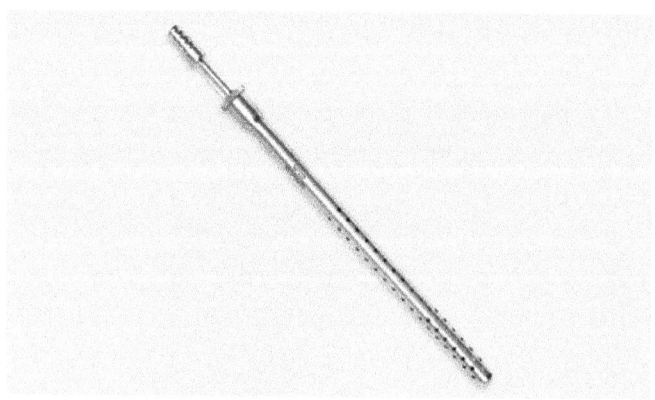

Fig. 4.30: Poole suction tube.

Frazier Suction Tip (Fig. 4.31)
Used primarily in ENT and neurosurgery. Usually angled.

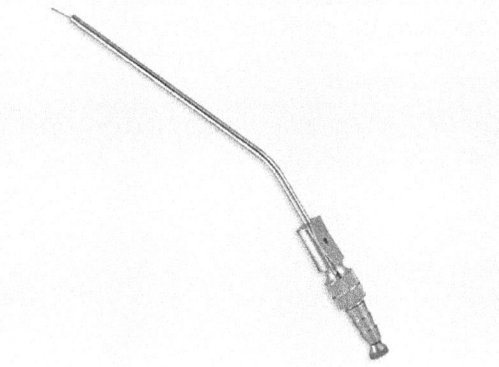

Fig. 4.31: Frazier suction tip.

Malleable Retractor (Fig. 4.32)
Can be bent and customized. Also used to protect intestines during abdominal closure.

Fig. 4.32: Malleable retractor.

Rake Retractor (Fig. 4.33)
Hand-held retractor with sharp teeth used to hold back surface structures.

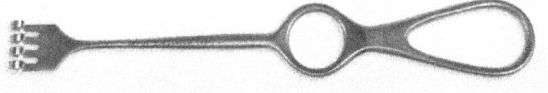

Fig. 4.33: Rake retractor.

Staplers and Clips

Used for reanastomosis of viscera, vessel ligation, and excision of specimens. Can be one-time use, reloadable, manual, or electronically powered. Staples come in multiple sizes.

Linear Stapler (Fig. 4.34)

Creates a linear staple line; no cutting function. Used in ligation and anastomosis. May be curved.

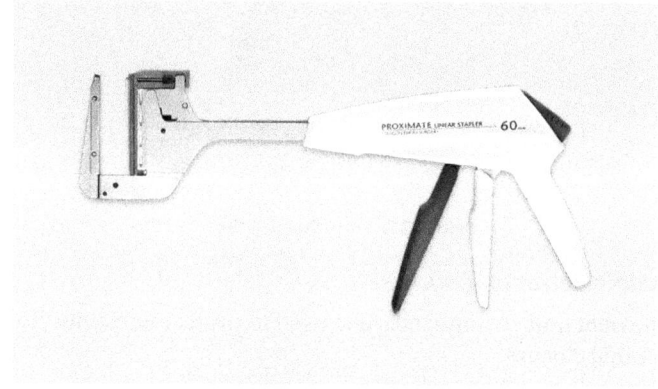

Fig. 4.34: Linear stapler.

Linear Cutter (Fig. 4.35)

Creates a linear cut and immediately staples both free edges. Used in separation and anastomosis.

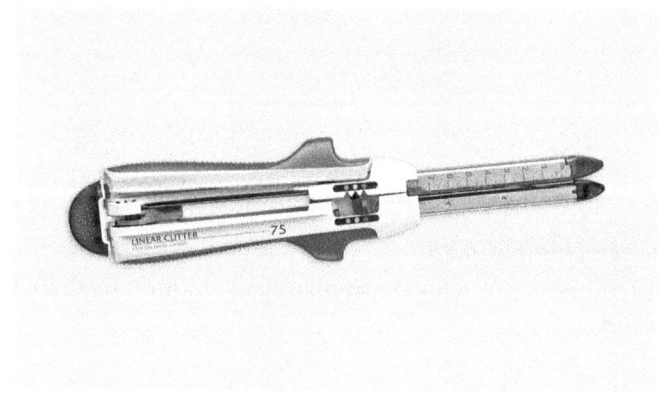

Fig. 4.35: Linear cutter.

Circular Cutter (Fig. 4.36)

Performs circular cut and staple. Used in reanastomosis of hollow viscera (e.g., large bowel).

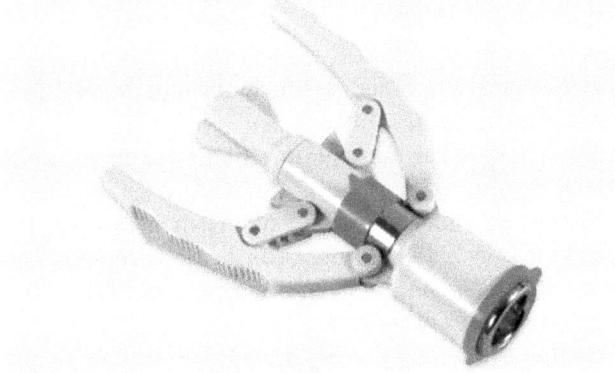

Fig. 4.36: Circular cutter.

Clips (Fig. 4.37)

Used in the ligation of vessels, maybe metal or absorbable material. Open and lap applicators.

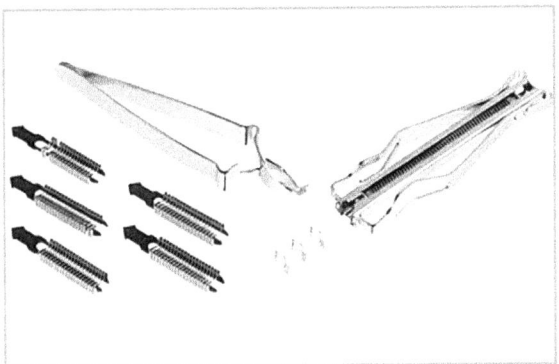

Fig. 4.37: Clips.

PREANESTHETIC CHECKUP

Preanesthetic Assessment

The preanesthetic assessment provides information needed to:
- Select the type of anesthesia to be administered and plan anesthetic care.

- ❖ Identify any medicine sensitivities.
- ❖ Safely administer the appropriate anesthetic
- ❖ Enquiry about any relevant medical history.

Duties of the Anesthetist

The duties of the anesthetist are listed below:
- ❖ An anesthesiologist or other qualified individual should conduct the preanesthetic assessment.
- ❖ Anesthetic care is carefully planned and documented in the anesthetic record.
- ❖ The plan considers information from other patient assessments and identifies the anesthetic to be used, the method of administration, other medications and fluids, monitoring procedures, and the anticipated postanesthetic care.
- ❖ The anesthetic planning process includes educating the patient and his or her family or her decision-maker regarding the risks, potential complications, and options related to the planned anesthesia and postoperative analgesia. This discussion occurs as part of the process of obtaining consent for anesthesia. The anesthesiologist or the qualified individual who will administer the anesthetic provides this education.
- ❖ Since anesthesia carries a high level of risks, its administration should be carefully planned. A preanesthetic assessment should be conducted and recorded.

When to Carry Out an Anesthetic Assessment

- ❖ An anesthetic assessment of a patient for elective surgery should be performed a day before the anesthesia is administered.
- ❖ An anesthetic assessment of a patient for emergency surgery should always be done before the patient is taken to the theatre.
- ❖ The medical assessment of surgical patient is documented before the start of the anesthesia.
- ❖ Interpret and act on any abnormal findings (e.g., blood pressure, hemoglobin, blood glucose, etc.) of the patient.

Other Requirements

The preoperative assessment will require a clinical check up by the surgeon prior to the operation. The surgical team should ensure that the patient fully understands the procedures and that the consent form is signed.

Reception of the Patient in the OT

The patient is taken to the OT on a patient trolley with side rails in position. The patient should be accompanied by a nurse and a porter. At the reception area in the OT, the OT nurse receives the patient in a polite and friendly way. The nurse escorting the patient should give his/her report to the receiving nurse and the information regarding the patient's identification and type of operation is checked. After handing over the patient, the escorting nurse must sign on the progress report.

The following is recommended:
- The person who receives the patient should introduce themselves to the patient and ask the patient for his/her name and what kind of operation they have come for.
- Patient with chronic illness should be asked if they took their medications (e.g., high blood pressure and diabetes treatment and how many hours prior to operation).
- Determine the condition of the infusion line.
- Determine whether or not preoperative dietary and fluid restrictions have been maintained. If not inform the anesthetist. Aspiration for gastric contents during induction of anesthesia is a danger.
- If applicable, check whether the anatomical site of the operation is clearly spelt out.
- Check whether the patient's vital signs were taken prior to coming to theatre.
- Ensure that the surgical safety check list is attached to the patient's file.

Types of Anesthesia

General Anesthesia

Anesthesia is produced as the central nervous system is affected. Association pathways are broken in the cerebral cortex to produce more or less complete lack of sensory perception and motor discharge. Unconsciousness is produced when blood circulating to the brains in adequate amount of the anesthetic agent. General anesthesia results in the unconscious, immobile, quite patient who does not recall surgical procedure.

Definition

General anesthesia is the administration of agents by intravenous injection or inhalation that renders the patient unconscious or obtunded.

Description

This anesthetic method is commonly employed. The depth and duration of anesthesia are regulated according to the type of anesthetic employed and the amount of the agent(s) administered. In addition to numerous intravenous and inhalation anesthetics, a large number of other agents, including muscle relaxants, tranquilizers, and narcotics, are employed. Rarely is a single drug used, although for limited procedures, a single agent (e.g., ketamine) may be employed. Intramuscular injection and rectal instillation of a primary agent are rarely used. During all general anesthetics, the patient must be well oxygenated and the patency of the airway maintained. The anesthesia provider must also maintain the patient's cardiovascular system and other vital functions.

Preparation of Patient for General Anesthesia

The patient is supine, with the safety strap in place across the thighs (about 3 inches above the knees). Care is taken not to compromise circulation by securing the restraint too tightly. The head support, a donut, pillow, or head frame is adjusted or removed at the discretion of the anesthesia provider. For procedures performed in the supine or lithotomy position that are of short duration, i.e., those in which profound muscle relaxation is not usually required, patency of the airway is managed with a mask and oral (or nasal airway or by means of a laryngeal mask airway (LMA).

Following induction, the insertion of an endotracheal tube will be required if the patient's position is to be other than supine or lithotomy, for a prolonged procedure in the supine position, for surgeries that affect respiration, or when profound muscular relaxation is needed. A variety of types and sizes of endotracheal tubes is available. Most often the endotracheal tube is placed transorally, but it may also be inserted transnasally or via an established tracheostomy.

Spinal Anesthesia

Spinal anesthesia is produced by making a spinal intrathecal injection of a heavy or light solution of anesthetic agent such as cinchocaine, lignocaine and bupivacaine. In spinal anesthetic the drug mixes with the cerebrospinal fluid and bathes a portion of the spinal cord and nerve roots, thereby rendering part of the body analgesic as well as paralyzing the muscles. The extent of its desired action is determined by the anesthetist and depends upon the volume of solution, the specific gravity of the solution and the position of the patient during and immediately after injection.

Local Anesthesia

Regional nerve block (e.g., brachial plexus block or ankle block) is achieved by depositing an anesthetic agent immediately adjacent to a larger peripheral nerves). This anesthetic is used primarily for surgery on the extremities. Intercostal nerve block is administered for local pain control, such as for a patient with a fractured rib or herpes zoster. A field block is used for limited abdominal surgery (e.g., gastrostomy or inguinal herniorrhaphy).

Local anesthesia refers to the injection of the anesthetic agent into, or immediately adjacent, to the site of surgery, anesthetizing smaller nerves directly. In topical anesthesia, the anesthetic agent (cream, gel, or liquid) is absorbed through the tissues (usually mucous membrane) to anesthetize the area immediately beneath where it is being applied, ophthalmic or gingival or the agent is applied to the tissue overlying a larger nerve trunk that courses close to the surface (e.g., glossopharyngeal nerve block). These anesthetic modalities (local or topical) may be administered by the surgeon (without the presence of an anesthesia provider); however, when the patient is medically fragile, or when general anesthesia or deep sedation is employed, an anesthesia provider is required. When the patient receives "conscious sedation," a perioperative registered nurse (RN), in addition to the circulator, is required to monitor the patient. Hyaluronidase (wydase) may be added to an injectable agent to promote more rapid spread and resolution of the local edema related to the injection. Epinephrine (adrenalin) added to the anesthetic solution will prolong the effect of the anesthetic solution. It is the injection of local anesthetic agent into the tissues through which the incision will be made.

Definition

An anesthetic agent may be applied by injection about the peripheral nerve trunk, by injection adjacent to or directly into the surgical site, or by application directly to the surface to be treated.

Preparation

The patient is positioned to expose the site of the proposed injection or application. In local or topical anesthesia, this site is often identical to the site of the surgery, whereas in regional anesthesia, the site of injection may be remote from that of surgery.

▌ SKIN PREPARATION

Regional

Skin preparation is done before the block is established, most often by the person performing the block (anesthesia provider or surgeon). The circulator may be requested to preparation the skin; the preparation begins at the site of injection, extending for an appropriately wide margin circumferentially.

Local

Skin preparation for the injection and the surgery are usually the same.

- **Topical:** Usually none is required, but an occlusive dressing is recommended for the transdermal application of EMLA™ or LMX™ (anesthetic agents in a cream formula).
- **Presentation of local anesthetics:** Local anesthetic is supplied as xylocaine plain or xylocaine with epinephrine (adrenaline). Advantages of xylocaine with adrenaline:
  - Causes constriction of blood vessels
  - Prevents rapid absorption of the anesthetics
  - Prolongs the action
  - Prevents convulsion (e.g., of local anesthetics).

Advantages of Local Anesthesia

- Simple, economical and nonexplosive.
- Less postoperative complications
- Ideal for short and superficial operations.

The American Society of Anesthesiologists (ASA) recommends the following standards for basic intraoperative monitoring:

- An anesthesia provider must be present throughout the administration of all general and most conduction anesthetics.
- During the administration of the anesthetic, vital signs and EKG are to be continually monitored and evaluated.
- Oxygen saturation is determined by use of an oxygen analyzer, pulse oximeter, and observing skin and nailbed color.
- The patient's temperature can be evaluated with a forehead tape strip or transesophageal or urinary bladder temperature probe.

Anesthetic Agents

(Refer p. 319)

Stages of Anesthesia

There are four stages of anesthesia. Brief explanation and nursing intervention in these stages are as follows: onset starts from anesthetic administration to loss of consciousness. In this stage, client may be drowsy or dizzy and may experience auditory or visual hallucinations. Nursing action in this stage will include, close operating room doors, keeping room quiet, and stand by to assist client **(Table 4.5)**.

Table 4.5: Stages of anesthesia.

Stage	Biological response	Patient reaction	Nursing action
Induction (relaxation)	• Amnesia • Analgesia	• Feels drowsy and dizzy • Exaggerated hearing decreased. Sensation of pain. May appear inebriated	• Close or doors check proper positioning of safety belt have suction available and working • Keep noise in the room to a minimum • Provide emotional support for the patient by remaining at his or her side
Excitement	Delirium	Irregular breathing, increased muscle tone and involuntary motor activity, may move all extremities, may vomit, hold breath or struggle (patient is very susceptible to external stimuli such as a loud noise or being touched)	• Avoid stimulating the patient • Be available to protect extremities or to restrain the patient • Be available to assist anesthesiologist with suctioning
Operative surgical anesthesia	Partial to complete sensory loss progression to complete intercostals paralysis	• Quiet, regular thoracoabdominal breathing, jaw relaxed • Auditory and pain sensation lost • Moderate to maximum decrease in muscle tone • Eyelid reflex is absent.	• Be available to assist anesthesiologist with intubation • Validate with anesthesiologist appropriate time for skin scrub and positioning of patient • Check position of patient's feet to ascertain they are not crossed
Danger	Medullary paralysis	• Respiratory muscles paralyzed and respiratory distress respiratory arrest provide • Pulse rapid and thread • Respirations cease	• Be available to assist in treatment of pupils fixed and dilated • Cardiac or emergency drug box and defibrillation • Document administrations of drugs

Excitement

Starts from loss of consciousness to loss of eyelid reflexes. Here there will be an increase in automatic activity, irregular breathing. In such a case the client may struggle. In this stage, nurse has to remain quietly as client's side, assist anesthetists if needed.

Surgical Anesthesia

This stage starts with loss of eyelid reflexes, to loss of motor reflexes and depression of vital functions. Here client is unconscious, muscles are relaxed and no blink or gag reflexes. In this stage, begins preparation (if indicated) only when anesthetists indicate stage III has been reached and the client is under good control.

Danger (Death) Stage

Vital functions too depressed may lead to respiratory and circulatory failure. In this stage, the client is not breathing, and he may or may not have a heartbeat. If arrest occurs, nurse responses immediately to assist establishing airway, provides cardiac arrest tray, drugs, syringes, long needles, assist surgeon with closed or open cardiac massage.

General Anesthesia

Can be administered by inhalation or intravenously. An inhalation agent will include nitrous oxide, halothane (fluothane), enflurane (enthrone) and isoflurane (porane) and the intravenous drugs are thiopental sodium (pentothal), fentanyl citrate droperidol (innovar) and ketamine hydrochloride. The selections of anesthetic agents are according to decision of the anesthesiologist. But continuous monitoring of side effects of the drugs, vital signs are essential.

Anesthetic Equipment's and Monitoring Needs

At least one anesthesiologist should be in the team involved in planning an OT. It is imperative that certain mandatory considerations with respect to the anesthetic equipment and monitors be planned during the planning and design stage itself. Personal, practice and cost preferences may influence the plans.

Communications

Telephones, intercom and code warning signals are desirable inside the OT. One phone per OT and one exclusively for use of anesthesia personnel is desirable. Intercom to connect to control desk, pathology and other OTs as well as use of paging receivers (bleeps) is also ideal.

A code signal, when activated, signals an emergency state such as cardiac arrest or need for immediate assistance.

Catering
Basic services such as preparation of beverages and some snacks, use of vending machines may be planned, augmented by provision of hot and cold meals from main hospital kitchen.

Cleaning
The construction materials selected for the OT complex should aim to minimize maintenance and cleaning costs.

Data Management
Customized network connections should be put in place or a conduit should be planned. A well-designed system can provide automated records, materials management, quality improvement and assessment, laboratory tracking, etc. The software for OT management is costly and hospitals are generally slow to adapt to changes. Customized OT software can be designed for individual needs.

Operating Theatre Satellite Pharmacy
Access to the OT areas and outside should be possible. It should have a laminar flow hood, a refrigerator, space for drug storage locked containers for controlled substances computer, desk area for paper work and pharmaceutical literature. Special kits for specific surgeries may also be arranged. The pharmacy may open for 1 to 24 hours based on need but it is desirable that an after hour system is planned.

Statutory Regulations
The design and planning of an OT complex will need compliance with mandatory regulations related to local administration such as Municipal Corporation, Government, Pollution Control Board, Fire Safety Department, Water supply and Drainage department, etc.

Usual areas of deficiency in OTs (existing OTS):
- No reception area.
- No separate rooms for:
  - Surgeons
  - Anesthesiologist
  - Jr. Doctor
  - OT attendants
- Not enough number of change rooms for different class of people.
- Inappropriate size and type of doors etc.

- Lack of laminar flow and mandatory air exchange systems in OT.
- Lack of standard OT protocol.
- No separate central sterile supply department (CSSD).
- Waiting area-recovery-not well equipped-lack of basic amenities.
- The authority for standardization recommendations are available in various surgical, anesthesia and nursing manuals with regard to the planning and establishment of operation theatres/complexes. The hospital can get accredited by the joint commission on accreditation of healthcare organizations (JCAHO), a professionally sponsored program that stimulates a high quality of patient care in healthcare facilities. There is also an accreditation option that is available for ambulatory surgery centers accreditation association for ambulatory healthcare (AAAH).

Monitoring and Recording the Physiological Status
During Anesthesia and Surgery

- Each patient's physiological status should be monitored and recorded during anesthesia and surgery.
- The anesthetist monitors and records the physiological status of the patient during anesthesia, and enters the anesthetic, medication and intravenous fluids used in the patient's anesthetic record.
- The anesthetist should have access to the patient care notes and know the findings of the medical examination. It is important that each health professional has access to the records of other care providers.

Anesthetic Machine and Other Anesthetic Apparatus

It is important that the anesthetic machine is checked before the administering of any anesthetic, to ensure that all the necessary items are available.

Ensure that the following items are on the anesthetic machine:
- Laryngoscope with different size blades. Make sure the laryngoscope is clean and in working condition.
- A big and a small McGill's (adult and pediatrics) forceps for the insertion of the intratracheal tube.
- A straight artery forceps to clamp the tube. This clamp must be marked for the use of the anesthetic machine only to prevent a mix up with the surgical instruments.
- A pair of scissors for the cutting of plaster.
- A set of McGill's connections.
- A catheter introducer to insert the intratracheal tube.

- ❖ Also ensure that the following items are in the drawer of the anesthetic machine:
    - Enough airways of different sizes
    - Hypodermic syringes of varied sizes
    - An ambu bag
    - Different size intratracheal tubes
    - Different size masks
    - Sufficient cut zinc oxide plaster for the sticking of the tubes, etc.
    - A tube of local lubricant gel (e.g.,. lignocaine)
    - Stethoscope
    - Nasal gastric (NG)—tube with different sizes
    - Chloramphenicol eye ointment
    - Sand bags
    - Suction nozzle (Yankauer)
    - Kidney dish with water
- ❖ Make sure the anesthetic tubes are correctly connected to the machine. Also check that the different gas cylinders have gas and a cylinder key is present.
- ❖ An empty cylinder must be replaced with a full one. The empty cylinder is marked "empty" with white chalk and is removed from the operation theatre.
- ❖ Check that the suction apparatus is in good working condition and connected to a suction tube and a suction catheter is connected.
- ❖ After every administered anesthesia, the used airways, intratracheal tubes and masks must be placed in a plastic bag. A new/clean airway, intratracheal tube and mask are used for every new patient. All used anesthetic items are removed from the operating theatre after the last operation.
- ❖ A new, sterile suction catheter must be used for every patient. Special anesthetic items must be kept ready, in case the anesthetist needs them.
- ❖ Ensure the defibrillating machine is available and checked daily. It is the responsibility of the anesthetist to check the anesthetic machine and all other apparatus before she/he administers the anesthesia. The anesthetic machine must be cleaned if it is soiled during the administration of anesthesia.

INFECTION CONTROL IN OT

Introduction

Postoperative infections do sometimes occur, even with the most careful and well-trained surgical team. Good units have an infection rate of about one case in a thousand or less. It is reasonable to assume that any infection developing within the first postoperative week has been contracted at the time of the operation. Even an isolated case of postoperative infection should make the surgeon and the surgical team review all their techniques, equipment and procedures. If several infections occur close to each other an even more radical overhaul to theatre procedures is required. Any irrigating fluids should be discarded and a new batch obtained. All made up disinfectant solution should be discarded and new ones made, and the sterilizer changed or a new method of sterilization tried. If available an infection control officer or a microbiology department will help to trace the source of an infection. The following is a list of the more common possible sources of infection during surgery.

Sources of Infection

From the Patient

- ❖ Conjunctivitis
- ❖ Blepharitis
- ❖ Dacryocystitis
- ❖ Septic lesion near the eye.

From the Staff

- ❖ Septic lesions
- ❖ Poor scrubbing up
- ❖ Contaminated gloves
- ❖ Failure to observe three no touch technique three by the surgeon or assistant, or touching the lids or lashes with instruments entering the eye.
- ❖ Prolonged manipulation during the operation.

From the Theatre Equipment

- ❖ Contaminated irrigating fluid
- ❖ Faulty sterilizer
- ❖ Faulty sterilizing technique
- ❖ Contamination or inactivation of disinfectant solutions.
- ❖ Broken or defective packaging for an IOL or instrument which is factory sterilized.

Infection Process

An infection is an invasion of the body by pathogens, or microorganisms capable of producing disease. The development of an infection occurs in a cyclical process that depends on the following six elements.

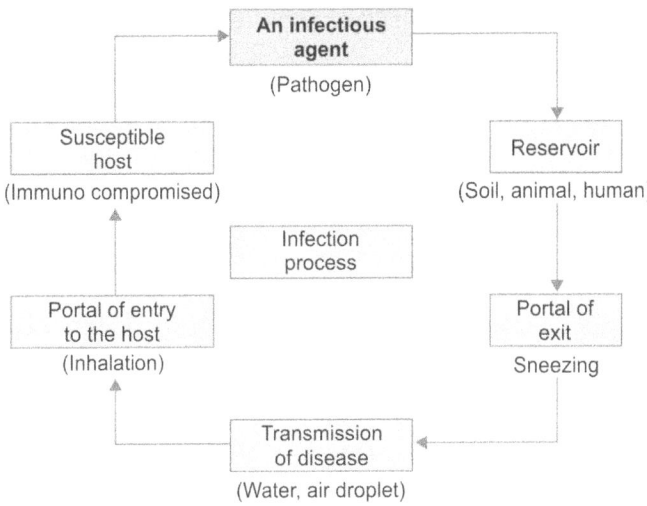

Fig. 4.38: Process of Infection.

An infection will develop if this cyclical chain remains intact. To prevent the spread of microorganisms, the cycle must be interrupted. Nurses use respective practices to break the chain, so that infection will not occur **(Fig. 4.38)**.

Infection Agent

The pathogenic organism includes bacteria, viruses, fungi and protozoa and more prevalent agents that are capable of causing infection.

Reservoir

The reservoir for growth and multiplication of microorganisms is the natural habitat of the organism. The possible reservoir that supports organism pathogenic to human includes other humans, (e.g., TB syphilis, HIV, HBV), animals (Rabies-dog), food (*Clostridium botulinum*) water, milk and inanimate object e.g., soil, gas gangrene, tetanus).

Portal of Exist

The exit from the reservoir is the point of escape for the organism. The organism cannot extend its influence unless it moves away from its original source. There usually a primary exist route for each type of organism. In human common escape route are as follows:
- Skin and mucus membrane (e.g., *S. aureus*, cause yellowish drainage. *P. aeruginosa* cause greenish drainage).

- Respiratory tract (e.g., *Mycobacterium tubercle* cause *tuberculosis*).
- Castro urinary tract.
- GI tract.
- Reproductive tract (e.g., STDs, HIV).
- Blood-serum hepatitis.

Modes of Transmission

An organism may be transmitted from its reservoir by various means of routes. Some organism can be transmitted by more than one route.

Contact

- Direct contact, e.g., *Staphylococcus, T. Palladium,* herpes simplex.
- Indirect contact, e.g., *Measles virus,* HBV, *Enterococcus* and *Pseudomonal* organism.
- Droplet contact, e.g., influenza virus, *M. tuberculosis*.

Air

Droplet nuclei, e.g., influenza virus, *Pneumococcus,* V-Z virus, Dust, e.g., *Aspergillus* and organism.

Vehicles

- Contaminated items, e.g., *M. tuberculosis*
- Liquids:
  - Water, e.g., *Vibrio cholerae*
  - Drugs solution, e.g., *Pseudomonas* organism
  - Blood, e.g., hepatitis B virus
  - Food, e.g., *Salmonella, Staphylococcus, Enterobacter,* etc., and *Klebsiella* organism.

Vectors

1. Insects, e.g., mosquitoes—e.g., *falciparum*
2. Fleas, ticks, e.g., *Rickettsia typhi* and *R. prowazekii*
3. Cows, Dogs, e.g., *Brucella* organism **(Table 4.6)**

Portal of Entry

The portal of entry is the point at which organism enters the host. The entry route often is the same as the exits route. The urinary, respiratory, gastrointestinal, reproductive tract and the skin are common entry points.

Table 4.6: Types of micro-organism.

Agents	Organism	Affected organs	Infections
1. Bacteria	• *Escherichia Coli* • *Staphylococcus aureus* • *Mycobacterium tuberculosis* • *Neisseria gonorrhoeae*	• Colon • Skin • Lungs • GI tract • Eye	• Enteritis • Wound infection • *Tuberculosis* • Gonorrhea • Conjunctivitis
2. Viruses	• Hepatitis A virus • Hepatitis B virus	• Feces, blood, urine • Body fluids and excretion	• Infection hepatitis • Serum hepatitis
3. Fungi	• *Aspergillus* organism • *Candida albicans*	• Mouth, Skin, GT • Soil, dust	• Aspergillosis • Thrush, dermatitis
4. Protozoa	*Pl falciparum*	Mosquito	Malaria

Susceptible Host

For microorganism to continue to exists, they must find a source that is acceptable (a host) and overcome any resistance mounted by the host defenses. Susceptibility is the degree of resistance and individual has to pathogens. An organism or parasite potential to produce disease depends on a variety of factors which includes following:

❖ Number of organism or parasites
❖ Virulence of organism or its ability to cause disease
❖ Competence of a person's immune system ability to enter and survive in the host.
❖ Length and intimacy of the contact between a person and the microorganisms.
❖ Susceptibility of the host.

Course of Infection

An understanding of the course of infection by the stage in the development of an infection is necessary if the nurse is to intervene and disrupt the infection cycle. An infection progresses through the different phases which include incubation period, prodromal stage, full stage of illness, convalescent phase.

Incubation Period

Incubation period is the interval between the invasion of the body by the pathogen or entrance of pathogen into the body and the appearance of the first symptoms of infection, e.g., chickenpox 2-3 weeks, common cold 1-2 days, tetanus 2-21 days.

Prodromal Stage

A person is the most infectious during this stage. It is an internal from onset of nonspecific signs and symptoms (malaise, low grade fever, fatigue) to more specific symptoms. During this time, microorganisms grow and multiplies and client is more capable of spreading disease to others.

Full Stage of Illness

Full stage of illness is an interval when client manifests signs and symptoms specific type of infection. The presence of specific signs and symptoms indicates the full stage of illness. The types of infection determine the length of illness and the severity of manifestations. Symptoms that are limited or restricted to a discrete area are referred to as localized symptoms, whereas systematic symptoms as manifested throughout the entire body.

Convalescent Period

Convalescent period represents recovery from the infection. It is an interval when acute symptoms of infection disappear and the person return to healthy state-length of recovery depends on severity of infection and clients general state of health; recovery may take several days to months.

Defenses Against Infection

The body has normal defenses against infection. Normal body flora that resides inside and outside of the body protect a person from several pathogens. Each organ system has defense, mechanism that minimize exposure to infectious microorganism as follow:

- **Skin:** In skin intact multilayered surface is a body's first line of defense against infection, i.e., it provides barrier to microorganism. The shedding of the outer layer of skin all removes organism that adhere to skin outer layers. The sebum contains fatty acid that kills some bacteria. These factors that may alter defense are cut abrasions, puncture wounds, areas of laceration; failure to bathe regularly and excessive bathing reduces sebum.
- **Mouth:** Intact multilayered mucosa of mouth provides mechanical barriers to microorganism. Saliva produces in the mouth, washes away particles containing microorganism and it contains microbial inhibitor, e.g., lysozyme, factors that alter defense are lacerations, trauma, extracted teeth, poor oral hygiene, and dehydration.

- **Respiratory tract:** Cilia lining upper airway, coated by mucous will trap inhaled microbes and sweep them outward in mucous to expectorated or swallowed. Microphages of the respiratory tract engulf and destroy microorganism that reach lungs alveoli. The factors that may alter defense here are smoking high concentration of oxygen and carbon dioxide, decreased humidity, cold air, etc.
- **Urinary tract:** The flushing action of urine flow washes away microorganisms on lining of bladder and urethra. An infect multilayered epithelium of the tract provide barrier to microorganism. The factors which may alter defense here are obstruction to normal flow by any means.
- **Gastrointestinal tract:** Here the acidity of the gastric secretions chemically destroys microorganism incapable of surviving low pH. The rapid peristalsis in small intestine prevents retention of bacterial content. The factors which alter defense here are administration of antacids, delayed motility resulting from impaction of fecal content in large bowl or mechanical obstruction by masses.
- **Vagina:** At puberty, normal flora causing vaginal secretion to achieve low pH, which inhibits growth of many microorganisms.

In addition, the inflammatory response is a protective vascular and cellular reaction that neutralizes pathogens and repairs body cells.

Normal flora, body system defenses and inflammation are all nonspecific defenses that protect against microorganism regardless of prior exposure. The immune system is composed of separate cells and molecules resistant to disease. Certain responses of the immune system of nonspecific, whereas others are specific defenses against specific pathogens. If any of the body's defenses fails, an infection can quickly progress to a serious health problem. The factors which affecting immunological defense mechanism is as follow:

- Increasing age
- Stress
- Poor nutrition
- Inherited condition
- Type of disease process
- Environments

Nosocomial Infections

The term 'nosocomial' is taken from the Greek word nosocomium meaning healthcare facility. A nosocomial infection is one that is acquired in a hospital or other health agency. This is a far-reaching and serious problem. A hospital is one of the most likely places for

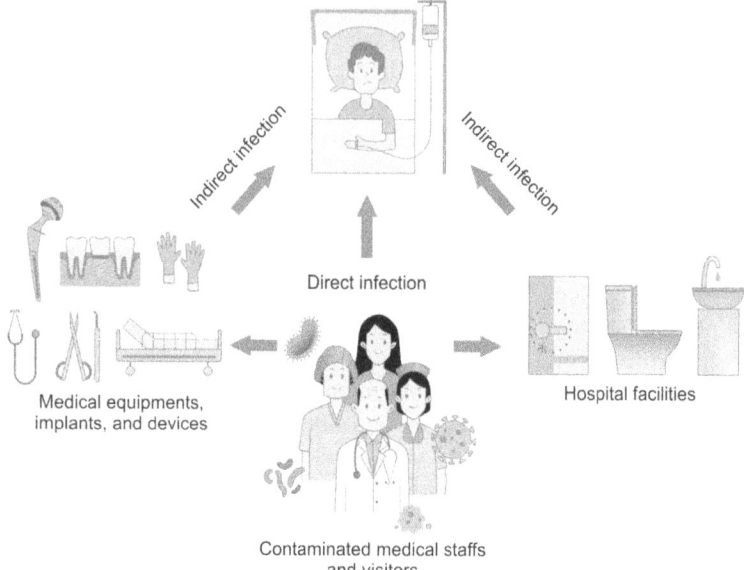

Fig. 4.39: Nosocomial infection.

acquiring an infection because it harbors a high population of virulent stains of microorganisms that are usually resistant to antibiotics. Nosocomial infections not only extend hospital care for the patient but also increase cost for both patient and hospital. Iatrogenic infection is a type of nosocomial infection resulting from the diagnostic or therapeutic procedure, e.g., insertion of catheter in urinary tract may develop infection **(Fig. 4.39)**.

Types of Hospital—Acquired Infections

- ❖ **Bloodstream infections:** These include bacteremia and septicemia. They are generally caused by the introduction of intravascular catheters/cannulas.
- ❖ **Pneumonia:** Ventilator-associated pneumonia in ICU patients, patients with prior respiratory tract pathology. Smokers, patients who have undergone abdominal/thoracic surgery are usually affected.
- ❖ **Urinary tract infection:** It is usually caused by introduction of exogenous organisms, urinary tract catheter or urinary tract instrumentation.
- ❖ **Gastrointestinal infections:** It can occur by consumption of contaminated food and cause food poisoning manifested by vomiting. Diarrhea or dysentery.

❖ **Skin and soft tissue infections:** It can occur following surgical procedures and contamination or burn wounds and secondary infection of traumatic wounds , e.g., causative micro-organism.
  - *Bloodstream infections:* Coagulase—negative *staphylococci, Enterococci,* Fungi, *Staphylococcus aureus, Enterobacter* species, *Pseudomonas* species, *Acinetobacter* species.
  - *Urinary tract infections:* Gram negative enteric bacteria, *enterococci* fungi like *Candia* species.
  - *Surgical site infections: Staphylococcus aureus, Pseudomonas* species, coagulase negative *staphylococci, enterococci, E. coil.*

Hospital Infection Control Program

Nosocomial infection is responsible for a substantial number of patients acquiring infection in healthcare set-ups. There are significant expenses involved in treating these infections. In some cases, the duration of hospital stay is increased and may also aggravate the patient's condition resulting in death. Therefore, it is a:

❖ **Amount of a soil or organic matter present:** Soil protects microbes and may inactive the disinfectant solution.
❖ **Contact time:** Disinfectant requires direct contact with the agent for a specific time.
❖ **Concentration of solution:** The more concentrated the solution has the greater is its killing capacity. The solution must be used at the concentration specified by the manufacturer to be most effective. Therefore, the manufacture's dilution instructions must be followed.

Classification of Patient Care Items

Earle H. Spaulding developed a classification system in 1968 to determine the appropriate processing method to attain the desired level of disinfection required for patient care items. This system was adopted and later modified by the centers of disease control and prevention (CDC).

❖ **Critical items:** Must be sterile because they enter sterile tissue, break the mucosal barrier, or come into contact with the vascular system. For examples, include surgical instruments, catheters, needles, implants, etc.
❖ **Semicritical:** Items come into contact with no intact skin and mucous membranes and require high-level disinfection, although they may also be sterilized. For examples, include respiratory

therapy equipment, anesthesia equipment, bronchoscopes, colonoscopies, gastroscopes, sigmoidoscopes, and cystoscopy.
* **Noncritical:** Items are used in contact only with intact skin. Intermediate or low-level disinfection is adequate. For examples, include blood pressure cuffs, furniture, linens, bedpans, and eating utensils.

Levels of Disinfection

Disinfectants vary in their ability to kill microorganisms. The levels of disinfection described are low, intermediate, and high.

High-Level Disinfectants are Effective Against

* All vegetative bacteria
* Viruses
* Fungi, and
* Tuberculosis/TB

Most high-level disinfectants have a demonstrated level of activity against bacterial spores. High-level disinfectants are used primarily for such semicritical items are:
* Laryngoscopes
* Respiratory therapy and anesthesia equipment
* Flexible fiberoptic endoscope.

Intermediate-Level

Disinfectants are more powerful and kill more resistant microorganism than low-level disinfectants. In addition to vegetative bacteria, fungi, and lipid-involved viruses, they are effective against *Mycobacterium tuberculosis* and nonlipid viruses. They are not effective against resistant bacterial spores. Chlorine, iodophors, phenolics, and alcohol belong to this group.

Low-Level Disinfectants

Kill most vegetative bacteria, fungi, and lipid-enveloped viruses, but do not kill spores or nonlipid viruses. They are less active against the *Mycobacterium tuberculosis* and some gram-negative rods, such as *Pseudomonas*. These disinfectants are typically used to wipe down items that will contact only intact skin or for environmental surface disinfection.

Methods of Disinfection

Many products and methods are used to disinfect instruments. A few are described below.

Chemical Disinfectants

Formaldehyde (37% aqueous; 8% alcohol)
❖ Kills microorganism by coagulating protein in the cells.
❖ The solution is effective at room temperature.
❖ It has a pungent odor and is irritating to the eyes and nasal passages.
❖ Its vapors can be toxic.

Hydrogen peroxide interacts with cell membranes, enzymes, or nucleic acids to disrupt the life functions of microorganisms.
❖ **Alcohol:** Ethyl or isopropyl, 70–95%, kills microorganisms by coagulation of cell proteins.
❖ **Chlorine compounds** kill microorganisms by denaturation of protein. It is not most commonly used in a 2% solution.
  ▪ *Iodophor:* A complex of free iodine with detergent, kills microorganisms through a process of oxidation of essential enzymes.

Physical Disinfectants

❖ **Boiling/pasteurization:** It is a method of thermal disinfection that involves immersion of precleaned items into water heated to approximately 75–100°F for 30 minutes.
  ▪ *Boiling method:*
    ♦ Cannot be depended on to kill spores.
    ♦ It is a nontoxic, high-level disinfection process.
  ▪ *Guidelines for boiling:*
    ♦ Never put focally contaminated instruments in the boiler.
    ♦ Instruments to be boiled should totally be submerged.
    ♦ Timing should be counted when the water comes to its full boil.
    ♦ Change the water in the boiler every day or every two days since as the water boils it leaves a scum of impurities which will satin the inside of the boiler and spoil the instrument.
    ♦ Boil the instrument separately.
    ♦ Inspect the boiler from time-to-time and keep it in good condition.
    ♦ Do necessary repairs before anything goes really wrong.

Guidelines for the Use of Instrument Disinfectants

❖ Use the disinfectant in a well-ventilated room.
❖ Make sure that items have been thoroughly cleaned before attempting disinfection.
❖ Disassemble all removable parts of the item.

- Thoroughly dry the item before placing it in the disinfectant.
- Mix the disinfectant as recommended on the label. Improper mixing can lead to injury of the patient, the instrument, and the person working with the solution. Read the directions for the specific precautions.
- Completely immerse all parts of the item in the solution, ensuring that all lumens, creases, joints, and channels are in contact with the solution and that no trapped air bubbles are present.
- Do not leave the item in the disinfection solution for and undetermined time. The solution may damage the item and may also become a source of contamination.
- Close the container to prevent evaporation of the solution.
- Thoroughly rinse the item in at least two fresh rinse solutions to ensure adequate removal of the disinfectant (use sterile water and then alcohol).
- Thoroughly dry the disinfected item with a sterile towel, and place it in a dry, covered until ready for use.

Disinfection of Articles

Concurrent disinfection: It is the disinfection of the contaminated articles immediately, then and there, during the course of illness. It includes cleaning of the nursing isolation unit daily with effective disinfectants.

Disinfectants of linen and contaminated articles should be done before these are removed from the unit. Incinerate all waste, and dispose of the excreta safely. Stool and urine of typhoid patients should be treated with lime, 1:4, for 4 hours, and then, disposed of. It can be burned after mixing with saw dust.

Terminal disinfection: After the patient has recovered from a communicable disease, the disinfection of the room and articles used by him is done after his discharge from the unit or transfer or death. Fumigation is done with sulfur and formalin for this purpose.
- **Fumigation with sulfur:** The room should be filled with steam from a kettle. Place sulfur in an earthen ware which is kept in a large container with water. Pour methylated spirit over the sulfur, put the sulfur afire and close the room.
- **Fumigation with formalin:** Potassium permanganate crystals and formalin are used for this purpose mix and place them in metal bowl. For 100 cu feet, 140 gm of $KMNO_4$ and 250 mL of formalin are to be used. The room should be closed completely and sealed for 24 hours for effective disinfection.

Care of Instruments

Surgical instruments are expensive and represent a major investment. Surgical procedures have become more complicated and intricate and, as a result, instruments have become more complex, more precise in design, and more delicate in structure. Abuse, misuse, inadequate cleaning or processing, or rough handling can damage and reduce the life expectancy of even the most durable instrument, and the cost of repair or replacement becomes unnecessarily high. Instruments can last for many years if they are handled or maintained properly. Careless handling of the surgeon's tools (instruments) result in frustration for surgeon and great financial loss to the department or hospital.

The skills of the surgeon are hampered if he/she is forced to work with interior equipment such as:
- Scissors that is dull
- Clamps that won't stay closed over bleeding vessels
- Needle holders that pop open to release the needle into the wound
- Forceps whose teeth do not mesh (fit) together properly.

It is the nurse's responsibility to care for the proper handling and maintenance of the instruments. Guidelines which help increase the lifespan of instruments and ensure their proper function include:

During Surgery
- Handle instrument gently
- Do not throw them into basins
- Keep the sharp surfaces of cutting instruments away from other metal surfaces that could dull them.
- Do not soak them into saline solution
- When feasible, wipe blood to cake and dry on the instrument.
- Use the correct instrument for the job at hand, e.g.
- Heavy needles will damage delicate needle holders
- Wire sutures must be cut with wire cutters, not suture scissors.
- Use towel clips and not hemostats for securing drapes.

After Surgery
- Decontaminate/clean instruments as soon as possible. Do not allow blood to try on them.
- Use accepted techniques when sterilizing instruments.
- Separate sharp or delicate instruments from others when processing.

❖ Process all instruments from a surgical case, whether or not they have been used.

Note: Lubrication of instruments before they are wrapped is important. Lubrication in water-soluble antimicrobial solution prevents hinges and box locks from becoming stiff and protect sharp surfaces of the metal.

Decontaminating and Cleaning of Instruments

Decontaminating is the first-step in handling used instruments and supplies. Immediately after use, all instruments should be placed in an approved disinfectant such as 0.5% chlorine solution for 10 minutes to inactivate most organisms, including HBV and HIV. It is a process that makes inanimate objects **safer** to be handled by staff **before** cleaning. Decontamination is performed in a designated area, not in the OR, immediately after completion of the surgical procedure. For achieving satisfactory decontamination:

❖ Make fresh solution every morning, or more often if the solution becomes cloudy.
❖ Use plastic, noncorrosive containers for decontamination. This prevents sharp instruments from getting:
  - Dull due to contact with metal containers
  - Rusted due to chemical reaction that can occur between two different metals when placed in water.
❖ Do not soak metal instruments in water for more than 1 hour, even if they are electroplated, to prevent rusting.
❖ Do not mix chlorine solutions with either formaldehyde or with ammonia-based solutions as toxic gas may be produced.

Decontaminating Used Instruments and Other Items

❖ Keep surgical or examination gloves after completing the procedure.
❖ Place all instruments in 0.5% chlorine solution for 10 minutes immediately after completing the procedure.
❖ Decontaminate any surface contaminated during the procedure by wiping them with a cloth soaked in 0.5% chlorine solution.
❖ Immerse gloved hands in 0.5% chlorine solution.
❖ Remove gloves by turning inside out. If disposing of gloves, place them in a leak proof plastic container.
❖ If reusing gloves, soak in 0.5% chlorine solution for 10 minutes.
❖ Remove instruments from 0.5% chlorine solution after 10 minutes and immediately rinse them with sterile cool water to remove residual chlorine before being thoroughly cleaned.

❖ Two buckets can be used in the procedure areas or operating rooms, one filled with 0.5% chlorine solution and the other one with water, so instruments can be placed in the water after 10 minutes to help prevent corrosion.

Steps for Making a 0.5% Chlorine Solution

- ❖ **Decontamination:** A 0.5% chlorine solution (Barakina/hypochlorite sodium) can be made from readily available under different brand names in different concentration, e.g., "Ghion" available in Ethiopia contains 5% chlorine. Manufacturers of widely used brand Cedex, contains 5% chlorine.
- ❖ **Formula for making a dilute solution from concentrated solutions:**
  - Determine the concentration (% concentration) of the chlorine solution.
  - Determine the desired concentration (% dilution).

Once instruments and other items have been decontaminated, they can safely be further processed. This consists of cleaning and finally either high-level disinfection or sterilization.

Cleaning is the removal of all visible dust, soil, and other foreign material from the instruments. The primary **purpose** of cleaning is to decrease the amount of organic matter and soil and the associated microorganisms on instruments can be cleansed manually or with a machine.

Disinfection of Operation Theater

It should be emphasized that general operation theater layouts, operating room etiquette, sterilization of instruments, sterile surgical protocol are all highly important and relevant factors, which directly affect the incidence of postoperative infections in any setting. Proper protocols need to be put in place for proper adoption of these simple procedures by all theater staff.

Aldehydes are the most commonly used agents for high-level disinfection of the theater environment. Formaldehyde is the commonly used agent. Formaldehyde gas is generated from liquid formalin utilizing potassium permanganate crystals. 40% formalin liquid is added to potassium permanganate crystals to generate gas. Alternately, formalin liquid can be dispersed by a sprayer like device in the theater environment. After a contact time of at least 6-8 hours, the formaldehyde needs to be neutralized by using ammonia, allowing at least 2 hours contact time for ammonia to neutralize the formaldehyde prior to the use of theater. Aldehydes are potentially carcinogenic and it is therefore recommended that other agent such as hydrogen peroxide, hydrogen peroxide with silver nitrate, peracetic acid and other chemical compound of formaldehyde should be used in place of the currently prevalent practice of using formaldehyde. These agents are dispersed with the aid of a fogger-like device inside the theater environment. The contact time is about an hour and the theater can be used immediately after the contact time.

Fumigation of Operation Theater

Fumigation is a process of disinfection by exposure to the fumes of vaporized germicides. Formalin (formaldehyde) is a commonly used agent to sterilize the OT and wards. It is very irritant to eye, mucus membrane and skin. That's why it is neutralized with ammonia. The exposure period is 3–6 hours. After fumigation all the doors must be kept closed. Then it is used for the operation. Our main aim is to give a sterilized environment to the patient. By this process all the articles which we use in OT are also sterilized by this method.

Problem for the hospital as well as for the patients. If remedial measures are not in place to tackle the menace of nosocomial infections, some hospitals have implemented a hospital infection control programme which seeks to prevent and control nosocomial infection.

The aim of the hospital infection control program is to disseminate information, carry out surveillance activities, investigate, prevent and control nosocomial infections in hospitals.

The Infection Control Program Should Include

- ❖ Organized reliable surveillance and control activities.
- ❖ One infection control doctor for every major health facility.
- ❖ A trained hospital epidemiologist.
- ❖ A system for reporting surgical wound infection rates and other infections back to the practicing surgeons and physicians.
- ❖ Continuing education of medical staff.
- ❖ Control of infectious disease outbreaks.
- ❖ Protection of employees from infections.
- ❖ Advice on new products, devices and producers pertinent to infection control.
- ❖ Instruction on all necessary control measures in the event of an outbreak or other infection control emergency.

The implementation of the infection control program in the hospital is supervised by the infection control committee. This committee consists of:
- Musicologist
- Epidemiologist or infectious disease physician
- Surgeon
- Personnel from medical and nursing staff
- Infection control nurse
- Representatives from OTs, CSSD, ICUs
- Hospital administrator having experience and training in infection control.

The Functions of the Committee

- **To gather relevant data pertaining to microbial flora** in high-risk areas such as OTs, ICUs, dialysis and oncology units. Details regarding organism identification, antibiotics susceptibility patterns and evolving trends in hospital flora are provided by the microbiology laboratory which is best equipped to identify outbreaks of infection.
- **To carry out surveillance:** Surveillance is mainly targeted in those areas where risk of infection can be problematic and antibiotics resistance more prevalent (e.g., ICUs, OTs, postoperative wards).
- **To enforce good infection control practices:** This requires that certain key concepts (e.g., standard precautions), knowledge about nosocomial pathogens, their reservoirs, modes of transmission and preventive measures to control infection are widely disseminated and practiced.

Hospital Infection Control Policy

Every hospital must have an infection control team which formulates a policy for control of nosocomial infection. The team members include the medical superintendent who heads the team, the microbiologist who is the infection control officer, heads of various clinical departments, blood bank, nursing superintendent and head supporting service such as housekeeping, laundry, and operation theatre. This team is concerned with introducing, modifying and maintaining policies in the following:
- Isolation of patient with communicable disease
- Admission of infected patients
- Aseptic techniques and practice
- Standardization of supplies
- Antibiotic management

This includes information of an antibiotic control policy: This policy outlines the first- and second-line antibiotics that can be administered for treatment of infections and helps prevent indiscriminate usage of antibiotics which contributes to the spread of drug resistant organism. This policy must be revised on a regular basis at least once in 6 months.

Infection Control Policies in Theatre Areas

Sharps Use and Disposal

- Ensure removable blades can be easily detached using an appropriate device.
- Use an appropriate size and type of 'sharps' bin/box for the area and anticipated volume of usage.
- Do not place 'sharps' bin/boxes in areas where there may be an obstacle to environmental cleaning.
- **Avoid overfilling:** The sharps containers must be closed securely when three quarters full.
- Used needles must be reheated.

Blood Spillage

- **Larger spills:** Sprinkle with chlorine releasing granules (NaDCC as 'Presept' or approved brands) until the fluid is absorbed.
- **Small blood splashes or drops:** Wipe up using fresh hypochlorite solution 10,000 ppm available chlorine (as per manufacturer's instructions on container: 'PreSept' or approved brand); apply solution using disposable paper towels.
- Leave the granules to solidify of paper towels with hypochlorite solution for a contact time of 2–5 minutes.
- Clear up using scoop (granules) or with disposable paper towels and dispose of as clinical waste. Wipe the area clean using hypochlorite solution.
- Rinse well using detergent and hot water (hypochlorite is corrosive). Dry using paper towels.

Universal Precautions

The devastating spread of acquired immunodeficiency syndrome and hepatitis B virus of the past decade has resulted in the creation of critically important documents and recommendations for the protection of health care workers and patients. These documents define the healthcare workers and patients, identify the risks to the worker and establish practices and recommendations to prevent the transmission of blood-borne disease.

The basic guidelines for universal precautions are as follows:
- All surgical patients are considered contaminated. In other words, all surgical patients are considered to be carriers of blood-borne pathogens.
- All personnel must wear gloves when handling blood, body fluids or contaminated surgical supplies.
  Contaminated supplies are those that have touched any body fluids. These supplies include instruments, linen waste, or any other type of item that is used in patient care or treatment.
- Gloves must be worn by personnel when they perform or assist in the performance of care that involves touching the patients' mucous membranes or nonintact skin surfaces.
- During all surgical procedures, with the possible exception of microsurgery, all team personnel must wear protective goggles or a face shield. Ordinary eyeglasses may suffice for protective eye wear as long as the eyeglasses are fitted with side shields that completely protect the eye. Goggles or other protective eye wear must be disinfected following each case.
- Face masks must be worn during every surgical case and properly disposed of following each case.
- Whenever it is anticipated that excessive amount of body fluids will be encountered during a surgical case, all team personnel must wear barrier gowns that prevent the penetration of these fluids to the skin of the team member.
- Any sharp item including scalpel blades, needles, pointed instruments or any other item that could penetrate skin, must be handled with extreme caution to prevent accidental puncture.
- All personnel must wash their hands thoroughly after contact with body fluids, even if gloves were worn during the contact.
- When discarding contaminated sponges during surgery, the receiving container must be placed close to the patient and operating team.
- Soiled linen and waste must be discarded in appropriate containers and not allowed to contact clean uncontaminated areas. Linen hampers must be leaking proof.
- Any tissues, blood or body fluid specimen or any specimen that has contacted patient blood or body fluids, must be secured in a leak proof container. Specimen may be placed in two separate containers. The outside container must be prevented from touching the tissue, specimen, or other body fluids.
- Personnel responsible for the decontamination of surgical suits following an operative procedure must don protective barrier attire

including gloves, mask, and waterproof apron when contact with body fluids is anticipated.
- When blood or body fluids are spilled an effective disinfectant agent must be poured carefully over the spill before cleanup.
- When an employee suffers any injury resulting from puncture or interruption of skin by a contaminated object, the injury must be immediately reported and follow-up care begun according to hospital policy.
- All operating room employees should be vaccinated against hepatitis B virus.
- Any employee whose exposed skin surface is not intact and is oozing exudates must be excluded from operating room duty until the condition is healed.

BASIC IDEAS OF DIFFERENT IV FLUIDS

There are three types of IV fluids: (1) Isotonic, (2) hypotonic, (3) hypertonic.

Isotonic Solutions

Isotonic solutions are IV fluids that have a similar concentration of dissolved particles as blood. An example of an isotonic IV solution is 0.9% normal saline (0.9% NaCl). Because the concentration of the IV fluid is similar to the blood, the fluid stays in the intravascular space and osmosis does not cause fluid movement between compartments. For an illustration of isotonic IV solution administration with no osmotic movement of fluid with cells. Isotonic solutions are used for patients with fluid volume deficit (also called hypovolemia) to raise their blood pressure. However, infusion of too much isotonic fluid can cause excessive fluid volume (also referred to as hypervolemia) **(Fig. 4.40)**.

Hypotonic Solutions

Hypotonic solutions have a lower concentration of dissolved solutes than blood **(Fig. 4.41)**. An example of a hypotonic IV solution is 0.45% normal saline (0.45% NaCl). When hypotonic IV solutions are infused, it results in a decreased concentration of dissolved solutes in the blood as compared to the intracellular space. This imbalance causes osmotic movement of water from the intravascular compartment into the intracellular space. For this reason, hypotonic fluids are used to treat cellular dehydration. For an illustration of the osmotic movement of fluid into a cell when a hypotonic IV solution is administered, causing

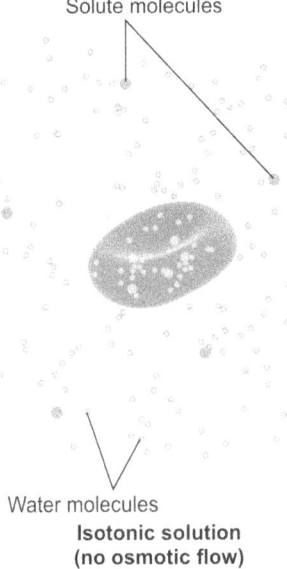

Fig. 4.40: Lack of fluid movement when isotonic IV solution is administered.

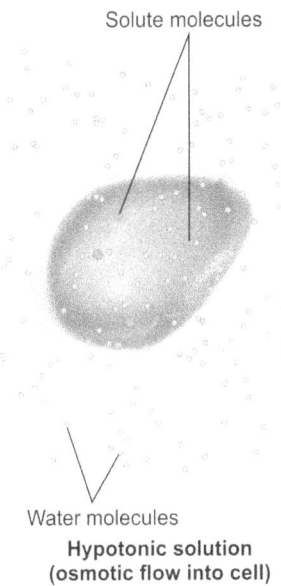

Fig. 4.41: Hypotonic IV solution causing osmotic movement of fluid into cell.

lower concentration of solutes (pink molecules) in the bloodstream compared to within the cell.

However, if too much fluid moves out of the intravascular compartment into cells, cerebral edema can occur. It is also possible to cause worsening hypovolemia and hypotension if too much fluid moves out of the intravascular space and into the cells. Therefore, patient status should be monitored carefully when hypotonic solutions are infused.

Hypertonic Solutions

Hypertonic solutions have a higher concentration of dissolved particles than blood. An example of hypertonic IV solution is 3% normal saline (3% NaCl). When infused, hypertonic fluids cause an increased concentration of dissolved solutes in the intravascular space compared to the cells. This causes the osmotic movement of water out of the cells and into the intravascular space to dilute the solutes in the blood **(Fig. 4.42)**. For an illustration of osmotic movement of fluid out of a cell when hypertonic IV fluid is administered due to a higher concentration of solutes (pink molecules) in the bloodstream compared to the cell **(Fig. 4.43)**.

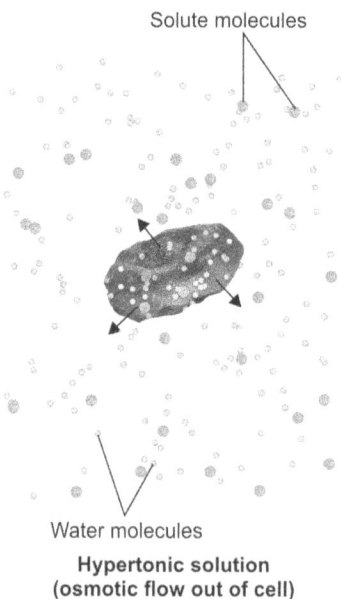

Hypertonic solution
(osmotic flow out of cell)

Fig. 4.42: Hypertonic IV solution causing osmotic fluid movement out of a cell.

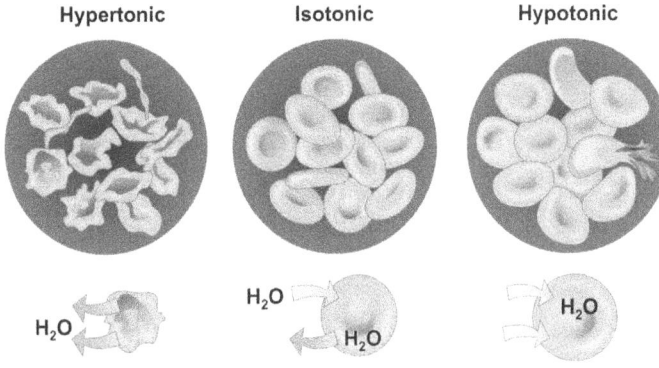

Fig. 4.43: Comparison of osmotic effects of hypertonic, isotonic, and hypotonic IV fluids on red blood cells.

When administering hypertonic fluids, it is essential to monitor for signs of hypervolemia such as breathing difficulties and elevated blood pressure. Additionally, if hypertonic solutions with sodium are given, the patient's serum sodium level should be closely monitored. For a comparison of types of IV solutions, their uses, and nursing considerations **(Table 4.7)**.

Table 4.7: Comparison of IV solutions.

Type	IV solution	Uses	Nursing considerations
Isotonic	0.9% normal saline (0.9% NaCl)	Fluid resuscitation for hemorrhaging, severe vomiting, diarrhea, GI suctioning losses, wound drainage, mild hyponatremia, or blood transfusions	Monitor closely for hypervolemia, especially with heart failure or renal failure
Isotonic	Lactated Ringer's solution (LR)	Fluid resuscitation, GI tract fluid losses, burns, traumas, or metabolic acidosis. Often used during surgery	Should not be used if serum pH is more than 7.5 because it will worsen alkalosis. May elevate potassium levels if used with renal failure
Isotonic	5% dextrose in water (D5W) *starts as isotonic and then changes to hypotonic when dextrose is metabolized	Provides free water to help renal excretion of solutes, hypernatremia, and some dextrose supplementation	Should not be used for fluid resuscitation, because after dextrose is metabolized, it becomes hypotonic and leaves the intravascular space, causing brain swelling. Used to dilute plasma electrolyte concentrations

Contd...

Contd...

Type	IV solution	Uses	Nursing considerations
Hypotonic	0.45% sodium chloride (0.45% NaCl)	Used to treat intracellular dehydration and hypernatremia and to provide fluid for renal excretion of solutes	Monitor closely for hypovolemia, hypotension, or confusion due to fluid shifting into the intracellular space, which can be life-threatening. Avoid use in patients with liver disease, trauma, and burns to prevent hypovolemia from worsening. Monitor closely for cerebral edema
Hypotonic	5% dextrose in water (D5W)	Provides free water to promote renal excretion of solutes and treat hypernatremia, as well as some dextrose supplementation	Monitor closely for hypovolemia, hypotension, or confusion due to fluid shifting out of the intravascular space, which can be life-threatening. Avoid use in patients with liver disease, trauma, and burns to prevent hypovolemia from worsening. Monitor closely for cerebral edema
Hypertonic	3% sodium chloride (3% NaCl)	Used to treat severe hyponatremia and cerebral edema	Monitor closely for hypervolemia, hypernatremia, and associated respiratory distress. Do not use it with patients experiencing heart failure, renal failure, or conditions caused by cellular dehydration because it will worsen these conditions
Hypertonic	5% dextrose and 0.45% sodium chloride (D50.45% NaCl)	Used to treat severe hyponatremia and cerebral edema	Monitor closely for hypervolemia, hypernatremia, and associated respiratory distress. Do not use it with patients experiencing heart failure, renal failure, or conditions caused by cellular dehydration because it will worsen these conditions

Contd...

Contd...

Type	IV solution	Uses	Nursing considerations
Hypertonic	5% dextrose and lactated Ringer's (D5LR) D10	Used to treat severe hyponatremia and cerebral edema	Monitor closely for hypervolemia, hypernatremia, and associated respiratory distress. Do not use it with patients experiencing heart failure, renal failure, or conditions caused by cellular dehydration because it will worsen these conditions

Osmolarity is defined as the proportion of dissolved particles in an amount of fluid and is generally the term used to describe body fluids. As the dissolved particles become more concentrated, the osmolarity increases. **Osmolality** refers to the proportion of dissolved particles in a specific weight of fluid. The terms osmolarity and osmolality are often used interchangeably in clinical practice.

NEEDLES, SUTURES AND KNOTS

Definition

The term "Suture" describes any strand of material utilized to approximate tissues.

Suturing refers to sewing together two structures using suture threaded on a needle.

Ligating or ligaturing refers to tying a ductal structure such as blood vessel simply by means of a suture thread.

Suturing Goals

- Provide adequate tension for wound closure but loose enough to prevent tissue ischemia and necrosis.
- Protecting underlying tissues from infection or other irritating factors.
- Preventing postoperative hemorrhage.
- Permitting healing by primary intention.
- Preventing bone exposure resulting in delayed healing and bone resorption.
- Permit proper flap position.

Ideal Suture Qualities

- Minimal tissue reaction
- Smoothness—minimum tissue drag
- Easily sterilizable
- Adequate tensile strength
- Ease of handling—minimum memory
- Knot security
- Cost effectiveness
- Favorable absorption profile
- Resistance to infection

Suture Material Types (Table 4.8)

- **Behavior—tissue:** Absorbable/Nonabsorbable
- **Structure:** Monofilament/multifilament
- **Origin:** Natural/synthetic

Table 4.8: Suture material.

Absorbable	Nonabsorbable
Catgut	Silk, linen, cotton
Chromic catgut	Horse/human hair
Dexon (polyglycolic acid)	Nylon or ethilon
Vicryl (polyglactin)	Polyester (mersilene/ethibond)
PDS (polydioxanone)	Polypropylene (prolene)
Collagen	Stainless steel, aluminum wire
Maxon (Polyglyconate)	Clips
Monocryl (poliglecaprone)	Staples, skin tapes, adhesives

Absorbable-Natural

- **Plain catgut:** Light, derived from submucosa of sheep intestine or serosa of beef intestine.
    - Used for ligating superficial blood vessels and subcutaneous fatty tissues.
- **Chromic catgut:** Yellow, treated with chromium salt.
    - It may be used in the presence of infection and in cancer cases.

Absorbable-Synthetic

- **Polyglactin (vicryl):** Purple, copolymer of lactide and glycolide.
    - Minimal tissue reaction. Used in general soft tissue approx. intestinal anastomosis, vessels ligation in all surgical specialties.

- ❖ **Dexon (polyglycolic acid):** Purple/cream, homo polymers of glycolide.
  - Avoid in adipose tissue and losses tensile strength more rapidly than vicryl.
- ❖ **Others:** For example, polyglyconate (maxon), polydiaxone (PDS), poliglecaprone (monocryl).

Nonabsorbable-Natural

- ❖ **Surgical silk:** Black, derived from the cocoon of the silkworm larvae, trigger inflammatory reactions, undergo proteolysis and undetected by 2 years.
  - Used in ligating major blood vessels, tendons repair etc.
- ❖ **Surgical steel and wires:** High tensile strength and Hold knots very well
  - Used in orthopedic, neurosurgery and thoracic surgery.
- ❖ **Others:** For example, virgin silk, cotton, linen.

Nonabsorbable-Synthetic

- ❖ **Nylon:** It is a polyamide polymer, blue/white.
  - 81% tensile strength at 1 year and 66% at 11 years
  - Elicits minimal tissue reaction
  - Has good memory
  - Pliable when moist
  - Premoistened form is used in cosmetic plastic surgery.
  - Its elasticity makes it useful for skin closure and herniorrhaphy
- ❖ **Others:** For example, polypropylene (prolene), polyester fiber (mersilene/dacron/ethibond).

Monofilament

- ❖ Grossly appears as single strand of suture material; all fibers run parallel minimal tissue trauma. Resists harboring microorganisms.
- ❖ Ties smoothly
- ❖ Requires more knots than multifilament suture
- ❖ Possesses memory
- ❖ **Examples:**
  - Monocryl
  - PDS, prolene
  - Nylon

Multifilament

- ❖ Fibers are twisted or braided together
- ❖ Greater resistance in tissue

Table 4.9: Suture degradation.

Suture material	Method of absorption	Time to absorb
Catgut	Proteolytic enzymatic digestive process	Days
Vicryl	Hydrolysis	Weeks
PDS	Slow hydrolysis	Months
Silk/Nylon	Gradual encapsulation by fibrous connective tissue	Years

- ❖ Provides good handling and ease off tying
- ❖ Fewer knots required
- ❖ **Examples:**
  - Vicryl (braided)
  - Chromic (twisted)
  - Silk (braided)

Suture Size (Table 4.9)

- ❖ Sized according to diameter with "0" as reference size numbers alone indicate progressively larger sutures ("1", "2", etc.)
- ❖ Numbers followed by a "0" indicate progressively smaller sutures ("2-0", "4-0", etc.)
- ❖ Smaller ←————————→ Larger ..... "3-0"... "2-0"... "1-0"... "0"... "1"... "2"... "3"..... [Thick] [Thin]

Needle-Anatomy (Fig. 4.44)

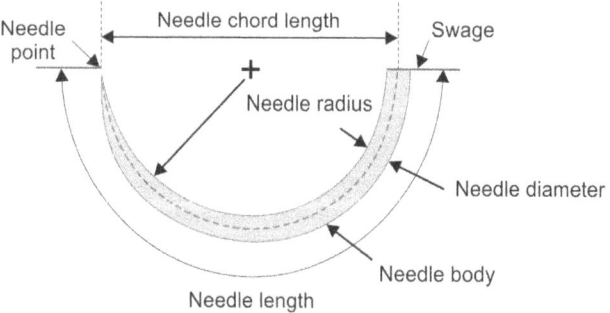

Fig. 4.44: Needle (Anatomy).

Needle Shapes
See **Table 4.10**.

Table 4.10: Needle point-geometry.

		Taper-point (round)	• Suited to soft tissue • Dilates rather than cuts
		Reverse cutting	• Very sharp • Ideal for skin • Cuts rather than dilates
		Conventional cutting	• Very sharp • Cuts rather than dilates • Creates weakness allowing suture tear out
		Taper-cutting	• Ideal in tough or calcified tissues • Mainly used in cardiac and vascular procedures

Ideal Suture-Needle

❖ High quality stainless steel
❖ Smallest diameter possible
❖ Stable in the grasp of needle holder
❖ Sharp enough to penetrate tissues with minimal resistance and trauma.
❖ Sterile and corrosive resistant.

Use of Needle Holders

❖ Loading needle
❖ Needle passing through skin.

Technique

❖ Needle should be grasped with the needle holder approximately 1/3 distance from the eye and 2/3 from the point.
❖ Needle should be placed perpendicular to surface being entered and pushed through tissues following curvature of the needle and rotating the wrist.
❖ Needle enters 2–3 mm away from the margin of the flap and exists at the same distance on the opposite side.

- The two ends of the suture are then tied in a knot and cut 0.8 cm above the knot.
- Knot should never lie on incision line.
- Never close under tension.

The Suture Packaging

1. Strand size
2. Material
3. Strand length
4. Product code
5. Color
6. Needle circle
7. Point type
8. Needle length
9. Needle code with with life size picture

Suture Techniques

- Simple sutures
- Mattress sutures
- Subcuticular sutures

Simple-Interrupted

- Suturing is passed through both edges at an equal depth and distance from the incision and knot is tied.
- Common and stronger.
- Each suture is independent and loosening of one suture will not produce loosening of other.

Simple-Continuous

- Useful in pediatrics
- Rapid
- Easy removal
- Provides effective hemostasis
- Distributed tension evenly along length
- Can also be locked with each stitch.

Mattress-Vertical

- It has a far-far-near-near order of bites.
- The knot is perpendicular to the wound edge.
- Useful in maximizing wound eversion, reducing dead space and minimizing the tension across the wound.

Mattress-Horizontal

- Used for high-tension wounds or wounds with fragile skin.
- The knot is parallel adjacent to the wound edge.
- Useful in maximizing wound eversion, reducing dead space and minimizing the tension across the wound.

Suture Removal

- **Face:** 2-3 days
- **Scalp:** 5 days
- **Trunk:** 7 days
- **Arm or leg:** 7-10 days
- **Foot:** 10-14 days

Recent advances staples adhesives tapes-steristrips:
- Formed from high quality
- A sterile, liquid topical skin adhesive
- Use of tissue adhesive adjunct stainless steel
- Reacts with moisture on skin surface (benzoin) to form a strong, flexible bond
- Suitable for skin closure
- Only for approximately skin edges of wounds
- Rarely used for primary closure.

Surgical Knots

Square or Reef Knot

- A square knot formed by wrapping the suture around the needle holder once in opposite directions between ties.
- Three ties are recommended.
- The two-hand square knot is the easiest and most reliable for tying most suture materials.
- It may be used to tie surgical gut, virgin silk, surgical cotton and surgical stainless steel.

Surgeon's or Friction Knot

- It is formed by two throws of suture around the needle holder on the first tie and one throw in the opposite direction on the second tie.
- The surgeon's or friction knot is recommended for tying braided synthetic absorbable suture, Vicryl*/Ethibond* polyester suture, Ethilon* nylon suture, Mersilene* polyester fiber suture, Nurolon* nylon.

Granny's or Slip Knot

❖ Granny's knot involve a tie in one direction followed by a tie in the same direction and third tie in the opposite direction to square the knot and hold it permanently.
❖ It has the tendency to slip when subjected to increasing pressure.
❖ It is not recommended.

■ CAUTERIZATION (CAUTERY)

Cauterization (cautery) is a medical practice or technique of burning a part of a body to remove or close off a part of it. It destroys some tissue in an attempt to mitigate bleeding and damage, remove an undesired growth, or minimize other potential medical harm, such as infections when antibiotics are unavailable.

The practice was once widespread for the treatment of wounds. Its utility before the advent of antibiotics was said to be effective at more than one level:
❖ To prevent exsanguinations
❖ To close amputations

Cautery was historically believed to prevent infection, but current research shows that cautery actually increases the risk for infection by causing more tissue damage and providing a more hospitable environment for bacterial growth. **Actual cautery** refers to the metal device, generally heated to a dull red glow, that a physician applies to produce blisters, to stop bleeding of a blood vessel, and for other similar purposes.

The main forms of cauterization used today are **electrocautery** and **chemical cautery** both are, e.g., prevalent in cosmetic removal of warts and stopping nosebleeds. Cautery can also mean the branding of a human.

Cauterization has been used to stop heavy bleeding since antiquity. The process was described in the Edwin Smith Papyrus and Hippocratic Corpus. It was primarily used to control hemorrhages, especially those resulting from surgery, in ancient Greece. Archigenes recommended cauterization in the event of hemorrhaging wounds, and Leonides of Alexandria described excising breast tumors and cauterizing the resulting wound in order to control bleeding. The Chinese *Su wen* recommends cauterization as a treatment for various ailments, including dog bites. Indigenous peoples of the Americas, ancient Arabs, and Persians also used the technique.

Tools used in the ancient cauterization process ranged from heated lances to cauterizing knives. The piece of metal was heated over fire and applied to the wound. This caused tissues and blood to heat rapidly to extreme temperatures, causing coagulation of the blood and thus controlling the bleeding, at the cost of extensive tissue damage. In rare cases, cauterization was instead accomplished via the application of cauterizing chemicals like lye.

Cauterization continued to be used as a common treatment in medieval times. While mainly employed to stop blood loss, it was also used in cases of tooth extraction and as a treatment for mental illness. In the Muslim world, scholars Al-Zahrawi and Avicenna wrote about techniques and instruments used for cauterization.

The technique of ligature of the arteries as an alternative to cauterization was later improved and used more effectively by Ambroise Paré.

Electrocautery

Electrocauterization is the process of destroying tissue (or cutting through soft tissue) using heat conduction from a metal probe heated by electric current. The procedure stops bleeding from small vessels (larger vessels being ligated). Electrocautery applies high frequency alternating current by a *unipolar* or *bipolar* method. It can be a continuous waveform to cut tissue, or intermittent to coagulate tissue.

The electrically produced heat in this process inherently can do numerous things to the tissue, depending on the waveform and power level, including cauterize, coagulate, cut, and dry (desiccate). Thus electrocautery, electrocoagulation, electrodesiccation, and electrocurettage are closely related and can co-occur in the same procedure when desired. Electrodesiccation and curettage is a common procedure.

Unipolar

In unipolar cauterization, the physician contacts the tissue with a single small electrode. The circuit's exit point is a large surface area, such as the buttocks, to prevent electrical burns. The amount of heat generated depends on the size of contact area, power setting or frequency of current, duration of application, and waveform. A constant waveform generates more heat than intermittent. The frequency used in cutting the tissue is higher than in coagulation mode.

Bipolar

Bipolar electrocautery passes the current between two tips of a forceps-like tool. It has the advantage of not disturbing other electrical body rhythms (such as the heart) and also coagulates tissue by pressure. Lateral thermal injury is greater in unipolar than bipolar devices.

Electrocauterization is preferable to chemical cauterization, because chemicals can leach into neighboring tissue and cauterize outside of intended boundaries. Concern has also been raised regarding toxicity of the surgical smoke electrocautery produces. This contains chemicals that, through inhalation, may harm patients or medical staff.

Ultrasonic coagulation and ablation systems are also available.

Chemical Cautery

Many chemical reactions can destroy tissue, and some are used routinely in medicine, most commonly to remove small skin lesions such as warts or necrotized tissue, or for hemostasis. Because chemicals can leach into areas not intended for cauterization, laser and electrical methods are preferable where practical. Some cauterizing agents are:

- ❖ Silver nitrate is the active ingredient of the lunar caustic, a stick that traditionally looks like a large match. It is dipped in water and pressed onto the lesion for a few moments.
- ❖ Trichloroacetic acid
- ❖ Cantharidin is an extract of the blister beetle that causes epidermal necrosis and blistering. It is used to treat warts.

Nasal Cauterization

Frequent nosebleeds are most likely caused by an exposed blood vessel in the nose, usually one in Kiesselbach's plexus.

Even if the nose is not bleeding at the time, a physician may cauterize it to prevent future bleeding. Cauterization methods include burning the affected area with acid, hot metal, or lasers. Such a procedure is naturally quite painful. Sometimes, a physician uses liquid nitrogen as a less painful alternative, though it is less effective. A physician may apply cocaine in the few countries that allow it for medical use. Cocaine is the only local anesthetic that also produces vasoconstriction, making it ideal for controlling nosebleeds.

More modern treatment applies silver nitrate after a local anesthetic. The procedure is generally painless, but after the anesthetic wears off, there may be pain for several days, and the nose may run for up to a week after this treatment.

Nasal cauterization can cause empty nose syndrome.

Infant Circumcision

Cauterization has been used for the circumcision of infants in the United States and Canada. The College of Physicians and Surgeons of Manitoba advises against its use in neonatal circumcision. This method of circumcision resulted in several infants having their penises severely burned, with at least seven male children being reassigned as female.

CHAPTER 5

Hand Hygiene and Prevention of Cross Infection

Chapter Outline

- Hand Hygiene and Method of Handwashing
- Prevention of Cross Infection
- Stages of Infection
- Nature of Infection
- Chain of Infection
- Universal Precaution
- Asepsis
- Hand Hygiene
- Personal Protective Equipment
- Biomedical Waste Management

■ HAND HYGIENE AND METHOD OF HANDWASHING

Handwashing is important in every setting, including hospitals. It is an effective infection control measure, as it prevents spread of microorganisms. For routine client care, the centers for disease control and prevention (CDC) recommends a vigorous handwashing under a stream of water for at least 10 seconds using soap **(Fig. 5.1)**.

Handwashing should be done:
- When there are known multiple resistant bacteria.
- Before invasive procedures.
- In special care units, such as nurseries, Intensive care units (ICUs) and offthe-shelf (OTs).

Purpose

- To remove transient and resident bacteria from fingers, hands and forearms.
- To prevent the risk of transmission of infection to patients.
- To reduce the risk of transmission of infection organisms to oneself.
- To prevent cross infection among patients.

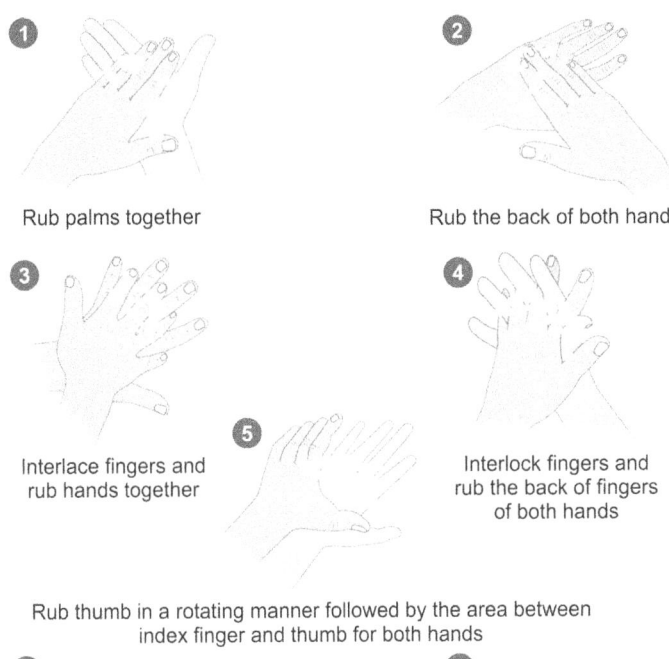

Fig. 5.1: Steps of handwashing.

Equipment/Articles

Articles	Rationale
Soap in a soap dish	Soap contains antibacterial agents and has a lasting bacteria static effect
Nail brush	To clean nails
Running water	To rinse soap and thoroughly wash hands
Towel	To dry hands

Steps of Procedure

Steps	Rationale
File the nails short; ensure that nails are free of nail polish	Short nails are less likely to harbor resident and transient microorganisms
Remove all jewelry and wrist watch	Microorganisms can be inside the settings of jewelry and under rings. Removal facilitates proper cleaning of hands and arms
Turn on the water to adjust the flow so that water is lukewarm	Warm water removes less of the protective oil of the skin than hot water
a. **Medical asepsis:** Wet the hands thoroughly by holding the hands lower than the elbows so that water flows from arms to finger tips	It allows water to flow from the least contaminated area (elbow) to the most contaminated area (hands)
b. **Surgical handwashing:** Wet hands and forearms liberally, keeping arms and hands above elbow level during the entire procedure	Water run by gravity from fingertips to elbows. Keeping hands elevated allows water to flow from least to the most contaminated area
Apply liberal amounts of soap into hands and later hands and arms using hand brushes	Soap emulsifies the oil and lowers the surface tension of water, facilitates the removal of micro-organisms, dust and oils. Brushes are used to enhance mechanical friction during handwashing
Thoroughly wash and rinse the hand using firm rubbing and circular movements to wash the palm, back and wrist of each hand. Interlace the fingers during handwashing	The circular action helps to remove micro-organisms mechanically. Running water and friction used in cleaning are the mechanical action of cleaning
Dry arms and hands thoroughly from fingers to wrists and forearms. Discard the towel in a proper container	Drying helps in removing moisture, prevents chapping and roughening of skin. Drying from cleaner to least clean area prevents contamination
Turn off the water tap using a paper towel or using an elbow	Handle is contaminated. Use of a paper towel or washed hands

■ PREVENTION OF CROSS INFECTION

Introduction

When a microorganism enters into the body tissue and multiplies there and has the ability to cause diseases in the person is known as infectious agent. In case when there is no symptom in the patient after entry of microorganism into the body, then the condition is called asymptomatic illness.

Definition

It is the infection of a patient with a disease other than that for which he had been admitted. In short patient gets the infection from someone during his stay in the hospital cross infection usually occurs in the hospital.

STAGES OF INFECTION

There are various steps by which microorganisms cause the disease in human beings.

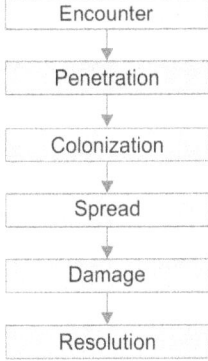

Encounter

There are various routes by which microorganisms come in contact with a person like through direct contact, ingestion and through transplacental **(Table 5.1)**.

Table 5.1: Infection contact.

Direct contact	Infection is transmitted through direct contact if an individual comes in contact with body fluids or tissues of infected person, e.g., • Open wounds • Mucus membrane • Blood saliva • Urine
Oral route	The microorganisms ingested through contaminated food or water
Droplet route	The microorganisms enter in the body through coughing or sneezing or during aerosol generating procedures like during suctioning or intubation

Contd...

Contd...

Airborne route	The microorganism enters into the person through dust particles or the small particles that which float in the air
Indirect route	The microorganism enters in the patient's body through an object which is infected like medical equipment or instruments contaminated with microorganisms
Vector born route	The infections which are caused by animals or insects

Penetration

For penetration into the human tissue, the microorganism must cross the surface barrier.

Colonization

When the microorganism enters into the human body, it starts multiplying over there. For the growth of the microorganism, it requires favorable conditions like temperature, pH and nutrition.

Spread

The invading microorganisms may spread by one or more routes: direct extension through surrounding destroys cells to cause damage. They can cause sublethal damage or alter cellular function.

Damage

Microorganism causes damage to the human host by various mechanisms like:
- Bulk effects.
- Toxins released by the bacteria.
- Altered function of the host.
- Response of the host to infection.

Resolution

The host response usually begins with an inflammatory reaction and is followed by a humoral or cell mediated immune response.

■ NATURE OF INFECTION

Communicable disease is the infectious process transmitted from one person to another.
- If pathogens multiply and cause clinical signs and symptoms, the infection is symptomatic.
- If clinical signs and symptoms are not present, the illness is termed asymptomatic.

- Hand hygiene is the most important technique to use in preventing and controlling transmission of infection.
- All persons have microorganisms on their skin, but usually no disease results.
- Disease or infection results, only if the pathogens grow or multiply and alter normal tissue function.
- An infectious disease transmitted directly from one person to another is considered a contagious or communicable disease.
- Infection is amongst the main reasons that lead to preventable morbidity and mortality in the community as well as in the long-term healthcare.

CHAIN OF INFECTION

Chain of infection is a process of infection that begins when an agent leave its reservoir through portal of exit and is conveyed by mode of transmission then enters through an appropriate portal of entry to infect a susceptible host.

- **Infectious agent:** Infectious agent is also known as causative agent. Agent can be physical, chemical, biological and has the ability to cause disease. There are various types of microorganisms that have the ability to cause diseases like bacteria, viruses, fungi, protozoa and parasites.
- **Reservoir of infection:** It is the place where the microorganism resides, thrives, and reproduces, i.e., food, water, toilet seat, elevator buttons, human feces, respiratory secretions, etc.
- **Portal of exit from reservoir/host:** It is the place where the microorganism leaves the reservoir, such as the respiratory tract (nose, mouth), intestinal tract (rectum via stool), urinary tract, or blood and other body fluids.
- **Modes of transmission:** Mode of transmission is the means by which an organism transfers from one carrier to another by either direct transmission or indirect transmission.
- **Portal of entry:** The opening where an infectious disease enters the host's body such as mucus membranes, open wounds, or tubes inserted in body cavities like urinary catheters or feeding tubes.
- **Susceptible host:** It is a person who is at risk for developing an infection from the disease. Factors include young people and elderly people, chronic diseases such as diabetes or asthma, conditions that weaken the immune system like HIV, certain types of medications, invasive devices like feeding tubes, and malnutrition.

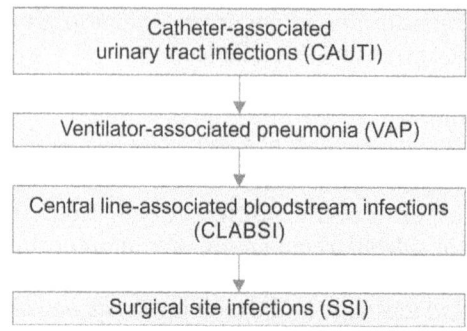

Fig. 5.2: Hospital acquired infection.

Healthcare-associated Infections (Hospital Acquired Infection)

Healthcare-associated infections are also known as hospital acquired infections or nosocomial infections. As the name suggests, hospital acquired means the infection that the patient gain or acquire during his/her hospital stay while receiving treatment for other disease condition **(Fig. 5.2)**.

Catheter-associated Urinary Tract Infections

Catheter-associated urinary tract infections (CAUTI) are one of the most common types of healthcare associated infections. The one of the risk factors for CAUTI is long term use of indwelling catheters.

The CAUTI are defined as "the urinary tract infections in the patient with current urinary tract catheterization or the patients who are catheterized within the past 48 hours."

Clinical Signs and Symptoms

- Patient has at least one of the following signs and symptoms:
- Fever (>38°C) in a patient that is ≤65 years of age
- Tenderness in the suprapubic area
- Costovertebral angle pain or tenderness
- Urinary frequency
- Urinary urgency
- Dysuria

Ventilator-associated Pneumonia

Ventilator-associated pneumonia (VAP) is defined as pneumonia that develops within 48–72 hours of endotracheal intubation. The features of VAP include.

- The presence of infiltrates in the chest, which are evident on chest X-ray.
- Signs of systemic infections like fever and changes in the WBC count.
- Changes in sputum characteristics and identification of the growth of microorganisms.

Sign and Symptoms
- Fever (>38.0°C or >100.4°F)
- Leukopenia (≤4,000 WBC/mm^3) or leukocytosis (>12,000 WBC/mm^3).
- For adults >70-year-old, altered mental status with no other recognized cause.
- Consolidation in lungs.

Prevention
In prevention of VAP, prevention bundle play a major important role. Nowadays every hospital has bundles.

Central Line-associated Bloodstream Infections (CLABSI)
CLABSI are the common healthcare-associated infections. A CLABSI is defined as the infection that develops within 48 hours of central line insertion.

Host Factors that Increase the Risk of CLABSI
- Chronic illnesses like hemodialysis, malignancy, gastrointestinal tract disorders and pulmonary hypertension.
- Patients who are immunosuppressed like the patients who are having organ transplantation and diabetes mellitus.
- Malnutrition in patients total parenteral nutrition.
- Advance age loss of skin integrity in patients like the patient with burns.
- Long hospital stay before line insertion.

Clinical Manifestation
- Fever and chills due to infections.
- Pain, swelling, discharge and redness at the insertion site.
- Poor blood flow and no back flow in the central line is the indicator of infection.

Surgical site infections (SSI) are one of the major reasons for hospital morbidity. It results increase in the ICU admission rates, doubling the mortality rates and increase the overall length of the hospital stay. The SSI are the infections that occur in the incision site, which are created by an invasive surgical procedure.

Risk Factors

There are two risk factors that predispose the patient for SSI, one is the patient factors and other is the operating factors:

Patient factor	Operating factor
Advance age	Preoperative shaving on site of incision, and length of operation
Poor nutritional status	Foreign material in surgical site
Disease condition like diabetes mellitus, renal failure and immunosuppressant state	Insertion of surgical drain
Smoking	Poor closure of wound

Signs and Symptoms

The signs and symptoms of surgical site infections appears in 5-7 days postoperatively, although it can develop up to 3 weeks after surgery especially if a patient has prosthesis. The common clinical features of surgical site infections include:

* Erythema
* Localized pain at the incision area
* Pus or discharge from the wound
* Wound dehiscence
* Fever

UNIVERSAL PRECAUTION

For universal precautions, protective barriers reduce the risk of exposure to blood, body fluids containing visible blood, and other fluids to which universal precautions apply. For example, protective barriers include gloves, gowns, masks, and protective eyewear.

Definition

"Universal precautions is the term applied to treating all blood, tissues and some body fluids as potentially infections. The appropriate level of precautions necessary is determined according to the extent of possible exposure to blood and body fluid and not because of the speculation of the infectious status of the patient."

Tiers of Universal Precaution

There are two types of tiers:

Standard Precaution (Tire 1)

- **Hand hygiene:** Refer p. 397
- **Gloves:** For touching blood, body fluids, secretions, excretions, nonintact skin, mucous membranes or contaminated areas.
- **Masks, eye protection or face shields:** If in contact with/sprays or splashes of body fluids.
- **Gowns:** To protect your clothing.
- **Contaminated linen:** Place in leak-proof bag so no contact with skin or mucous membranes.
- **Respiratory hygiene/cough etiquette:** Provide client with tissues and containers for disposal; stand ~3 feet away from coughing; use masks.

Transmission-Based Precaution (Tier 2)

- Contact = private room or cohort clients, gloves and gowns
- Droplet = private room or cohort clients, mask is required
  - Strep, pertussis, mumps, flu
- Airborne = private room, negative airflow, hepa filtration; N95 respirator mask required
  - TB, chickenpox, measles
- Protective environment = private room, positive pressure room; hepa filtration; gloves, gowns, mask (controversial); No flowers or potted plants.
  - Stem cell transplant.

Barrier Nursing

Barrier nursing is a nursing technique by which a patient with an infectious disease is prevented from infecting other people is called barrier nursing. Nosocomial infections is present worldwide and affect both developed and countries.

Techniques of Barrier Nursing

Isolation

The isolation is defined as any of the various interventions usually termed as isolation precautions adopted within a healthcare facility (HFC) for the control of infection and for the prevention of communicable disease from a patient to other patients, healthcare personals and visitors.

Handeling of Sharps Safely

- All sharps should be discarded directly into an appropriate sharps box immediately after use.
- Syringe needles should not be bent, broken or re-sheathed or prior to disposal.
- Syringe needles should not be detached from a syringe and should be disposed of as one unit.
- Handling should be kept to a minimum and sharps must not be passed from hand-to-hand.

Handling of Linen and Disposal

- The linen of the patient suffering from severe acute respiratory syndrome (SARS), pulmonary tuberculosis should be handled carefully.
- Follow bed making and linen changing techniques.

Waste Disposal

Disposal of waste is an important procedure to be followed by an individual in a community. Health professionals need to have a basic knowledge of the subject since improper disposal of waste constitutes a health hazard. Health professionals may be called upon to give advice in some special situations, such as coping with waste disposal problems when there is a disruption or breakdown of community health services in natural disasters.

Risk Assessment and Staff Health

There are specific steps to carrying out a risk assessment:
- Identify the hazards
- Identify who or what could be injured
- Evaluate the risk
- Evaluate probability
- Record and identify parties included
- Review and inform

Step 1: Research—identify what failures or incidents can cause damage.
Step 2: Identify who or what could be injured or displaced by such a failure or event—patients, staff or the public.
Step 3: How critical would the damage be if the defect took place.
Step 4: How likely is this problem to happen?
Step 5: Create a remedy or procedure to work around the adverse event and identify the responsible parties.

Step 6: Review the corrective action plan with staff to make sure they understand and can fulfil their responsibilities in the event of a defect occurring.

Healthcare professionals are at high-risk of infections. Immunization of healthcare professionals is important to prevent the transmission of infection. Maintenance of self-hygiene is important like handwashing, oral hygiene and nail care. Hands and nails are the major source of infection.

Aseptic Techniques
- Aseptic technique reduces the risk of healthcare associated infections.
- Aseptic technique is required for all invasive procedures.
- Aseptic technique has been shown to significantly improve the practice of clinicians performing procedures and reduce the risk of infection.

Responsibilities of Nurse in Barrier Nursing
- The medical equipment should be only for the patient who is under barrier nursing like disposable bedding and PPE should also be disposable.
- The medical equipment used for the patient like syringe pump, infusion pump, thermometer and stethoscope should be decontaminated thoroughly after use.
- Restrict the number of visitors. In case the visitors are permitted, proper infection control policies need to be followed.
- Make sure that isolation area is equipped with consumable and cleaning products.

Transportation of Infectious Patient
- The area where the patient is transferred need to be informed prior to shifting so that the equipment and appropriate precautions can be arranged.
- Ensure segregation facilities.
- Do not place the patients in the communal waiting area with known or suspected infections.

ASEPSIS

Asepsis is a condition in which no living disease-causing microorganisms are present. Asepsis covers all those procedures designed to reduce the risk of bacterial, fungal or viral contamination, using sterile instruments, sterile draping and the gloved 'no touch' technique.

Definition

❖ Asepsis is the state of being free from disease-causing contaminants (such as bacteria, viruses, fungi, and parasites) or preventing contact with microorganisms.
❖ The term asepsis often refers to those practices used to promote or induce asepsis in an operative field in surgery or medicine to prevent infection.

Levels of Aseptic Techniques

Cleaning Process

The unclean environmental surfaces in the clinical environment play a major role by acting as a good medium for harboring the microorganism and thus causing and spreading the infections that are specifically termed as the healthcare-associated infections (HAIs). For example, the commonly occurring hospital environmental contamination is due to the *Clostridium difficile* spores.

Environmental Cleaning

Environment cleaning can be defined as the removal of the inanimate inorganic as well as the organic matter from the surfaces or objects in an environment. This is usually achieved with the help of either detergents or some products possessing an enzymatic action. Sterilization and disinfection followed by the cleaning process makes it more effective.

Risk assessment (*Source:* Reproduced directly from provincial infectious disease advisory committee (PIDAC), 2018): Before implementing the environment cleaning procedures, the environment should be assessed for the risk involvement specific to that particular environment in the following "three steps" to get a risk score for that environment.

Equipment Cleaning

The types or levels of cleaning of the medical equipment can be well understood on the basis of the "Spaulding's principle" which classifies the medical equipment based upon the intended usage of the equipment (**Table 5.2**).

Spaulding's Principle (Dr EH Spaulding, 1968)

This principle states that the level of exposure of medical equipment to the patient's body determines the level of infection transmission onto the medical equipment and thus the medical equipment can be classified on the basis of the Spaulding's principle that

Table 5.2: Levels of cleaning.

Categories	Description
Critical equipment	• That invade the sterile tissue, or the vascular system are defined as the critical items, e.g., surgical instruments, implants, vascular devices, urinary catheters and cardiac catheters • They need to be sterilized (surgical asepsis)
Semi critical equipment	• That come in contact with the mucous membranes or nonintact skin are defined as the semi-critical items, e.g., anesthesia equipment, respiratory equipment, vaginal ultrasound probes, transesophageal echocardiography (TEE) probes, laryngoscope blades and endoscopic equipment. • These equipment require high-level of disinfection • (Surgical asepsis)
Noncritical equipment	• Which come in contact with the intact skin but not with the mucous membrane, e.g., bedpans, stethoscopes, blood pressure cuffs, bedside tables, bed rails, portable pumps, toys and crutches • These are cleaned by low-level of disinfection (medical asepsis)

further facilitates easier and accurate selection of the cleaning and disinfection processes with regard to the medical equipment.

Spaulding's Classification

The different categories of the medical equipment based on the Spaulding's principle are depicted.

Aseptic Processes

There are two types of aseptic processes used in a healthcare facility **(Table 5.3)**:
1. Medical asepsis
2. Surgical asepsis

Medical Asepsis

Medical asepsis, also known as "clean technique" is aimed at controlling the number of microorganisms. Medical asepsis is used for all clinical patient care activities.
❖ Routine hand rubs:
  ▪ The hands must be washed as per the right procedure.
  ▪ The nails must be trimmed.
  ▪ All the jewelry must be removed.

Table 5.3: Methods of aseptic processes.

Points of difference	Cleaning	Medical asepsis	Surgical asepsis
Objective	To reduce the risk of contamination, sterile instruments or sterile cleaning liquids are not required	To protect the site like wound site or the medical equipment being used like catheters etc. from sepsis	To protect the surgical wounds or inside of the patient which list in the operation theatre from any procedural infection
Gloves	Nonsterile	Sterile/Nonsterile depending on the task	Only sterile strictly
Nontouch technique	Followed	Followed	Followed
Dressings	Sterile	Sterile	Sterile
Cleansing liquids	Nonsterile	Sterile	Sterile
Work surface	Clean	Clean	Clean
Paper towel	Sterile	Sterile	Sterile

- Storage of equipment should be done aseptically so as to avoid any contamination.
- Preparing equipment by disinfecting them properly before use.
- Use of gloves and aprons is must.
- Maintaining a sterile environment is a must.
- Equipment disposal should be as per the biomedical waste (BMW).
- Management standards.

Surgical Asepsis

Sterile technique is used to prevent the introduction or spread of pathogens from the environment into the patient.
- Surgical hand rub (long rub antiseptic), i.e., the hands must be rubbed for longer time period as compared to the medical hand wash.
- Usage of sterile towel for hands drying.
- The field of operation must be properly sterilized before the surgical procedures.
- Sterile gowns and masks must be worn by the healthcare workers inside the operation theatres. Sterile gloves must be worn by the healthcare personnel inside the theater following appropriate procedure of wearing and the removal.

- ❖ The surgical supplies must be all sterile.
- ❖ The skin of the patient to be incised must be properly sterilized prior to incision for the surgical procedure.

HAND HYGIENE

Handwashing (or handwashing), also known as hand hygiene, is the act of cleaning hands for the purpose of removing soil, dirt, and microorganisms. If water and soap is not available, hands can be cleaned with ash instead.

Ignaz Semmelweis introduced handwashing standards after discovering that the occurrence of puerperal fever could be prevented by practicing hand disinfection in obstetrical clinics. He believed that microbes causing infection were readily transferred from patients to patients, medical staff to patients and vice versa.

Indication of Handwashing

- ❖ Visibly soiled or contaminated with blood or body fluids.
- ❖ After using washroom.
- ❖ Before and after having foods.

Types of Handwashing

Antiseptic Hand Hygiene

Antiseptic hand rubbing (or hand rubbing) applying an antiseptic hand rub to reduce or inhibit the growth of microorganisms without the need for an exogenous source of water and requiring no rinsing or drying with towels or other devices.

Antiseptic Hand Wash

This is the washing of the hands done by using the antimicrobial soap/solution and water. The antimicrobial soaps include chlorhexidine, iodine and iodophors, chloroxylenol (PCMX) and triclosan, etc.

Alcohol-based Handrub (ABHR)

This includes the use of alcohol-based antiseptic hand rub, e.g., hydrox hand rub. The use of ABHR has many advantages for hand hygiene purpose.

Steps for ABHR

Duration of the entire procedure 20–30 seconds:
- ❖ **Step 1:** Apply ABHR product in a cupped hand, covering all surfaces.
- ❖ **Step 2:** Rub hands palm to palm.

- **Step 3:** Right palm over left dorsum with interlaced fingers and vice versa.
- **Step 4:** Palm to palm with fingers interlaced.
- **Step 5:** Back of fingers to opposing palms with fingers interlocked.
- **Step 6:** Rotational rubbing of left thumb clasped in right palm and vice versa.
- **Step 7:** Rotational rubbing, backwards and forwards with clasped fingers of right hand in left palm and vice versa.

Medical Handwashing

The hand when washed with soap and water usually removes dirt, dead skin, organic matter and most of the transient microbes on the hands. The handwashing before the general procedures is called routine handwashing. Wet the hand and apply soap, rub all the surfaces, rinse the hand and then dry thoroughly with a single use towel or tissue paper.

Procedure for Medical Handwashing

Sl. No.	Step	Rational
1.	Collect the articles (soap, towel, water supply). Do not allow yourself to touch the washing area	For smooth functioning to prevent contamination as sink is considered contaminated
2.	Remove the ornaments or jewelry, nails should be short	Microorganisms may collect in the jewelry and nails
3.	Turn on the tap and wet your hands with water, regulate the temperature	For easy application of soap and temperature regulation to prevent burns. Warm water opens pores
4.	Take the soap from soap dispenser, if soap bar is used after application rinses it under water. Apply soap with firm circular motion, in such manner that all hand surfaces should be covered	Rinsing soap helps to remove the microorganisms from the surface. To wash off microorganisms
5.	Rub your hand palm	To wash of microorganisms
6.	Place right palm over left dorsum with figure interlaced and vice versa. Rub palm to palm with finger interlaced	
7.	Then rub the backs of finger to opposing palms with finger interlocked. Clean the knuckles thoroughly	

Contd...

Contd...

Sl. No.	Step	Rational
8.	Do rotational rubbing of the left thumb clasped in right palm and vice versa	Paying attention to area that are commonly missed and microbes grow
9.	Perform rotational rubbing in backward and forward manner using clasped finger of right hand in left palm and vice versa. Thereafter working on the wrist	
10.	Rinse hand thoroughly with water and hold the hands down	To remove dirt
11.	Afterwards dry your hands thoroughly with a single use towel	So that hand does not get contaminated with used towel
12.	Turn off the tap or faucet by using tissue paper or towel	To save water

PERSONAL PROTECTIVE EQUIPMENT

The PPE is a "specialized clothing or equipment worn by an employ for protection against the infectious materials", —*Occupational safety and health administration (OSHA)*.

Gowns

The gowns can be of two types:
1. Isolation gown
2. Surgical gown

Isolation Gown

- Long-sleeved, fluid resistant, single-use, disposable (preferably).
- Designed to prevent contamination of HCW's arms, body's exposed areas and clothing from blood and body fluids and other potentially infectious material.

Surgical Gown

Surgical gowns are sterile and are fluid resistant:
- Are with sleeves tapering gently toward the wrists or end with elastic ties around the wrists.
- Ought to be without the large droopy sleeves to avoid accidental contamination.
- Are used during surgery or procedures.
- Should be accompanied by a plastic apron over the cloth or paper gown.

Wearing Sterile Gown

Steps	Rationale
Open the pack of sterile gown	Prevent contamination of gown. Outer side of pack is considered contaminated
Do handwashing	Wash off microbes
Pick the sterile gown from the crease near the neck	
Hold the gown away from you. Let the gown unfold freely, it should be in a way that it should not touch anything. Put the hands inside the shoulder of gown. Do not touch the outside of the gown take your hands gown to the sleeves of a sterile gown	Openings should be in such a way that the opens side should face the individual wearing it. If the gown is open other way around than it is considered to be contaminated
Ask the other staff to hold the ties without touching the outside of the gown. Pull the gown upward side so that the neckline of the uniform in front and back covered	Other staff should touch the inner side of the gown and tie the gown, outer side is considered to be sterile
Ask the other staff to hold the long end of the waist tie of your gown, using sterile gloves or a sterile forceps or drape	This prevents contamination of sterile area

Aprons

Plastic apron provides a waterproof barrier along the front of the body, protecting the skin of the healthcare worker from contamination with the blood and other body fluid during patents care (e.g., during cesarean section or vaginal delivery) cleaning and handling of textiles and other soiled items.

Masks and Respirators

Many different types of masks can be used to cover the mouth and nose. The mask and the respirator mask if worn accurately offers protection to the wearer from infectious droplets and air particles.

Type of Mask

1. Procedure mask/isolation masks
2. N 95 respirator mask.

Steps of Wearing the Respirators

Step 1: Cup the respirator in one hand, with the nosepiece at the fingertips, allowing the headbands to hang freely below your hand.

Step 2: Position the respirator under the chin with the nosepiece up. Pull the top strap over your head, resting it height at the top of the back of your head. Pull the bottom strap over your head and position it around the neck, below the ears.

Step 3: Perform a user 'fit test'. Place fingertips from both hands at the top of the metal nose clip. Slide fingertips down both sides of the metal strip to mold the nose area to the shape of your nose.

Step 4: Perform user 'seal check'. At a minimum, a seal check should be perform by the wearer of a respirator each time a respirator is worn to minimize air leakage around the face piece. If either taste fails, adjust the respirator and perform seal check again.

- **Positive pressure seal check:** Put on the respirator and exhale gently while blocking the paths for exhaled breath to exit the face piece. A successful check is when the face piece is slightly pressurized before increased pressure causes outward leakage.
- **Negative pressure seal check:** Put on the respirator and inhale sharply while blocking the paths for inhaled breath to enter the face piece. A successful check is when the face piece collapses slightly under the negative pressure that is created with inhalation.

Protective Eyewear

The eye protection is necessary for the procedures involving generation of splashes, sprays of blood and body fluids while dealing with the patients or BMW management. It includes the following:

- Goggles
- Safety glasses
- Face shields
- Masks with attached shield.

Effective Usage of Eye Protection

- Put on eye protection after putting on the isolation gown and mask (if used) but before putting on gloves.
- Removal of face shield, goggles, and mask can be performed safely after gloves have been removed. The ties, ear pieces, and/or head band used to secure the equipment to the head are considered 'clean' and safe to touch with bare hands. If the ties, earpiece, and/or head band are found to be contaminated, they should be removed using gloved hands and the skin/face should be rinsed using ample running water and soap. The front of a mask, goggles and face shield is considered contaminated.

Gloves

Procedure of How to Wear a Glove

Steps	Rationale
Open the outer cover of gloves and perform hand hygiene	Prevent cross contamination
Open the inner packing of the sterile gloves packet	To clear the working area and prevent contamination of sterile gloves
Put on the first sterile gloves pick the gloves from the inner side to prevent the contamination of the gloves from the outside	This will maintain the sterile field. Don't unfold the folded cuff
Pick up the second sterile gloves carefully by inserting the gloved fingers under the cuff and holding the gloved thumb closed to the gloved palm	
Adjust each glove, so that it fits properly; pull the cuff up by sliding the fingers inside the cuff	

Procedure of How to Remove Gloves

Steps
Pick one glove from the wrist level, without touching the skin of the forearm and take it away from the hand and allow the gloves to turn inside out (maintain glove to glove, skin to skin)
Afterwards hold the removed glove in a gloved hand
Slide the fingers of the bare hand inside the glove and wrist
Remove the second glove by rolling it down, and fold into the first glove
Discard the gloves

The glove pyramid (WHO): To aid decision making on when to wear (and not to wear) gloves is depicted in:

Sequence of Removing the PPE

Steps	Description
Step 1: Second pair of gloves	• Grasp the outside of the glove with gloved hand of opposite side • Take out the glove • Then hold the removed glove in gloved hand and then take out the glove over first glove • Discard the gloves in the appropriate container

Contd...

Contd...

Steps	Description
Step 2: Goggles or face shield, cap (if used)	Hold the goggles or face shield by head band or thorough earpieces and place in designated place
Step 3: Gown	• Unfasten the ties • Take out the gown away from neck and shoulders • It should turn inside out • Fold the gown in a bundle and discard in appropriate bin
Step 4: Shoe cover	• Hold the highest part of shoe cover behind ankle • Remove the shoe cover of the first shoe and place foot in a clean area • Take out the shoe cover of second shoe and then place foot in clean area
Step 5: Mask or respirator	• Using your gloved hand • Pick side of the mask with both hands • Carefully pull it from the face • Discard it in appropriate bin
Step 6: First pair of gloves	• Hold the outside of glove with opposite hand and take it off • Just hold the removed glove in the opposite gloved hand • Slide fingers of ungloved hand under remaining glove at wrist • Take the glove off over first glove and discard them
Step 7	Perform hand hygiene

BIOMEDICAL WASTE MANAGEMENT

❖ Solid waste generated during the diagnosis, testing, treatment, research or production of biological products for humans or animals (WHO).
❖ Nosocomial infections in patients from poor infection control practices and poor waste management.
❖ Drugs which have been disposed of, being repacked and sold off to unsuspecting buyers.
❖ Risk of air, water and soil pollution directly due to waste, or due to defective incineration emissions and ash.
❖ Risk of infection outside hospital for waste handlers and scavengers, other peoples.

Source of Biomedical Waste

Classification of Biomedical Waste

Types of waste	Description
Pathological	It includes the body parts, tissues, organs and body fluids removed during the surgery and autopsy
Blood and blood product	It involves blood, serum, plasma and blood products
Culture and infectious agents	It includes the microbiological waste like specimens from the laboratories
Contaminated waste	It involves the needles, scalpels blades broken glasses and glass syringes
Isolation waste	The waste which is generated from the area where patient is kept in separate area in order to prevent others from the cross infections
Animal waste	The waste which is generated from the animals those who are intentionally exposed to pathogens in research or in biological production

Biomedical Waste Management

Definition

The strictly appropriate and sequentially stepwise, verified handling and disposal of the infectious waste generated via any healthcare facility or activity, in order to safeguard the health of the concerned personnel, patients, public at large, the immediate and distant environment and the earth's biosphere is known as the biomedical waste management.

Seven Steps of BMW Management

Step 1: BMW-Segregation

Definition: BMW segregation means the separation of the mixed waste specifically at its point of generation a per the color coding specified under the 'BMWM Rule Schedule-1, 2016'.

Segregation feature:

Segregation features	Descriptions
Point of generation	The BMW must be segregated at the point of its generation by the person who generated it, into specified color-coded bags or containers
BMW waste segregation posters	The wards and the waste storage places must be provided with the appropriate BMW waste segregation posters for reference if required

Contd...

Contd...

Segregation features	Descriptions
Color coded bags/bins	The points of generation of BMW waste must have an adequate supply of the color-coded bags/bins
Specification of bags	The color-coded plastic bags must be specified according to the Annexure-1 of the Plastic Waste Management Rules, 2016
PPE	Appropriate PPE must be made available to the HCWs who are responsible for segregating the BMW

Step 2: BMW-Collection

Definition: Collection is the process of taking away the segregated BMW from its every point of generation in an HCF to be transported to the storage area within the HCF.

Step 3: BMW-Transportation (In-house/Intra-mural)

- ❖ Transportation trolleys must be used for the in-house (intramural) transportation.
- ❖ Route of in-house transportation:
    - Should not be moved through the high-risk areas.
    - The movement of supplies and the waste should be done via different routes.
    - Should not be moved through the areas having large number of patients and visitors.
    - The storage area (central waste collection room) must be easily approached through the waste movement route.

Step 4: BMW-Storage (Central Waste Collection Room)

- ❖ Must be away from the high traffic areas.
- ❖ Space must be sufficient.
- ❖ Should be under lock and key.
- ❖ No general waste should be stored here.

Step 5 and 6: BMW-Treatment and Disposal

- ❖ The BMW has to be strictly treated and disposed of by the common biomedical waste treatment facility (CBWTF) only and not within the HCF.
- ❖ Only in case, the CBWTF is not available within the 75 km distance around the HCF or if a distant CBWTF is also not available to provide its services, then the BMW can be disposed of in the captive treatment and disposal facility or by authorized deep burial.

Hazards Associated with Hospital Waste

Between 75% and 90% of the waste produced by healthcare providers is comparable to domestic waste and usually called 'nonhazardous' or 'general healthcare waste. It comes mostly from the administrative, kitchen, housekeeping functions at healthcare facilities and may also include packaging waste and waste generated during maintenance of healthcare buildings. The remaining 10–25% of healthcare waste is regarded as 'hazardous' and may pose a variety of environmental and health risks.

Meaning

Exposure to hazardous healthcare waste can result in disease or injury. The hazardous nature of healthcare waste may be due to one or more of the following characteristics:

- It contains agents
- It is genotoxic
- It contains toxic or hazardous chemicals or pharmaceuticals.
- It is radioactive
- It contains sharps

Persons at Risk of BMW Hazards

All individuals exposed to hazardous healthcare waste are potentially at risk. The main groups at risk are the following:

- Medical doctors, nurses, healthcare auxiliaries, and hospital maintenance personnel.
- Patients in healthcare establishments or receiving home care; visitors to healthcare establishments.
- Workers in support services allied to healthcare establishments, such as laundries, waste handling, and transportation; workers in waste disposal facilities (such as incinerators), including scavengers.

Health Hazards

- **Infection:** Healthcare waste contains potentially harmful microorganisms, which can infect hospital patients, health workers, and the general public.
- **Drug-resistant microorganisms:** Other potential infectious risks may include the spread of drug resistant microorganisms from health facilities into the environment.
- **Needle-stick injury:** A person who experiences one needle-stick injury from a needle used on an infected source patient has risks

of 30%, 1.8%, and 0.3%, respectively, of becoming infected with HBV, HCV, and HIV. The waste handlers are at immediate risk of needle-stick injuries and exposure to toxic or infectious materials.
* **Environmental hazard:** Treatment and disposal of healthcare waste may pose health risks indirectly through the release of pathogens and toxic pollutants into the environment.
* Poisoning and pollution through wastewater; and by toxic elements or compounds such as mercury or dioxins that are released during incineration.
* Incineration of waste has been widely practiced, but inadequate incineration or the incineration of unsuitable materials results in the release of pollutants into the air and of ash residue.

Other Hazards
* Radiation burns.
* Sharps-inflicted injuries.
* Poisoning and pollution through the release of pharmaceutical products, in particular, antibiotics and cytotoxic drugs.

# CHAPTER 6

Basic Life Support and Cardiopulmonary Resuscitation

Chapter Outline

- Code blue
- Resuscitation Techniques or Basic Life Support
- Procedure of CPR
- Advanced Trauma Life Support (ATLS)

CODE BLUE

The term "code blue" is a hospital emergency code used to describe the critical status of a patient. Hospital staff may call a code blue if a patient goes into cardiac arrest, has respiratory issues, or experiences any other medical emergency. Hospitals typically have rapid response teams ready to go when they get notified about a code blue.

Hospital Emergency Code

Most hospitals rely on a standardized coding system to communicate an emergency. These codes are not limited to medical events. There is currently no national standard set for emergency codes, so you may see some variance among those used in hospitals. Using hospital codes allows staff to quickly communicate the status of a situation with minimal words.

Code blue typically lets hospital staff know a patient requires resuscitation because of a medical emergency.

- **Code blue:** Adult medical emergency that does not allow movement of the patient.
- **Code blue pediatric:** Medical emergency in a child that does not allow movement of the patient.
- **Code blue neonate:** Medical emergency in an infant that does not allow movement of the patient.

These are a few ways that hospitals use code blue codes. A code blue sub-category could also alert staff to render aid to a patient who's having a stroke without specifying the patient's age.

When Is a Code Blue Called?

A doctor or nurse typically calls code blue, alerting the hospital staff team that's assigned to responding to this specific, life-or-death emergency. Members of a code blue team may have experience with advanced cardiac life support or in resuscitating patients. The team may also include specialists like an anesthesiologist or internal medicine doctor **(Fig. 6.1)**.

A code blue may be called in situations where the patient is experiencing:
- Cardiopulmonary arrest
- Mental status changes
- Chest pain
- Presyncope
- General worries about a patient's status
- Doctors and nurses are the ones who typically confirm a patient's status by checking for vitals like a pulse or signs of breathing. They might call code blue if the patient is not getting enough oxygenated blood pumping through their body due to respiratory distress or a cardiac arrest. They might also call code blue if the patient is breathing but their condition is critical.

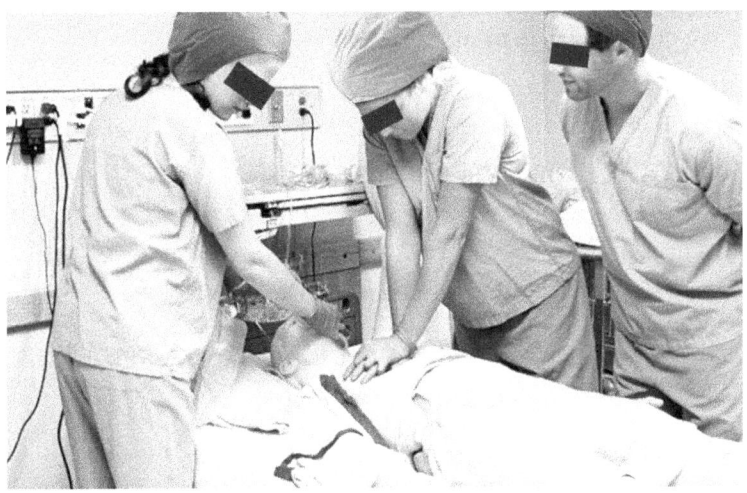

Fig. 6.1: Code blue.

- If a patient has a do not resuscitate (DNR) order on file, the hospital staff must respect its legal boundaries. That usually precludes issuing a code blue. Patients with a DNR typically do not receive any cardiopulmonary resuscitation (CPR) efforts or any form of advanced cardiac life support (ACLS).

What Happens During a Code Blue?

A hospital's response to a code blue call varies depending on the patient's condition. Medical doctors typically take charge of a code blue situation. If a doctor or nurse issued the call because the patient's heart stopped or they couldn't find signs of breathing, they start performing CPR.

Other efforts may include intubating the patient. That involves inserting an endotracheal tube (ET) through a patient's mouth or nose and into their trachea. Because the tube must pass through the vocal cords, patients won't be able to speak until the ET is removed by staff. Intubation aids in resuscitation efforts during a code blue by opening the patient's airway and helping them breathe.

If a patient's heartbeat is irregular, staff may decide to employ an automated external defibrillator (AED) to re-establish a stable heart rhythm. If that does not help, doctors may administer medications like epinephrine to start the patient's heart or naloxone to get them breathing. Hospitals often have rules established about what drugs to use during medical emergencies.

RESUSCITATION TECHNIQUES OR BASIC LIFE SUPPORT

The ABCs of basic life support are:
- **A:** Airway
- **B:** Breathing
- **C:** Circulation

Airway

Open the airway. Position the victim on his/her back.
- **Check breathing:**
  - Hear and feel any breath by placing your ear above casualty's mouth.
  - See movements along the chest and abdomen.
- **Open the airway:**
  - Clear any debris (broken teeth, vomits, mucus or foreign matter) out of his/her mouth that got into the mouth during injury.

- Airway are opened by two methods:
  1. Head tilt: Tilt the victim's head backward as far as possible by placing one hand on victim's forehead and using either the neck lift or chin lift with the other hand.
  2. Jaw thrust: In case of suspected cervical or spinal injury pull back the mandible with fingers of hands carefully without tilting the head backward or turning it from side-to-side.

Breathing

Restore breathing by mouth-to-mouth or mouth-to-nose ventilation (when victim is lying on his/her back) or artificial ventilation when the casualty is lying face down.

Mouth-to-Mouth Ventilation

- ❖ Open the airway by removing any debris or obstruction.
- ❖ Take a deep breath, open your mouth wide, pinch the victim's nostrils with your fingers, and seal your lips around the victim's mouth.
- ❖ Looking around the chest below into the casualty's lungs until you can see the chest rise to maximum expansion.
- ❖ Remove your mouth well away from the casualty for taking in the fresh air. Watch the chest wall and repeat inflation. Give the first four inflations as quickly as possible without waiting for complete lung deflation between breaths.
- ❖ Check the casualty's pulse to make sure that the heart is breathing.
- ❖ In case of normal heart breathing, continue to give inflations at normal breathing rate (16-18 times per minute) until natural breathing is restored. When the casualty is breathing normally. Place in the recovery position.

Mouth-to-Nose Ventilation

- ❖ Mouth-to-nose ventilation is applied when it is not possible to open casualty mouth due to injury, etc.
- ❖ Close the casualty's mouth with your thumb and seal your lips around the casualty's lungs as in case of mouth-to-mouth respiration.

Schaffer's Method (When Casualty is Lying Face Down)

- ❖ Rest the casualty's forehead on the back of overlapped hands and turn the face to one side.
- ❖ Kneeling by the side of casualty just below his hip. Place your hands on the loins of the casualty (one on either side of backbone) with wrists almost touching and thumbs apart, close fingers together

at the side of loins and come vertically above the hands putting pressure of your body weight (not exceeding 60 lbs) for 2 seconds. This results in abdominal organs to be compressed against the ground and up against the diaphragm to force air out of lung (expiration).
- ❖ Now release the pressure to allow inspiration.
- ❖ Complete two phases of movements in 5 seconds (12 times a minute).
- ❖ Continue artificial is restored (or a doctor decides that further effects are no use).

Silvester Method

This method is used when the casualty is trapped on the back or there is external chest compression.
- ❖ Place a folded jacket or other padding beneath the shoulders so that the head is tilted back in the open airway position.
- ❖ Kneeling at the casualty's head, grasp the wrists and cross them over on the lower chest (clear of the abdomen). Look straight and press down firmly on the lower part of the casualty's chest with a steady. Even pressure for 2 seconds.
- ❖ Release the pressure, rock backwards and with a continuous sweeping movement, draw the casualty's arm-upwards and outwards as far as possible for 3 seconds.
- ❖ Repeat this sequence rhythmically, 12 times per minute.
- ❖ After four sequences, check for heartbeat. In the case of normal breathing, continue this method until natural breathing is restored. If the casualty is not responding, continue resuscitation with 15 chest compressions to two Silvester ventilation.
- ❖ If casualty begins to breath normally, place in the recovery position.

Circulation

Cardiopulmonary resuscitation (CPR): The use of artificial ventilation with external heart compression is called CPR. This should be started in all case of cardiac arrest (sudden death).

The signs and symptoms of cardiac and respiratory arrest are same, but the difference is that in cardiac arrest, there is no arterial pulse but in respiration arrest arterial pulse is present.

Indication

Loss of consciousness. Becoming pale with absence of pulse.
- ❖ Respiration is slow, labored or absent.
- ❖ No reaction of pupils to light.

Principle

The main principle of CPR is to prevent brain damage due to anoxia by restoring circulation within 4-5 minutes.

Causes of Cardiac Arrest

- Coronary obstruction
- Airway obstruction
- Pulmonary embolism
- Drowning
- Central nervous system depression
- Overdose of depressant drugs
- Hypertension
- Electric shock
- Cardiomyopathy
- Myocardial infection
- Foreign body obstruction
- Pneumothorax
- Head injury
- Increased intracranial pressure
- Hypothermia
- Retention of CO_2
- Electrolyte disorders.

Sign of Cardiac Arrest

- **Unconsciousness**—cerebral hypoxia causes decreased oxygen supply to cerebral cortex. Brain cells are very sensitive to decreased amount of O_2 causing confusion, disorientation and even unconsciousness.
- **Apnea**—absence of movement of chest and abdomen muscles due to absence of respiration.
- **Absence of cardiac and femoral pulse**—carotid pulse and femoral pulse are difficult to be located or absent.
- **Dilated pupils**—cerebral hypoxia can cause loss of muscle control of whole body even eyes, so eyes do not respond to light source and pupils remain dilated.
- **Cyanosis**—the decreased oxygen supply to the blood.
- **Fits/seizures**—this may also cause decreased oxygen supply in the blood and indeed to whole of body.

PROCEDURE OF CPR

- Lay the casualty on the back on a firm surface. Kneel alongside the casualty facing the chest and in line with the heart. Locate the

sternal notch and place the heel of your hand about two finger's width above the tip of sternum (xiphoid process) parallel to the long axis of the body. Cover this hand with the heel of your other and lock your fingers together.
* Keeping your arms straight and your elbows locked, apply firm heavy pressure so that sternum is depressed 4–5 cm.
* After each compression completely relax the pressure keeping your hands in the same position, compression and relaxation should be equal. Complete 15 compressions at the rate of 80 compressions per minute.

External Cardiac Chest Compression
* Now move back to the casualty's head, reopen the airway and give two breaths of mouth–to–mouth ventilation **(Fig. 6.2)**.
* Continue with 15 compressions of chest followed by two full ventilations, repeating heart check after the first minute. Thereafter check heartbeat after every 3 minutes.
* As soon as the heartbeat returns stop compression immediately and continue mouth-to-mouth ventilations until natural treating is restored.
* Now place the casualty in the recovery position.

CPR for Children (1–8 year)
The technique of giving CPR in children is same as in adults only the difference occurs in the depth of compression and the sensitiveness with which the procedure is done.
* As soon as cardiac arrest is suspected start giving CPR.
* Check for the airway clearance of the child if it is not clear, clear it immediately.

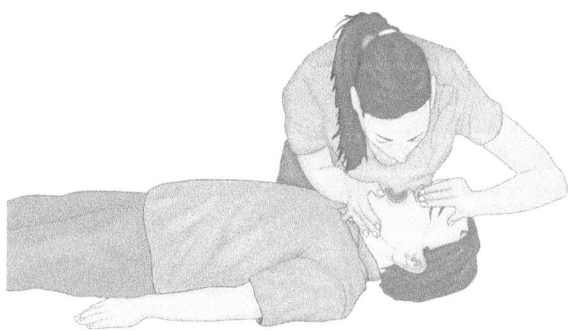

Fig. 6.2: Giving mouth-to-mouth breathing.

- Make the patient comfortable in supine position on some firm table or bed.
- Place hand two fingers width above the tip of the sternum.
- Press down chest so as to compress the sternum 1-15 inch.
- It should be maintained to 100-110 times/minute.
- The compression to ventilation (mouth-to-mouth breathing) is done in the ratio of 5:1.
- The procedure remains same even with two rescuers the ratio of compression to ventilation is followed as 5:1.
- Check the pulse from the cardiac artery and papillary response of the child to find out if the CPR is giving in effective manner.
- Do not stop CPR until the patient revives or is completely declared dead.

CPR Technique in Infants (0-1 Year)

CPR in the case of infants should only be given by some skillful person. Even if the procedure of giving CPR is the same, the unskillful person can even give some harm to the delicate body of the infant by a light mistake.

- The method of doing CPR is same for the infants as in children or adults just it needs to more care.
- Check for the unresponsiveness of infants.
- Now the rescuer needs to place the fingers correctly.
- The position of the two fingers should be in midline of the chest, one finger width below the nipple (only fingers are used to give CPR to infant).
- Open the airway of infant by tilting the head. Lifting the chin and Jaw thrust.
- Keep head tilled back, pinch nose shut, seat the mouth by your own mouth.
- Now give two slow puffs. Without giving much force avoid deep inspiration in case of mouth-to-mouth breathing in infants.
- Watch for the rise in chest.
- Check the pulse again.
- Continue CPR ventilation with five compressions.
- Even in two rescuers ventilation compression ratio follows 1:5 rule.

Signs of Successful CPR

- Lung expansion will occur each ventilation and pulse will be perceptible each time the sternum is compressed.
- The pupils will react to light or appear normal.

- ❖ Normal heartbeat will return.
- ❖ A spontaneous gasp or breathing will occur.
- ❖ Victims may move legs or arms; color of skin may improve.

Note:
- ❖ Elevate the fingers from the chest wall and interlock by fingers of other hand.
- ❖ No flexion should be elbows. Keep arms straight with elbow lock.
- ❖ Position shoulders at 90° to hands. Do not interrupt CPR for more than 5 seconds to any reason.
- ❖ Tongue cannot fall to the back of the throat.
- ❖ Never compress over the xiphoid process or the tip of sternum. Pressure on it may cause laceration of liver.

ADVANCED TRAUMA LIFE SUPPORT (ATLS)

- ❖ Advanced trauma life support (commonly abbreviated ATLS) is a training program for medical provider in the management of acute trauma cases, developed by the American College of Surgeons, similar programs exist for lower care providers such as paramedical. The program has been adopted worldwide in over 60 countries sometimes.
- ❖ Under the name of **early management of severe trauma,** especially outside North America, its goal is to teach a simplified and standardized approach to trauma patient originally designed for emergency situations where only one doctor and one nurse are present. ATLS is now widely accepted as the standard of care for initial assessment and treatment in trauma centers.
- ❖ The premise of the ATLS program is to treat the greatest threat to life first. It also advocates that the lack of a definitive diagnosis and a detailed history should not slow the application of indicated treatment for life-threatening injury. With the most time critical innervations performed early. However, there is no high quality evidence to show that ATLS improves patient outcomes as it has not been studied.

Primary Survey

The first and key part of the assessment of patients presenting with trauma is called the primary survey, during this time life-threatening injuries are identified and simultaneously resuscitation is begun.

Airway Maintenance with Cervical Spiral Protection
Airway Management
- The first stage of the primary survey is to assess the airway. If the patient is able to talk, the airway is likely to be clear if the patient is unconscious, he/she may not be able to maintain his own airway.
- The airway can be opened, adjuncts may be required. If the airway is blocked (e.g., by blood or vomit) the fluid must be cleaned out of the patient's mouth with the help of suctioning instruments. In case of obstruction pass an endotracheal.

Breathing and Ventilation
- The chest must be exanimate by inspection, palpation, percussion and auscultation. Subcutaneous emphysema and tracheal deviation must be identified if present. The aim is to identify and manage six life-threatening thoracic conditions as airway obstruction, tension pneumothorax, massive hemothorax, open pneumothorax, flail chest segment with pulmonary contusion and cardiac tamponade.
- Flail chest, tracheal deviation, penetration injuries and bruising can be recognized by inspection.

Circulation with Hemorrhage Control
Hemorrhage is the predominant cause of preventable postinjury deaths. Hypovolemic shock is caused by significant blood loss. Two large bore intravenous lines are established and crystalloid solutions may be given. If the person close not respond to this type of specific blood or O—if this is not available should be given. External bleeding is controlled by direct pressure. Occult blood loss may be from the chest abdomen, pelvis or from the long bones.

Disability/Neurologic Assessment
- During the primary survey a basic neurological assessment is made, known by the mnemonic AVPU (alert, verbal, stimuli response, painful stimuli response or unresponsive). A more detailed and rapid neurological evolution is performed at the end of the primary survey. This established the patient's level of consciousness, pupil size and reaction lateralizing sign and spinal cord injury level.
- The glasgow coma scale is a quick method to determine the level of consciousness and is predictive of patient outcome. If not done in the primary survey, it should be performed as part of more detailed neurologic examination in the secondary survey and altered level

of consciousness indicates the need for immediate re-evaluation of the patient's oxygenation, ventilation and perfusion status. Hypoglycemia and drugs including alcohol, may influence the level of consciousness, if these are excluded, changes in the level of consciousness should be considered to the due to traumatic brain injury until proven otherwise.

Exposure and Environmental Control

The patient should be completely undressed, usually by cutting off the garments. It is imperative to cover the patient with warm blankets to prevent hypothermia in the emergency department. Intravenous fluid should be warmed and a warm environment maintained. Patient privacy should be maintained.

Secondary Survey

When the primary survey is completed, resuscitation efforts are well established and the vital signs are normalizing, the secondary survey can begin. The secondary survey is a head-to-toe evaluation of the trauma patient, including a complete history and physical examination, including the reassessment of the vital sign. Each region of the body must be fully examined. X-rays indicated by examination are obtained. If at any time during the secondary survey is carried out as a potential life threat may be present. The person should be removed from the hard spine board and placed on a firm mattress as soon as reasonably feasible as the spine board can rapidly cause skin breakdown and pain while a firm mattress provides equivalent stability for potential spinal factors.

Tertiary Survey

A careful and complete examination followed by serial assessment helps recognize missed injuries and related problems allowing definitive care management. The rate of delayed diagnosis may be as high as 10%.

Index

Page numbers followed by *f* refer to figure and *t* refer to table.

A

Abdomen 178, 256
  boundaries of 229
  division of 227
  layers of 230f
  regions of 228f
Abdominal cavity 74, 232, 240
Abdominal operation 233
Abdominal pain 187
Abdominal wall
  anterior view of 238f
  fasciae of posterior 238
  muscles of 42, 42f, 230, 231f, 283
  posterior view of 238f
  structure of posterior 236
Acinetobacter species 355
Acquired immune deficiencies, temporary 147
Acquired infections 354
Acquired viral infection 147
Acrivastine 205
Actinomycetes 157
Acute inflammation 121, 124
Adam's apple 253, 254f
Addisonian pernicious anemia 208
Adductor group 44, 285
Adenoids 119
Adenosine diphosphate 98
Adhesion 123
Adhesive dressing 301
Adipose tissue 23, 270
Adrenal gland 84
  hormones of 84f
Adrenal medulla 275
Adrenaline 172, 341
Adrenocorticotropic hormone 82
Adson forceps 326f
Advanced trauma life support 416
Advanced triage 322
  principles of 322
Adverse drug reaction, common causes of 163
Aerosols 171
Airway 410
  maintenance 417
  management 417
Alcohol 166, 357, 418

Alcohol-based handrub 397
  steps for 397
Aldehydes 361
Alimentary system 47
Allergic diseases 146
Allergic reactions 170, 204
Allergic rhinitis 147
Allis and Babcock clamps 329, 329f
Alternative macrophage activation 125
Alveolar macrophages 125
Amino
  amides 217
  esters 217
Aminophylline 173
Ammonia 361, 362
Analgesia, stage of 210
Analgesics 168
Anaphase 20
Anaphylactic shock 135
Anatomical components 57
Anatomical spaces 44
Anemia, treatment of 205, 207
Anesthesia 312
  and surgery, during 346
  complications of 313
  dissociative 210
  gases used in 319
  machine 316
  provider 341
  risks of 313
  stages of 313, 342, 343t
  technique 286
  types of 314, 339
  work station 312
Anesthetic agents 319, 339, 342
Anesthetic apparatus 346
Anesthetic equipment's 344
Anesthetic machine 346
Anesthetic method 340
Anesthetics agent 209
Aneurysm rupture 100
Angiogenesis 129
Ankle block 341
Antacids 183, 184
Anterior abdominal wall 229, 231
  structure of 227
Antibiotic 152
  control policy, information of 364

Antibody 144
Antidepressants 185
Antidiarrheal agents 185, 186
Antifungal targets, main 195t
Antihistamine 171, 204
    indication of 204
Anti-inflammatory drugs 149 173
Antimicrobial 192
    agents, classes of 192
    dosing 200
    policies 203
    resistance 201
Anti-phospholipid antibody syndrome 100
Antitussive agent 171
    classification of 171
Antivirals 153
Aorta, abdominal 236
Aortic dissection 267
Aortic lymph nodes 240
Apnea 413
Apocrine glands 273
Apomorphine 179
Apoptosis 129, 130f, 133, 133f
Appendages 45
Appendicitis 295
Appendicular skeleton 27
Aprons 400
Aqueous humor 279
Arachnoid 246, 247
    mater 88, 89, 247
    trabeculae 89
    tube 248
Arm, muscles of 42, 283
Army-navy retractor 332, 332f
Arterial blood 76
Arterial supply 250, 279
Arterioles 115
Artery 115, 263
    and vein 115f
        comparison of 117t
Arthrology joints 35
    types 35
Articular cartilage 32
Articulations 33
Asepsis 393
Aseptic processes 395
    methods of 396t
Aseptic techniques 393
    levels of 394
Aspergillus 350
    fumigatus 158
Asthma 147, 387
    acute emergency of 205
Atracurium 219, 315, 320
Atrial systole 113
Atrioventricular valves 111
Atropine methonitrate 173

Auditory ossicles 27
Auriculotemporal nerve 251
Autoclave 308
Autoimmune diseases 146
Autoimmune disorders
    diagnosis of 148
    risk factors for 148
    treatment for 149
    types of 147
Automated external defibrillator 410
Autonomic nervous system 265
Avascular necrosis 131
Axilla 44
Azelastine 205
Azygos hemiazygos veins 263

B

Bacillus 157
Back, muscles of 41, 41f, 283
Baclofen 219, 222
Bacteria 157, 159t, 194, 201, 349, 351
    common targets in 195t
    resistance in 203t
Bacterial infections 274
Bambuterol 172
Barakina 361
Barbiturates 320
Barrier nursing 391
    techniques of 391
Bartholin's glands 76, 77
Basic life support 408, 410
Benzocaine 316
Benzodiazepines 164, 165, 191, 210, 320
Benzonatate 171
Benzoquinonium 219
Bernard-Soulier disease 100
Beta
    agonist 172
    propiolactone 155, 303
    stimulant, nonselective 172
Beta-blockers 191
Biceps 42, 283
Bicuspid valve 111
Biological indicators 309
Biomedical waste
    classification of 404
    collection 405
    hazards, risk of 406
    management 403, 404
        steps of 404
    segregation 404
    source of 404
    storage 405
    transportation 405
    treatment and disposal 405

Bipolar electrocautery 379
Blood 23
  clots, formation of 101f
  clotting 96
  coagulation of 138f
    system, disorders of 137
  components of 95
  composition and functions 94
  flow 312
  functions of 94
  glucose 338
  pressure 312, 338
    high 170
  spillage 364
  supply 241, 264, 271
  transfusion 141
  vessels 114, 249
    types of 114
Blood-borne disease, transmission of 364
Blood-serum hepatitis 350
Bloodstream infections 354, 355, 389
Bodok seal 317
Body
  cavity 227
  major muscles of 281
  temperature 274
    regulation of 274
Boiling 154, 302, 357
  points 212
Bone 257, 270
  compact 32
  irregular 31
  long 30
  major landmarks of 257
  marrow 119, 145
  microscopic structure of 30
  parts of 32
  short 31
  types of 30, 31f
Bony landmarks 251, 258
Bony part 236
Bookwalter retractor 333, 333f, 334, 334f
Boyle's machine 312, 316
Brachial plexus 243, 281
  block 341
Brachialis 42, 284
Brachioradialis 43, 284
Brain 33, 90, 90f, 179, 246
  anatomy of 91f
  left 91
  lobes of 92
  right 91
  structure of 86
  wall, cross section of 91f
Brainstem 90

Breast
  areola of 273
  fat necrosis of 132
Breathing 312, 411, 417
  intrapleural 64
  mechanism 62
  mouth-to-mouth 414f
Bronchi 60
Bronchial asthma 171
  drugs in 172
Bronchodilators 172
Brown adipose tissue 23
Brucella organism 350
Bubble boy disease 147
Buccinator 38, 281
Buclizine 204
Bupivacaine 316, 340
Burns 134, 288

C

Calcium channel blockers 191
Camper's fascia 229
Canal of Schlemm 279
Candida albicans 158
Capillaries 116
  carry blood 116
Carbamazepine 191
Carbohydrate 52
  digestion 53f, 53t
  step of 53
Carbon dioxide 108, 317
  output of 83
Cardiac arrest
  case of 412
  causes of 413
  sign of 413
Cardiac chest compression, external 414
Cardiac cycle 113
Cardiac dysrhythmias 136
Cardiac muscle tissue 25
Cardiac position 311
Cardiac system 107
Cardiac tamponade 267
Cardiac tissue 264
Cardiogenic shock 136, 136f
  causes of 136
Cardiopulmonary arrest 409
Cardiopulmonary resuscitation 137, 408, 410, 412, 414
  procedure of 413
  technique 415
Cardiovascular homeostasis 265
Cardiovascular stability, maintaining 299
Carisoprodol 219, 221
Carotid triangle 255

Carpal joints 37
Carpometacarpal joints 37
Cartilage 24
Caseous necrosis 131
Cauda equina 94
Caudal anesthesia 314
Cauterization 378
Cell
- cycle 17, 18f
- excitable 25
- layers, classification of 22f
- membrane 10
  - functions of 11
- organelles 10
- structure 10, 11f
Cellular structures 102
Central cough suppressant 171
Central emetics 179
Central line-associated bloodstream infections, risk of 389
Central nervous system 86
Central sterile supply department 304, 346
- activities of 305
- basic functioning of 302
- designing of 305
- layout of 306
- manager, role of 309
- planning of 305
- staffing of 308
- techniques 286
- workflow of 307
Central waste collection room 405
Centrally acting muscle relaxants 221
Centrosomes 16
Cerebellum 90, 247, 280
Cerebral cortex 280
Cerebral hemispheres 89
Cerebral hypoxia 413
Cerebrospinal fluid 88, 340
Cerebrum 90
Cervical 27, 281
- nerve 251
  - roots 250
- spiral protection 417
Cervix 79
Cetirizine 205
Chemical cautery 378, 380
Chemical disinfectants 156t
- in-use dilution of 304t
Chemical formula 212
Chemical indicators 309
Chemical sterilization 155, 303
- agents, classification of 155t, 303t
Chemotaxis 123
- defects of 124
Chest
- abdomen 417

pain 409
- voluntary muscles of 178
Chlophedianol 171
Chloramphenicol eye ointment 347
Chlorhexidine 397
Chlorine
- compounds 357
- solution 361
Chloroquine 191
Chloroxylenol 397
Chlorpheniramine 171, 204
Chlorpromazine 174
Chlorzoxazone 219, 221
Choline theophillinate 172
Chordae tendineae 111
Choroid 277, 279
Chromic catgut 372
Ciliary body 278
Cimetidine 191
Cinchocaine 340
Circular cutter 337f
Cisatracurium besylate 315
Cisterna chyli 239
Clamps 327
Clavicle bone 255, 256f
Clean technique 395
Cleaning, levels of 395t
Clips 337, 337f
Clitoris 77
Clonidine 165
Clostridium
- botulinum 349
- difficile spores 394
Clotting factor defects 100
Coagulase negative staphylococci 355
Coagulation disorders 139
Coagulative necrosis 130
Cocaine 380
Coccidioides 158
Coccobacilli 157
Coccus 157
Coccygeus 40, 282
Coccyx 27, 247
- periosteum of 248
Code blue 408, 409f, 410
- neonate 408
- pediatric 408
Codeine 171
Collagen fibres 270
Colle's fascia of perineum 230
Columnar epithelium 22
Coma 175
Common coagulation disorders 139
Common iliac nodes 240
Communications 344
Complement system 144
Complementary medicines 165, 166

Complications and death, causes of 300
Conductive tissue, strand of 112
Condyle 259
Connective tissue 23, 270
Consciousness, loss of 412
Contaminated linen 391
Control finger movements 43, 284
Conventional cutting needle 330, 330f
Coracobrachialis 40, 282
Cornea 276, 277
Corneal epithelium 277
Corneal reflexes, loss of 313
Coronary diastole 112
Coronary systole 112
Corpora cavernosa 76
Corpus callosum 91
Corticosteroids 149, 165, 173, 204, 205
Costal cartilage 28
Cough
    drugs for 171
    etiquette 391
Cranial nerve 276
    second 280
Cranium 251, 252f
Cremaster muscle 230, 232
Crests 259
Crile hemostat 328, 328f
Crista galli 89
Critical equipment 395
Critical temperature 212
Cross infection, prevention of 382, 384
Cryptococcus neoformans 158
Cubital fossa 44
Cuboidal epithelium 22
Cutaneous mycosis 158
Cutaneous tissues 268
Cyanocobalamin 209
Cyanosis 413
Cyclizine 204
Cyclopropane 317
Cytokine mediators 122
Cytokinesis 20
Cytomegalovirus 150, 197
Cytoplasm 11, 12f
Cytoplasmic granules 98
Cytotoxic drugs 407

D

Daltonism 103
Dantrolene 219
Data management 345
Deaver retractor 332, 332f
Debakey forceps 327, 327f
Deep dermis 46
Deep membranous layer 229
Deep vein thrombosis 300
Deficiency, treatment for 149
Dehydration 134
Delirium, stages of 210
Deltoid 40
Demerol 321
Dense connective tissue 23, 249
Deoxyribonucleic acid 75
    viruses 158
Dermal papilla 271
Dermatome 243
Dermis 270
Descending tracts 94
Desferrioxamine 207
Desflurane 315
Desloratadine 205
Dexon 373
Dextromethorphan 171
Diabetes 387
Diameter index safety system 318
Diapedesis 123
Diaphragm 40, 245, 261, 282
    sellae 89
    sulci 247
Diaphragmatic hernia 235
Diaphysis 32, 258
Diarrhea 169, 354
    symptoms of 186
Diastole 112
Digastric muscle 254
Digestion 52
Digestive tract 146
Dimenhydrinate 174, 204
Diphenhydramine 171, 204
Disability 417
Disinfectants, high-level 356
Disinfection
    concurrent 358
    levels of 356
    methods of 356
Disposable gloves
    removing 290, 292
    wearing 290
Disseminated intravascular coagulation 100
Disulfiram 187
Domperidone 174, 175
Dressing 300
    method of 301
Drowsiness 175
Drug
    accidental overdoses of 179
    administration, routes of 159
    adverse effects of 162
    antiasthmatic 172
    antifibrinolytic 141
    delivering 199
    related factors 163

resistant microorganisms 406
side effects of 162, 165
Dry powder mannitol 172
D-tubocurarine 220
Dura mater 88, 246, 247
  endosteal layer of 248
Dural venous sinuses 250
Dysentery 354
Dyspnea 311

E

Ear 101
  structure of 104f
Eccrine glands 273
Echinacea 166
Eczema 147
Elastic fibrocartilage 24
Elastic tissue 23
Elective urgent emergency 295
Electrocauterization 380
Electrocautery 378, 379
  applies 379
Electrolyte imbalance 187
Elimination 55
Emesis 56
Emetics 178
Empty nose syndrome 380
Encounter 385
Encourage activity 300
Endocardium 108, 110, 114
Endocrine
  reactions 107
  system 80
  organs of 81f
Endometrium 80
Endoplasmic reticulum 13
Endothelial cell contraction 122
Endothelial injuries 122
Endothelium cell 114, 123
Endotracheal intubation 212, 388
Endotracheal tube 410
Enflurane 315, 344
Enterobacter species 350, 355
Enterococcus 350
Enthrone 344
Environmental cleaning 394
Environmental hazard 407
Enzymes 53f
Eosinophils 125
Ephedriner 172
Epicardium 108, 109
Epicranial aponeurosis 250
Epidermis 268
Epidermophytosis 158
Epidural anesthesia 314

Epidural space 90, 247, 248
Epigastric hernia 235
Epinephrine 316
Epiphysis 32, 258
Epithelial tissue 21
  classification of 21f
Epithelium
  ciliated 22
  classification of 22f
Equilibrioception 107
Equipment 287, 383
  cleaning 394
  noncritical 395
  storage of 396
Erect position 311
Erythema 390
Esophageal cancer 267
Esophagus 178, 262
  portion of 265
Ethambutol 164
Ether 210
Ethyl morphine 171
Ethylene gas 155, 303
Etomidate 320
Evaporation 275
Exercise 274
Expectoration, drugs in 171
Expiration 62
  mechanism of 63
Expiratory reserve volume 66
Extensor carpi
  radialis longus and brevis 43, 284
  ulnaris 43, 284
Extradural spaces 248
Extrapyramidal reactions 175
Eye 101, 276
  anterior of 279
  protect 365
  protection 391
    effective usage of 401
  segment of 280f
  structure of 102f
Eyeball 252, 276, 279
Eyewear, protective 390, 401

F

Face
  auricular region 252
  mental region 253
  muscles of 38, 281
  nasal region 253
  orbital 252
  shields 391
Fail safe valve 318
Fallopian tubes 78

Falx cerebella 89, 248
Falx cerebri 89, 248
Famotidine 191
Fascia 236, 323
  iliaca 236, 238
  psoas 236
  superficial 229
  thoracolumbar 236
  transversalis 230
Fat necrosis 131
Fatty layer, superficial 229
Femoral condyles 259
Femoral hernia 233, 234f
Femoral pulse, absence of 413
Fentanyl 168, 214, 321
  citrate droperidol 344
Ferric
  ammonium citrate 206
  carboxymaltose 207
Ferrous
  fumarate 206
  gluconate 206
  succinate 206
  sulfate 206
Ferumoxytol 207
Fever 126, 390
Fexofenadine 204
Fibrinogen to fibrin, conversion of 98
Fibrinoid necrosis 131
Fibroblasts 270
Fibrocartilage 24
Fibrosis 124
Fibrous layer, outer 276
Fibrous tissue 23
First aid 134, 135, 137
  dressing in 301
Fish tapeworm infestation 208
Fits 413
Flash sterilizer 308
Flat bones 31
Flexor carpi radialis 43, 284
Fluid
  and electrolyte, replacement of 185
  into cell, osmotic movement of 367f
  movement, lack of 367f
Fluothane 344
Folic acid 208, 209
Fontanels 34
Food ingestion 274
  digestion, absorption and defecation, process of 52
Foot
  and toes 257
  joints of 38
Foramen 259
Forceps 325
  non-toothed 326
  toothed 326
Foreign substances, inhalation of 266
Formaldehyde 357, 361, 362
  gas 155, 303
Formalin 362
  fumigation with 358
Formoterol 172
Fowler's position 311
Frazier suction tip 335, 335f
Frequent nosebleeds 380
Friction knot 377
Function residual capacity 67
Fungal infections 157
Fungi 157, 195, 349, 351
  opportunistic 158
Furosemide 164

G

Gallbladder 51, 51f
Gangrenous necrosis 131
Gas 210
  exchange of 64
  flow, mechanism of 316
  gangrene 349
Gastrectomy 208
Gastric acid secretion, inhibition of 189
Gastric parietal cells 189
Gastritis, chronic 208
Gastrocnemius 44, 285
Gastrointestinal function, managing 299
Gastrointestinal infection 354
Gastrointestinal tract 353
  drugs in 174
Gastrostomy 341
General anesthesia 314, 339, 344
  drugs for 315
  preparation for 340
  stage of 210
Genitalia
  external 76
  internal 77
Glabrous skin 271
Glanzmann thrombasthenia 100
Glasgow coma scale 417
Glomerular filtration 72
Glove 390, 391, 402
  procedure of
    remove 402
    wear 402
  steps of 291f
Glutaraldehyde 155, 303
Gluteals 44
Glutes 285
Goiter 267

Golgi apparatus 14, 15f
Gowning, steps of 289f
Gowns 390, 391, 399
Granisetron 175, 176
Granny's knot 378
Granulomatous inflammation 125
Graves' disease 147
Gray matter 94
Great auricular nerve 251
Great vessels 245
Growth and development 34

H

H_1 blockers, classification of 204
Hageman factor 99
Hair 272
    color of 272
    follicles 45
    growth 272
        phases of 46
    removal 296, 297
    root, connects to 46
    structure of 272
Hairy skin 271
Halothane 211, 315, 344
Hamstrings 44, 285
Hand
    bones of 29
    hygiene 382, 391, 397
        antiseptic 397
    instruments 323
    rubbing 397
    wash, antiseptic 397
Handwashing 286, 382, 397
    indication of 397
    method of 382
    regular 152
    routine 398
    steps of 287f, 383f
    types of 397
Hazards 407
Head 259
Healing 126
    process, stages of 129f
Health
    hazards 406
    problems 313
Healthcare
    facility 391
        infection control in 153
    waste, disposal of 407
Healthcare-associated infections 153, 388, 394
Hearing 103
    organ of 104f

Heart 33, 245, 262
    blood flow
        through 113
        within 114f
    chambers of 110
    conduction system of 111, 112f
    disease 267
    gross anatomy of 108f
    layers of 109f
    rate 312
        resting 109
    structure of 107
    valves of 108, 110
    wall, structure of 109
Heartburn 169
Heat loss 274
Heat production 274
Helminths 198
Hematinics 205
Hematopoiesis 33
Hemoglobin 270, 338
Hemophilia 139
Hemorrhage 134, 300
    control, circulation with 417
Hemostasis
    disorders of primary 100
    disorders of secondary 100
    primary 97
    rapid 128
    secondary 98
Heparin 164
Hepatitis B virus 350
Hepatocytes 47
Hepatotoxicity 183
Hernia 232, 232f
    abdominal 182
    causes of 235
    clinical anatomy of 227
    common forms of 233
    prevention 236
    symptoms of 235
    types of 233, 235f
Herpes simplex virus 197
Hiatus hernia 233, 234f
Hinge joint 29
Hip
    ball and socket joint of 29
    joint 37
    muscles of 43, 284
Histamine 188
    H_2 antagonists 189
    inhibits action of 189
Hodgkin lymphoma 117
Homeostasis 268
Hormone 274
    human chorionic gonadotropin 79

increased release of 275
secrete 81f
Hospital acquired infection 388, 388f
Hospital emergency code 408
Hospital infection control
  policy 363
  program 355
Hospital waste, hazards with 406
Human anatomy 227
  branches of 4
Human body
  parts of 3
  vertebral column of 27
Human brain, parts of 92f
Human cell shape 10
Human digestive system 48f
Human eye 276
Human tissues, types 21
Hyaline cartilage 24
Hydrating agents 171
Hydrocodone 171
Hydrocortisone 173, 205
Hydromorphone 321
Hydroxyethyl theophyllinate 172
Hymen 77
Hyoid and auditory ossicles 27
Hyoscyamine 315
Hypersensitivity 187
Hypertonic fluids, osmotic effects of 369f
Hypertonic solutions 368
Hypochlorite 364
  sodium 361
Hypodermis 270
Hypoglycemia 418
Hypophysis cerebri 249
Hypothalamic thermostatic 275
Hypothalamus 81
  pituitary gland-adrenal gland 57
Hypothermia, prevent 418
Hypotonic IV fluids, osmotic effects of 369f
Hypotonic solutions 366

I

Iatrogenic infection 151
Ideal suture qualities 372
Iliac crest 257
Iliac nodes, external 240
Iliacus 43, 285
Illegal drugs 313
Illness, full stage of 352
Immune
  disorders 146
  properties 274
Immune system
  common disorders of 146
  of body, disorders of 142
  parts of 143, 143f
Immunity
  active 142
  innate 142
  passive 143
  types of 142, 142f
Immunization 150
Immunodeficiency, severe combined 147
Immunoglobulin therapy 149
Immunosuppressant drugs 149
Immunosuppression, high dose 149
Incisional hernia 233
Infant circumcision 381
Infection 148, 216, 267, 406
  agent 349
  chain of 387
  contact 385t
  control
    policies 364
    practices 363
    program 362
  course of 351
  defenses against 352
  laboratory 151
  modes of transmission of 150
  nature of 386
  nosocomial 353, 354f
  opportunistic 147
  prevention of 151
  process of 348, 349f
  reservoir of 387
  sources of 348
  stages of 385
  treating 193
Infectious agent 387
Infectious patient, transportation of 393
Inflammation 121, 128
  chronic 124
  phase 126
Inflammatory bowel disease 147
Inflammatory cells, chronic 125
Influenza virus 350
Ingestion 52, 150
Inguinal hernia 233, 233f
Inguinal herniorrhaphy 341
Inguinal ligament 257
Inhalation 150, 162
  anesthetics 210
  steroid 173, 205
Inner nervous tissue layer 276
Inspiration 62
  mechanism of 62
Inspiratory capacity 67
Inspiratory reserve volume 66

Instrument
   care of 359
   cleaning of 360
   disinfectants, use of 357
Insulin 164
Intercostal artery 242
   anterior 242
Intercostal muscle 40, 243, 282
   fibers, external 40, 282
Internal intercostal muscle 244
   fibers 40, 282
Internal occipital protuberance 89
Interventricular septum 112
Intestinal lymph trunks, left and right 239
Intestinal obstruction 295, 300
Intra-abdominal suction 334
Intraocular pressure 279
Intravenous anesthetics 213
Iodine 397
Iodophors 397
Ipratropium bromide 173
Iris 278
   scissors 325, 325f
Iron
   amount of 141
   calcium complex 206
   dextran 206
   poisoning, acute 207
   sucrose 207
   supplementation 141
Iron-deficiency anemia 207
Iron-sorbitol-citric acid complex 207
Ischiorectal fossa 45
Isoflurane 344
Isolation 391
   gown 399
Isoprenaline 172
Isopropyl group 213
Isotonic fluids, osmotic effects of 369f
Isotonic solutions 366

J

Jaundice 177
Jaw, osteonecrosis of 132
Joint
   acromioclavicular 35
   cartilaginous 35
   elbow 28, 36
   fibrous 35
   humeroscapular 35
   interphalangeal 37
   radioulnar 36
   sternoclavicular 35
   synovial 35

K

Kelly clamp 328, 328f
Keratin plates 271
Keratinized stratified epithelium 23
Ketamine 315, 320, 340
   hydrochloride 214, 344
Ketotifen 173
Kidney 69
   cross section of 71f
   functions of 71
   microscopic structure of 70
   organs with 69
   structure of 70
Kiesselbach's plexus 380
Kinesthesia 107
Klebsiella organism 350
Knee
   chest position 312
   joint 29, 37
Kocher clamp 328, 329f
Krause bulbs 271
Kupffer cells 125

L

Labia
   majora 76
   minora 77
Lamina, anterior limiting 277
Laryngeal mask airway 340
Laryngeal reflexes, loss of 313
Larynx 58, 59f
Latissimus dorsi 41, 283
Lens 278
Leptomeninges 89
Lesser occipital nerve 251
Leukocyte 123
   adhesion deficiency 124
   cellular events 122
   function, defects of 124
Leukocytosis 126
Leukotriene antagonist 173
Levator ani 40, 282
Levator palpebrae superioris 38, 281
Levocabastine 205
Levocetirizine 205
Lidocaine 185, 316, 319
Lignocaine 340, 347
Linctuses 162
Linear cutter 336, 336f
Linear stapler 336, 336f
Linen and disposal, handling of 392
Lipid 54
   digestion 54

Liquefactive necrosis 131
Liquid 210
Lithium 163
Lithotomy position 312
Liver 47
   disease 100, 139
   enzymes, elevation of 177
   functions of 48
Lobe
   anterior 82
   secretions, posterior 82
Lobules 47
Local anesthesia 217, 314, 341
   advantages of 342
   drugs for 316
   methods of 216
Local anesthetic
   presentation of 342
   proiaine 171
Local infiltration 216
Locking forceps 327
Loop of Henle 70
Loose areolar connective tissue 250
Loratadine 204
Low pressure system 318
Lower extremity, joints of 37
Lower limb 27, 29
   bones 29
   muscles of 43, 284
Low-level disinfectants 356
Lumbar lymph trunks, left and right 239
Lumbar vertebrae 231
Lumen 114
Lung 61, 61f, 145, 245
   capacities 67
   volume 65, 66
Luteotropin 82
Lymph 117
   drainage 77
   nodes 118, 144, 240
   presence of 118f
Lymph vessels 118, 144, 270
   pair of 239
Lymphatic supply 241
Lymphatic system 117, 144, 145f
Lymphocytes 118, 125
Lymphoma 267
Lysosome 15, 15f
Lysozyme 352

M

Macrophage 125
   activation, classical 125
Madurella mycetomatis 158
Malabsorption 208

Malleable retractor 335, 335f
Malleus 103
Mask 390, 391
   and respirators 400
   disposable 292
   putting of 292
   type of 400
   wearing 292
Masseter 38, 281
Mast cell stabilizers 173
Maturation phase 127
Mayo scissors 323, 324f
Meadiastinum, parts of 263
Measles virus 350
Mechanical indicators 309
Meclizine 204
Mediastinal tumors 267
Mediastinitis 267
Mediastinum 245, 261f, 262, 267
   anterior 262, 263, 265
   common conditions affect 267
   concept of 260
   middle 262, 263
   posterior 262, 263, 265
   superior 244, 262, 263
Medical asepsis 288, 384, 395
Medical emergencies 410
Medical handwashing 398
   procedure for 398
Medical interventions 152
Medications, types of 387
Medullary cavity 33
Megaloblastic anemia, treatment of 208
Meiosis 18, 18f
Meissner's corpuscles 271
Membrane functions 155
   interfere with 303
Meninges 88, 88f, 246
   function of 249
Meningococcal meningitis 89
Mental status changes 409
Meperidine 321
Mephenesin 219
Mepivacaine 316
Mepyramine 204
Mequitazine 205
Merkel's disc 271
Metabolic wastes 107
Metacarpophalangeal joints 37
Metaphase 20
Metaphysis 32
Metaxalone 219, 222
Metformin 191
Methocarbamol 219, 221
Methylxanthines 172
Metoclopramide 174

Metronidazole 186
Metzenbaum scissors 324, 324f
Microbial flora 363
Microfilaments 16
Micro-organism, types of 351t
Microscopic anatomy 4
Microsporum 158
Microtubules 16
Migration 128
Mitochondria 12, 13f
Mitosis 18, 18f
Mizoplastine 205
Modularly paralysis, stage of 210
Moist heat 154, 302
Monocular vision 276
Monofilament 373
Mononucleosis 147
Montelukast 173
Morphine 171, 320
Mouth 352
Mucoactive agent 172
Mucokinetics 172
Mucolytics 172
Mucosa layer 50
Multi-pseudopodal plugs 98
Muscle 243, 265, 270
    extends 231
    layer 50
    lies 231
    pair of 230
    parts of 283
    relaxant 219, 320
    tissue, types of 25f
Muscular tissue 24
Muscular triangle 255
Myasthenia gravis 266, 267
Mycobacterium tuberculosis 350, 356
Mycoplasma pneumoniae 157
Mycosis, superficial 157
Myocardial depression 320
Myocardial infarction 136
Myocardium 108, 110
Myology 38, 281
Myometrium 80
Myotome 243

N

Nails 271
Nalidixic acid 186
Nasal cannula 212
Nasal cauterization 380
Nasal cavity 57, 105f
Naturally quite painful 380
Nausea, treatment of 319

Neck
    anterior region of 253
    lateral region of 255
    muscles of 39, 281
    region, posterior 253
    triangles of 253
Necrosis 130, 130f, 133, 133f
    types of 131
Needle 329, 371
    anatomy 374
    holders, use of 375
    point-geometry 375t
    shapes of 331, 331f, 374
    stick injury 406
    types 329
Negative pressure seal check 401
Nephron 70
Nerve 263, 264
    blocks 315
    supply 77, 271
Nervous control 273
Nervous system 86, 87f, 274
Nervous tissue 25
Neuroleptanalgesia 210
Neurologic assessment 417
Neuropathy 209
Nitrofurantoin antagonizes 187
Nitrous oxide 211, 317, 319, 344
Nizatidine 191
Nonadhesive dressing 301
Nondepolarizing 320
Non-keratinized stratified epithelium 22
Non-nucleoside reverse transcriptase
    inhibitors 197
Nonopioid antitussive 171
Non-steroidal anti-inflammatory
    drugs 169, 170
    side effects of 169
Noscapine 171
Nose 57, 101
Nuchal region 253
Nucleoside reverse transcriptase inhibitors
    197
Nucleus 17f
Nurse in barrier nursing, responsibilities
    of 393
Nursing care 153

O

Obstructive conditions 136
Obturators 44
Occipital nerve, greater 251
Occipital triangle 255
Occupational safety and health
    administration 399

Omalizumab 173
Ondansetron 174, 175
Operating theatre
   deficiency in 345
   disinfection of 361
   fumigation of 362
   infection control in 347
   satellite pharmacy 345
   techniques, basics of 286
Opioids 320
   drug 168, 214
Opium preparations 186
Optic chiasma 280
Optic nerve 102, 280
Optic tracts 280
Oral cavity 58
Oral ingestion 159
Oral iron
   adverse effects of 206
   preparations 206
Orbicularis oculi 38, 281
Orbicularis oris 38, 281
Organic matter present 355
Organogram 309
Orphenadrine 219, 221
Oseltamivir 197
Osmolarity 371
Osmotic purgatives 181
Osmotic purges 181
Osteocytes 32
Osteology 26
Osteonecrosis 131
Ovary 78
   suspensory ligament of 78
Oxepin 171
Oxethazaine 316
Oxycodone 171
Oxygen 212
   cylinder 317
   failure alarm 318
   flush 317
   mask 212
   tents 212
Oxyhemoglobin 64, 270

P

Pain 107
   killing medication 149
Palmaris longus 43, 284
Pancreas 85
   body of 85
   head of 85
   parts of 86f
   tail of 85
Pancreatic islets 85

Pancreatic necrosis 132
Pancuronium 219, 220
Parathyroid glands 83
Parenteral iron 206
   adverse effects of 207
Parietal peritoneum 230
Parkinson's disease 175
Pasteurization 357
Patent airway, maintaining 299
Patient care items, classification of 355
Pectoral girdle 28, 29f
Pectoralis major 40, 282
Pellet implantation 161
Pelvic
   floor, muscles of 40, 282
   girdle 27, 29, 30f
   operation 233
Pelvis 417
Penetrating trauma 295
Pentazocine 168, 215
Pericardial cavity 109
Perimetrium 79
Periosteum 32, 250
Peripheral nervous system 86
Peritoneal tissue, extra 230
Peritonitis 295, 311
Personal protective equipment 153, 399
   sequence of removing 402
Pethidine 215
Phagocytosis 123
   defects of 124
Pharyngeal demulcent 171
Pharynx 58, 178
Pheniramine 204
Phenolphthalein 181
Phenothiazine 177
Phenytoin 185, 191
Pholcodine 171
Phosphodiesterase inhibitors 172
Phrenic nerves 244
   left and right 265
Physical examination, positions for 311
Physiology 4
Pia mater 88, 89, 246-248
Pin index safety system 317
Pink molecules 368
Piperazine, theophylline ethanoate of 173
Pituitary gland 82, 89
Plain catgut 372
Plasma 95
Plasmodium
   falciparum 198
   knowlesi 198
   malariae 198
   ovale 198
   vivax 198

Plastic bags 307
Platelet 96
    activation 98
    defects 100
Platelet-to-endothelial adherence 98
Platelet-to-platelet aggregation 98
Pleural cavity 65
Pleural sacs 260
Pneumococcus 350
Pneumonia 354
    ventilator-associated 388
Pneumothorax 246
Polyglactin 372
Polyglycolic acid 373
Poole suction tube 334, 334f
Popliteal space 45
Positive pressure seal check 401
Posterior abdominal wall 236, 237f
    muscles of 237
    nerves of 240
Postoperative care unit 298, 299
Potency 217
    immediate 217
Potential spinal factors 418
Pott's scissors 324, 324f
Preanesthetic assessment 337
Preanesthetic checkup 337
Preaortic nodes 240
Prednisolone 173, 205
Pressure reducing valve, second 318
Pressure regulator 317
Presyncope 409
Pretracheal lymph nodes 264
Prilocaine 316
Probenecid 187
Prochlorperazine 175, 176
Prodromal stage 352
Prolactin 82
Proliferation 128
Promethazine 171, 204
    theoclate 175, 176
Pronator quadratus 43, 284
Pronator teres 43, 284
Propofol 213, 315
Propoxyphene 171
Propranolol 185
Protease inhibitors 198
Protein 54
    digestion of 54t
Prothrombin to thrombin, conversion of 98
Protozoa 198, 349, 351
Pseudomonal organism 350
Pseudomonas 356
    organism 350
    species 355
Psoas 43
    abscess 239
    fascia 238, 239
    major 237
        muscles 237
    minor 238
Psoriasis 148
Pterygoid 38, 281
    muscles 250
Pulmonary branches 265
Pulmonary circulation 108
Pulmonary embolism 136, 300
Pulmonary toilet 246
Pulp necrosis 133
Pupils, dilated 413
Pure red cell aplasia 266
Pyramidalis 232

Q

Quadratus lumborum 41, 237, 238, 283
Quadriceps femoris 44, 285
Quality assurance 309
Quinidine 191

R

Rabies dog 349
Radiation 275
    necrosis 132
Range of motion 6f
Ranitidine 191
Rapacuronium 315
Re-breathing mask 212
Recovery room 300
Rectus abdominis 42, 230, 232, 283
Red blood cells 95, 369f
Re-epithelialization 129
Reflex
    action 274
    emetics 179
Regeneration phase 128
Regional anesthesia 314
Registered nurse 341
Relaxation phase 113
Relieving pain and anxiety 299
Renal papillary necrosis 132
Reproductive system 73
    female 76, 76f
    male 73, 74f
Residual volume 67
Resistance genes
    acquisition of 201
    transfer of 201
Resolution phase 128
Respiration 63f
    mechanism of 63
    muscles of 61

Respiratory diaphragm 241
Respiratory gas transport 65
Respiratory hygiene 391
Respiratory system 56
   anatomy of 57f
Respiratory tract 353
Respiratory volume 65, 66f
Resuscitation techniques 410
Retina 278
Retractors 332
Rheumatoid arthritis 148
Rhythm 312
Rib 28
   and sternum 28f
   false 28
   floating 28
   true 28
Ribonucleic acid viruses 158
Ribosome 13, 14f
Richardson retractor 333, 333f
Rickettsia typhi 350
Rocuronium 315
Roflumilast 174
Rotameter 318
Ruffini's ending 271
Ruptured aneurysm 295
Russian forceps 327, 327f

S

Sacral vertebra, second 249
Sacrospinalis 41, 283
Sacrum 27
Safe disposal, pharmacy for 168
Safety features 318
Salbutamol 172, 350
Sartorius 44, 285
Scalp 246, 250
   layers of 249
Scalpel 323
   blade 323f
Scarpa's fascia 229
Schaffer's method 411
Scissors 323
Sclera 276, 277f
Sclerocorneal junction 277
Scleroderma 148
Sclerosis, multiple 148
Scrotum 74
Sebaceous gland 273
Secretion 73
Seitz filter 156
Seizures 413
Self-retaining retractor system 333
Sella turcica 89
Semi critical equipment 395

Sense organs, beyond five 107
Sensory nerve cells 94
Sensory organ 268
   structure and functions of 101
Sesamoid bones 31
Severe acute respiratory syndrome 392
Sevoflurane 315
Sex hormones 148
Shaft, layers of 272
Shock 133, 300
   distributive 135
   hypovolemic 134, 417
   neurogenic 135
   septic 135
Short duration low potency 217
Shoulder
   and upper limb, muscles of 40, 282
   ball and socket joint of 28
   joint 350
Side effects, reduce risk of 167
Silastic implant 161
Silvester method 412
Sim's position 312
Simple epithelium 21
Sinoatrial node 111
Sinus 259
   histiocytes 125
Six-pack abs 256
Skeletal muscle relaxant 219
   classification of 219
Skeletal system 26, 26f
Skeleton, thoracic region of 28
Skin 106f, 145, 229, 249, 268, 352, 355
   appendages of 271
   blood vessels of 275
   functions of 46, 273
   glue 331, 332f
   histology 45
   layers of 268, 269f
   necrosis 132
   pigmentation of 270
   preparation 341
      intraoperative 297
      preadmission 297
   structure of 45, 46f, 268
   thick 271
   tissue 251
   types of 271
Skull 27
Slip knot 378
Small blood splashes 364
Small vessels, defects in 100
Smell 105
   sense of 105
Smooth muscle tissue 25
Sodium
   cromoglycate 173

ethyl thiobarbiturate 213
ferric gluconate 207
Soft tissue
   infections 355
   layers 249
Soil, amount of 355
Soleus 44, 285
Sounds emitted from organs, listen to 251
Spaulding's classification 395
Spaulding's principle 394
Spermatozoa 75
Spider bite necrosis 133
Spigelian hernia 235
Spills, larger 364
Spinal anesthesia 340
Spinal cord 88, 93, 93f
   structure of 86
   to muscles 94
Spinal nerves 94
Spirilla 157
Spirochaete 157
Spleen 119, 144
Staphylococcus 350
   aureus 355
Statutory regulations 345
Steam 171
   inhalation 172
Sterile draping 298
Sterile gown, wearing 400
Sterile matrix 272
Sterilization 154
   methods of 302
   preferred method of 304t
Sternocleidomastoid muscles 255
Sternum 28, 245f, 256
Stimulant purgatives 181
Stimulant purges 181
Stomach 49, 178, 184
   functions of 50
   pain 169
   parts of 49, 50f
   structure of 49
   walls of 49
Stool softners 181
Stratified epithelium 22
Stratum basale 269
Stratum cornium 270
Stratum granulosum 269
Stratum lucidum 269
Stratum spinosum 269
Streptococcus faecalis 154, 302
Subarachnoid 249
   space 90, 249
Subcutaneous immunoglobulin 149
Subcutaneous injection 161

Subcutaneous mycosis 158
Subcutaneous tissue 251, 268
Subdural spaces 248
Submandibular gland 254
Submandibular triangle 254
Submental triangle 254
Subsartorial canal 45
Substantia propria 277
Succinylcholine 219, 220, 315, 320
Suction nozzle 347
Sudden death 412
Sulfonamides 163
Sulfur, fumigation with 358
Supraclavicular triangle 255
Supraorbital nerve 251
Supratrochlear nerve 251
Surgeon tools 297
Surgery
   preoperative preparation for 295
   preparing for 296
Surgical anatomy 227
Surgical anesthesia 313, 344
   operative 343
Surgical asepsis 396
   principles of 293
Surgical gown 399
Surgical hand washing 288, 384
Surgical knots 377
Surgical scrubbing 286
Surgical silk 373
Surgical site
   infections 355, 389
      signs of 390
      symptoms of 390
   managing 299
   preparation 296
Surgical steel and wires 373
Suture 329
   degradation 374t
   material 372t
   removal 377
   scissors 323
   size 330, 374
   techniques 376
   types of 330, 331t
Sweat glands 272
Swelling 267
Sympathetic nerves 265
Synesthesia 107
Synthetic materials 330
Synthetic opiates 186
Systematic mycosis 158
Systemic lupus erythematosus 148
Systemic steroids 173, 205
Systemic toxicity 180, 188
Systole 112

T

Tapered needle 330, 330f
Taste 104
  buds 104
Telophase 20
Temperature 107
Temporalis 38, 281
Temporomandibular joint 35
Tentorium cerebelli 89, 248
Terbutaline 172
Teres major 41, 283
Terminal disinfection 358
Testes 74
Tetanus 349
Theatre equipment 348
Theophyllinate 172
Theophylline 185
  level 187
Thermoception 107
Thiopentone sodium 213
  chemically 213
Third occipital nerve 251
Thoracic aorta, descending 242
Thoracic aortic aneurysm 267
Thoracic artery, internal 264
Thoracic cavity 240, 241
  part of 260
Thoracic duct 242, 263
Thoracic mediastinum 261, 265, 266
  posterior 264
Thoracic wall 243
  muscles of 244f
  nerve supply to 243, 243f
  structure of 240
Thoraco-abdominal diaphragm 227
Thoracolumbar fascia 239
Thorax 255
  anatomy of 245
  muscles of 40, 282
  structure of 242f
Thrombosis 99
Thymus 119, 145, 263
  cancer 266
  gland 84
  protecting 262
Thyroid gland 82
Thyroid-stimulating hormone 275
Tibialis, anterior 44, 285
Tibiofibular joints 38
Tidal volume 66
Tinea
  barbae 158
  capitis 157
  cruris 158
  pedis 158

Tiotropium bromide 173
Tissue
  damaged by inflammation, healing of 128
  factor 99
  forceps 325, 325f
  structure and function, complete resolution of 124
Tizanidine 219, 222
Tongue
  muscles 27
  special senses 101
  taste buds of 105f
Tonsils 119
Total lung capacity 67
Touch 106
  sense of 106f
Toxicity 177, 180, 183, 185, 188, 191
  risk of 185
  selective 193
Toxoplasma gondii rubella virus 150
Trabeculae 32, 257
Trachea 27, 59, 60f, 263
Trained nursing staff 300
Transitional epithelium 23
Transmission, chain of 151f
Transmit sensory information 94
Transverse abdominis 42, 231, 283
Trapezius 41, 281, 283
Trauma, management of severe 416
Trendelenburg position 312
Triage
  advantages of 322
  principles of 321
  types of 322
Tributaries 239
Triceps 42, 284
Trichophytons 158
Tricuspid valve 111
Trigeminal nerve 251
Tripelennamine 204
Trochanter 259
Trunk, muscles of 41, 283
Tuberosity 258
Tubular necrosis, acute 132
Tunica albuginea 75
Tunica vasculosa 75

U

Ulcerative colitis 187
Ultrasonic coagulation 380
Ultrasonic washer 307
Ultraviolet radiation 155, 303
Umbilical hernia 233, 234f
Unconsciousness 413

Unipolar cauterization 379
Universal precaution 390
Upper extremity, joints of 35
Upper limb 28, 27
Ureters 68
Urinary bladder 69
Urinary retention 300
Urinary system 68, 68f
Urinary tract 353
    catheterization 388
    infection 354, 355
        catheter-associated 388
Urine 73
    formation 72, 72f
        process of 71
Uterine tube 78
    wall of 78
Uterus 79
    neck' of 79

V

Vacuoles 16
Vagina 77, 353
Valvular insufficiency 136
Vapor sterilization 154, 302
Vaporizers 318
Varicella-zoster virus 197
Vascular endothelial growth factor 122
Vascular leakage 122
Vasculitides 100
Vecuronium 219
Veins and
    lymphatics 263
    venules 116
Vena cava
    inferior 108, 236
    superior 244
Venous drainage 50, 77, 250
Ventilation 417
    mouth-to-mouth 411
    mouth-to-nose 411
Ventricular systole 113
Venturi mask 212
Vertebrae 27
Vertebral arches, joints of 35
Vestibular glands 76, 77
Vestibule 77
Vibrio 157
    cholerae 350

Virus 157, 158, 159t, 196, 349, 351
Visual information 276
Vital capacity 67
Vital signs 300
Vitamin 55
    B 209
        deficiency 209
    B_{12} 208
    K deficiency 100
        bleeding 139
    K supplements 141
Vitreous body 276
Vitreous humor 276
Volatile agents 319
Voluntary bonding, managing 299
Vomeronasal organ 106
Vomiting 178
von Willebrand's disease 100, 139
Vulva 76
V-Z virus 350

W

Warfarin 163, 185
Waste
    disposal 392
    incineration of 407
Wearing respirators, steps of 400
Weitlaner retractor 333, 333f
White adipose tissue 23
White blood cells 96, 144
Wound 288
    debridement 295
    dehiscence 390
    healing 126
        process 127f, 128
Wrist joint 36

X

Xiphoid process 245, 414

Z

Zafirlukast 173
Zanamivir 197
Zygomaticotemporal nerve 251

EU GSPR Authorised Reprsentative
Logos Europe, 9 rue Nicolas Poussin
1700, La Rochelle, France
Phone: +33 (0) 6 67 93 73 78
E-mail: contact@logoseurope.eu

www.ingramcontent.com/pod-product-compliance
Ingram Content Group UK Ltd.
Pitfield, Milton Keynes, MK11 3LW, UK
UKHW020039250426
12086UKWH00003B/392